Atrial Fibrillation,
a Treatable Disease?

Edited by

J. H. Kingma
N. M. van Hemel

Department of Cardiology,
St. Antonius Hospital,
Nieuwegein, The Netherlands

and

K. I. Lie

Department of Cardiology,
Thorax-center, University Hospital Groningen,
Groningen, The Netherlands

Springer Science+Business Media, B.V.

ISBN 978-0-7923-2008-1   ISBN 978-94-011-1816-3 (eBook)
DOI 10.1007/978-94-011-1816-3

Printed on acid-free paper

Developments in Cardiovascular Medicine

VOLUME 139

The titles published in this series are listed at the end of this volume.

ATRIAL FIBRILLATION, A TREATABLE DISEASE?

CONTENTS

FOREWORD

by Philippe Coumel

The atrium is a particularly convenient tool for the electrophysiologist in experimental as well as clinical conditions. Curiously, the atrium was relatively neglected during the early years of clinical electrophysiology when attention was focused on the atrioventricular junction, and then on the ventricle. At the junctional level, the progress of knowledge was very fast and fruitful. In the ventricle some disappointment came from therapeutic conclusions drawn from invasive as well as noninvasive investigations. This was partly due to concepts developed in a too straightforward way, making artificially-induced tachy-arrhythmias, or spontaneous trivial arrhythmias supposedly reliable surrogates of the real phenomena that finally lead to death. With these considerations in mind, one realizes how important it is to pay more attention to atrial fibrillation.

The ventricle and the atrium may develop identical electrophysiological mechanisms of arrhythmias such as reentry, automaticity and triggered activity. Although, the causal diseases are different at each level the fibrillation process represents something like the end of the road and poses the most difficult problems of comprehension and treatment. At this point, the atrium possesses considerable advantages over the ventricle. Two are of paramount importance. For the investigator the atrium has the advantage of being a two-rather than a three-dimensional tissue, which makes it very easy to explore precisely and completely, to map, to represent and to model with computers. For the clinician the atrium has the definite advantage not to be hemodynamically essential, so that fibrillation does not directly threaten life: the practical consequence is, that therapeutic errors that are catastrophic in the ventricle are forgivable in the atrium.

Although obvious, one must realize how much this difference in the hemodynamic consequences of fibrillation completely changes the situation from every viewpoint. As long as the first therapeutic mistake is the last one, for ventricular fibrillation the clinician is forced to have his therapeutic strategy based on theories which hypothesize the beneficial effects of his options. That they may be inadequate is initially difficult to establish and even more difficult to explain for numerous reasons: experiences cannot be reiterated in the same patient, no patient really matches another one, and fibrillation is just a final common stage that cannot be reliably considered as reproducible in an identical way. In the case of atrial fibrillation which does not kill the patient immediately, the opportunity is given to adapt the treatment and try to understand what went wrong in previous unsuccessful attempts.

Fibrillation may not be the right target in itself, and many etiological factors may lead to this state. The most important distinction is probably between primary and secondary fibrillations. Again, this applies to the ventricle as well as to the atrium, where the environmental electrophysiological conditions do not allow the surrounding myocardium to follow on a 1:1 basis. This situation is much easier to understand and to reproduce than primary fibrillation. This arrhythmia is mainly characterized by an escape of normal safety mechanisms. In both situations, be it primary or secondary fibrillation, in either experimental of clinical situations, the task of the electrophysiologists is simplified by the two-dimensional nature of the atrial tissue, and the observations from either field can be almost directly transposed to the other.

The importance of the role of the autonomic nervous system in arrhythmias is now recognized at both levels. In ventricular tachyarrhythmias this was principally due to convincing evidence provided by the consistent results of therapeutic interventions with ß-blockers. In the atrium, the message was given much earlier thanks to circumstances that permanently provide information on the vago-sympathetic balance. The atrial tissue has its autonomic influences closely reflected at any time by the sinus rhythm so that the autonomic nervous system can be permanently traced. Although discrepancies are conceivable between the sinus node area and the rest of the atria, this information certainly is more direct and reliable than extrapolating from sinus rhythm to the status of the vagosympathetic balance at the ventricular level.

Although, much of what is important at the ventricular level can be learned at the atrial level, not everything observed in the atrium can apply to the ventricle. With the extended use of implanted cardioverter defibrillator one can hope that in the future the opportunity will be given to manipulate drugs without the permanent threat of a lethal mistake and the even more damaging idea of having learned nothing from the mistake. This assumes that we have obtained the maximal amount of knowledge on fibrillation from the atrium, and to emphasize the importance of meetings and books such as the present one, in which the editors have offered me the privilege to express these ideas.

PREFACE

Atrial fibrillation is the most common arrhythmia after premature beats from the atria and the ventricles. Unlike many other cardiac conditions, the management of atrial fibrillation is not the prerogative of the cardiologist since many practitioners from other areas in health care are confronted with this arrhythmia.

As study tools seemed to be lacking in the electrophysiological laboratory, atrial fibrillation remained a disease managed by the clinical cardiologist, and not the electrophysiologist. However, from basic research the understanding of atrial arrhythmias has increased tremendously although only recently these new insights became translated to the clinic. The conference of which proceedings are included in this book, dealt with these newer insights and applications.

Van Hemel et al. discuss the pathophysiological basis of atrial fibrillation and flutter and from there the implementation of new surgical techniques such as the 'corridor' procedure directed to maintain sinus rhythm. To be able to modify the atria electrically, knowledge of their functional anatomy is essential, which appears more complex than that of the ventricles, the valves and the coronary circulation. Guiraudon, who was the first surgeon undertaking map-guided surgery of ventricular and later atrial arrhythmias, describes in detail the functional anatomy of the atria. This is followed by a chapter by Colette Guiraudon on pathological changes in the atria of patients with atrial fibrillation.

Allessie et al. bring us back to the pharmacology and teaches why Class I drugs are indeed effective for atrial fibrillation despite their negative dromotropic effects. However, efficacy decreases rapidly with prolonged use, which is in accordance with clinical observations. Van Gelder et al. describe the characteristics of patients with atrial fibrillation and their chance for maintenance of sinus rhythm after DC-cardioversion.

Atrial fibrillation is a tachycardia frequently accepted, and therefore only treated by agents like digitalis that reduce ventricular rate. However, in view of the decreasing efficacy of drugs over time with prolonged use and the electro-physiological and morphological changes occurring during longstanding atrial fibrillation, it becomes more and more clear that atrial fibrillation should be cured as soon as possible to prevent the electrophysiological and morphological sequelae which tend to sustain atrial fibrillation. DC cardioversion is a crude method requiring anesthesia and frequently leading to hospitalization. Therefore, efforts were made to design methods for acute pharmacological conversion as discussed by Suttorp et al. Maintenance therapy after cardioversion as discussed by Crijns et al. is frequently failing and often accompanied by side-effects. Therefore, intermittent and episodic therapy could be a valuable alternative. However, only a few steps have been made in the development of this concept as pointed out by Lie-A-Huen and Kingma.

A considerable number of our patients cannot be cured or treated pharmacologically. Two possible approaches to address this problem were discussed. An AICD for atrial fibrillation by Tonkin et al. and alternatively the Corridor procedure by Defauw. Whereas the AICD is still experimental, there is a growing body of evidence that surgery may be a solution in selected intractable cases.

Why should atrial fibrillation be treated at all other then by rate control, is the question of many practitioners? The answer is that several risks and untoward conditions are affecting the prognosis and quality of life in patients with atrial fibrillation. The role of the autonomic nervous system, discussed by Murgatroyd and Camm, is an essential determinant in these patients, and changes in autonomic tone may provoke atrial fibrillation. On the other hand, imbalance of the autonomic nervous system may also evolve from atrial fibrillation itself. Kalman et al. discuss the sympathetic mechanisms involved in atrial arrhythmias following coronary artery bypass surgery, whereas Suttorp et al. report on their large experience with antiarrhythmic drugs to prevent atrial fibrillation after this intervention. These authors have also evaluated cardiovascular risk factors of postoperative atrial fibrillation. When atrial tachycardias impose high heart rates on the ventricle, this may in the long run worsen left ventricular function. The so-called tachycardia induced cardiomyopathy should be recognized as a clinical syndrome that needs attention since it can be cured by proper management as can be concluded from the contribution of Wellens et al.

Atrial fibrillation is the most important risk factor in stroke, more important than hypertension, coronary heart disease etc. Therefore, treatment of atrial fibrillation also implies risk management for the prevention of stroke. The role of anticoagulant therapy in both paroxysmal and chronic atrial fibrillation is extensively discussed by Gosselink et al. by reviewing the outcome of recent trials and the perspectives of large ongoing trials. The impact is clear: the management of atrial fibrillation should always include proper anticoagulant treatment. The mechanisms which contribute to thrombus formation during atrial fibrillation are further elaborated with echocardiographic flow studies by Kamp et al.

Finally, when taking into consideration all different treatment modalities, careful selection of therapy in the individual patient is mandatory. This selection process, discussed by Kingma et al., implies that one should not easily resign to ordinary treatment by rate control with digitalis but that optimal therapy should be pursued, even by use of innovative approaches. The patient should be offered therapy commensurate with his needs, our new insights in old and new antiarrhythmic drugs and alternative forms of treatment.

J.H. Kingma

N.M. van Hemel

K.I. Lie

ACKNOWLEDGEMENTS

The conference titled 'Atrial Fibrillation, a Treatable Disease?', organized in Amsterdam on May 7, 1992, was made possible under educational grants from Riker 3 M Nederland B.V., Leiden, and Interpace Nederland B.V., Ruurlo, The Netherlands. Their support also permitted the publication of the Proceedings of this conference, presented in this book. The financial support of the Roger Crowson Foundation, Nieuwegein, The Netherlands, a young organization for clinical research of arrhythmias, is strongly appreciated.

The Editors gratefully acknowledge the skilful assistance of Mrs Gerda van der Kuijl in the preparation and completion of this book.

Chapter 1

FROM EXPERIMENT TO THERAPEUTIC INNOVATION

IN ATRIAL FIBRILLATION AND FLUTTER

Norbert M. van Hemel

Jacques M.T. de Bakker

Anand Ramdat Misier

Jo A.M. Defauw

Departments of Cardiology and Thoracic Surgery
St Antonius Hospital
Nieuwegein

Department of Experimental Cardiology
Academic Medical Center
Amsterdam

and

Interuniversity Cardiology Institute
Utrecht

The Netherlands

1

J. H. Kingma et al. (eds.), Atrial fibrillation, a treatable disease?, 1–22.
© 1992 *Kluwer Academic Publishers.*

INTRODUCTION _____

Since the application of computers in the experimental laboratory in the mid seventies, the facilities and scale of arrhythmia studies of cardiac muscle preparation and intact animal heart have impressively been expanded. Intracavitary mapping of both atria using 480 simultaneous recording electrodes is a good example of computer application shedding new light on the mechanism of atrial fibrillation[1]. However, one might have concern on the validity of these high technology experiments for clinical cardiology. Difference in the type of ventricular arrhythmias observed after myocardial reperfusion illustrates very well this disparity: ventricular fibrillation and tachycardia are the case in animal experiments, whereas accelerated idioventricular rhythm is today recognized a marker of reperfusion following thrombolysis in human coronary arteries[2,3].

Despite this dismatch, the experimental model offers the advantage that theories can be validated because of an artificial limitation of variables that are used to impede interpretation of the results of clinical studies. Furthermore, experimental studies provide the unique opportunity to determine the reproducibility of observations. Still more important and inspiring, they evoke the scientific pleasure of exploring new ideas, an ineradicable drive of mankind. In this context we prefer to quote M.B. Rosenbaum: 'The special intellectual satisfaction of connecting facts to each other constitutes the real fascination of knowledge and the true mother of ideas and hypothesis'[4].

In this study some concepts resulting from experiments on electrophysiology and arrhythmias that have influenced the pharmacologic and invasive treatment of atrial fibrillation and flutter will be discussed. It will be shown that today patients with atrial fibrillation and flutter indeed benefit from results of experimental studies and clinical trials. Furthermore, we will speculate on the therapeutical consequences of some new experimental theories.

THE SINUS NODE IN ATRIAL FIBRILLATION _____

For several reasons the role of the sinus node in atrial fibrillation and flutter is viewed in the clinic with particular interest. Firstly, a gradual exhaustion or damage, clinically manifest as impaired sinus node firing (sinus bradycardia, sinus arrest, sick sinus syndrome) might be anticipated due to chronic atrial arrhythmias. Using intracellular recordings, Allessie et al.[5] have demonstrated that the sinus node area is continuously penetrated with various depth of fibrillating wavelets coming from different directions. Because the core of the sinus node region is highly protected from the invading impulses, the automatic firing of the sinus node is, however, hardly suppressed. On the other hand, these authors showed that the sinus node could maintain atrial fibrillation by delivering of impulses during an episode of local atrial excitability. [5]. However, these experiments do not inform at all about the long-term influence of atrial fibrillation and flutter on the behaviour of the sinus node. Clinical experience with the sick-sinus syndrome has shown that chronic atrial fibrillation without any visible sinus node activity is the endstage in many patients but the time of occurrence of this arrhythmia remains unpredictable[6]. In addition, after 'corridor' operation the sinus node function was frequently insufficient in patients with preoperative chronic atrial fibrillation, despite extensive measures to avoid damage of the sinus node area and its vascular supply[7].

Secondly, paroxysmal atrial fibrillation or flutter frequently require drug therapy to suppress and prevent the arrhythmia. The continuous use of antiarrhythmic drugs, varying from ß-blocking agents to Class I drugs or amiodarone, might adversely influence the long-term behaviour of the sinus node by chronic suppression of impulse information[8]. Therefore, one might speculate on the potential side-effect of a gradual damage to the sinus node by chronic drug therapy for atrial fibrillation or flutter and clinically manifest as sick-sinus syndrome. As far as we know prospective studies to evaluate this drawback of antiarrhythmic drugs have not been conducted. An ideal situation would be the availability of antiarrhythmic drugs with exclusive effectiveness for atrial muscular tissue and not for the sinus or atrioventricular node.

Thirdly, irrespective of the mechanism of impaired sinus node firing in atrial fibrillation, an increase in the time window due to sinus bradycardia can strongly facilitate the conditions for atrial fibrillation to occur by an increase of dispersion of refractoriness[9]. Apart from a regular rhythm offered by atrial pacing, which guarantees a more physiologic cycle length than the extreme ones observed in sick sinus syndrome, the direction of atrial activation appears to be associated with atrial fibrillation. Recent studies of pacemaker patients with sick sinus syndrome have shown the superior effects of chronic atrial pacing to prevent atrial fibrillation when compared to ventricular pacing [10,11]. In addition, in atrial paced patients with preimplant pure sinus brady-cardia the incidence of atrial fibrillation after pacemaker implant was significantly lower than in patients with preimplant brady-tachycardia pattern[12]. This observation suggests the effectiveness of early atrial pacing with the aim to normalize the atrial cycle length to prevent and suppress atrial fibrillation in case of failing sinus node activity.

In conclusion, since only the acute behaviour of the sinus node is explored in experimental studies, questions concerning the chronic effect of atrial fibrillation on sinus node characteristics remain unclarified and await investigation. In the meantime, atrial pacing, sometimes with rate modulation, appears to be the therapy of choice to prevent or suppress atrial fibrillation in cases of failing sinus node firing. The development of antiarrhythmic drugs with specific action on atrial muscle is highly desired to prevent long-term suppression of the sinus node and possible damage of its function.

REFRACTORY PERIODS AND ATRIAL FIBRILLATION _____

In 1990 a task group of experimental and clinical investigators on arrhythmias designed a new matrix for the classification of antiarrhythmic drugs[13]. There are several reasons to improve the current classification system of Vaughan Williams, for example the need to have a more flexible categorization of arrhythmias, their mechanisms and the interaction of anti-arrhythmic drugs. With respect to atrial fibrillation, prolongation of the refracto-ry period (RP) was preferred as a 'beneficial counter measure, because it will reduce the number of simultaneously present wave fronts'[13]. The investiga-tors considered control of the refractory period as a 'vulnerable parameter', because this electrophysiologic parameter appears to be most accessible to drug therapy.

It is today a matter of dispute whether the atrial RP in patients with atrial arrhythmias differs from that of patients without those arrhythmias. Kühlkamp et al. could not measure significant differences in RP of the right atrium between patients with and without arrhythmias, determined at sinus rhythm and various paced cycle lengths[14]. Furthermore, in this study the values of atrial RP diminished gradually when the stimulation rate was increased. However, intra-atrial conduction times measured at various paced heart rates, were significantly longer in patients with atrial arrhythmias. Because the diameter of the left atrium was comparable in patients with and without arrhythmias, the prolonged intra-atrial conduction probably reflects a primary electrical abnormality. Attuel et al. have noted an absence of change in atrial RP following variation of stimulation rates[15]. At short cycle lengths of about 350 to 400 msec, the atrial RP was comparable in patients with arrhythmias and controls, but during deceleration (up to cycle length of 800 to 1.000 msec) the RP did not increase in contrast to arrhythmia-free patients. In addition, RP measured in atrial tissue obtained from patients with atrial fibrillation was usually shorter than that observed in controls, except at fast rates where postrepolarization refractoriness could be observed[16]. These findings are in agreement with the earlier observations of Cosio et al.[17]. Coumel et al. addressed the role of the autonomic nervous system for the genesis of atrial fibrillation by showing provocation of human atrial fibrillation following isoprote-ronol as well as adenosine triphosphate, which initiates strong vagal stimulati-on[8]. Shortening of the RP of atrial fibers was noted following strong vagal activity, which favours the development of reentry. However, concerning human atrial fibrillation, the hypothesis of vagal induced atrial fibrillation by shortening of atrial RP needs validation.

The evidence available today shows that a relatively short RP of atrial tissue can be observed in a subset of patients with atrial fibrillation which facilitates the initiation and maintenance of atrial fibrillation. Differences in observed atrial RP might be explained by discordant pacing protocols and dissimilarity of studied patient populations.

Because the extrastimulus method to determine atrial RP at many sites of the atria is time-consuming and frequently a source of atrial fibrillation in patients prone to this arrhythmia, Lammers et al. and Opthof et al. have used the average interval between local depolarizations during atrial fibrillation as an index for local refractoriness[18,19]. This approach is justified because atrial tissue is reexcited immediately following completion of the refractory period during atrial fibrillation. Ramdat Misier et al.[20] have found a very good correlation between RP determined with the extrastimulus method and atrial fibrillation intervals measured at 4 different epicardial sites of the human right atrium, which validates this technique for measurement of 'refractoriness' during atrial fibrillation.

To determine the difference in local 'refractoriness' and the degree of inhomogeneity of 'refractoriness' in patients with and without atrial fibrillation, a multiterminal grid with up to 64 electrodes was positioned over the epicardial right atrium of patients operated for drug refractory atrial fibrillation and a control group. In both groups antiarrhythmic drugs were discontinued at least 5 drug half-lifes and recordings were made prior to institution of extracorporeal circulation. In patients with drug refractory atrial fibrillation, 'corridor' surgery was carried out[21]. Shorter intervals of atrial fibrillation were recorded in patients with paroxysmal atrial fibrillation compared to control patients (Figure 1).

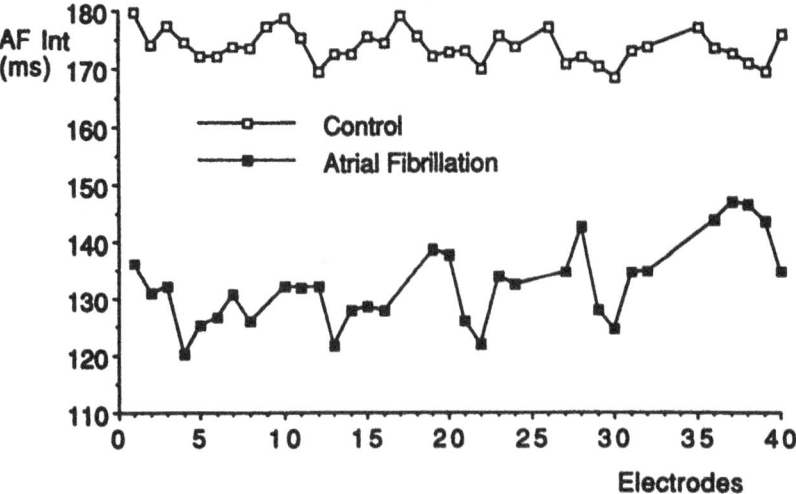

Figure 1. Atrial fibrillation intervals (AF Int) recorded simultaneously at 37 sites (electrodes) in a control patient and at 32 sites in a patient with paroxysmal atrial fibrillation (from: Ramdat Misier et al.[20] (with permission).

In addition, the dispersion of atrial fibrillation intervals or 'refractoriness' extended that of control patients but the dispersion was rather localized (Table 1).

Table 1. **Summary of recording sites, mean atrial fibrillation interval and variance in all patients from both groups**

	AF	Control	p Value
Patients (no.)	10	6	–
Recording sites (no.)	247	118	–
AF interval (ms)	152 ± 3	176 ± 8.1	<0.05
Variance (ms²)	31.2	11.5	<0.001

Values are mean values ± SEM; AF = atrial fibrillation.

Because both groups had normal atrial dimensions, the difference in 'refractoriness' and 'dispersion of refractoriness' cannot be attributed to differences in atrial tissue mass.

Dispersion of 'refractoriness' of atrial tissue has been earlier observed in animal studies. Alessie et al.[22] have found a difference of 40 msec of RP, and Zipes et al.[23] have reported differences in RP of 25 to 110 msec. In view of the wavelength theory, these studies on atrial RP suggest strongly that the shortened 'refractoriness' is an important risk factor for the initiation and perpetuation of atrial fibrillation. Moreover, the significant increase in dispersion of 'refractoriness' seems sufficient to create unidirectional block, which is one of the prerequisites for reentrant circuits. Allessie et al. have reported that a difference of RP of 11 to 16 msec in adjacent tissue was sufficient to establish unidirectional block following properly timed extrastimuli [24].

From these studies it can be concluded that 'refractoriness' of human atrial fibrillation cannot be measured by invasive studies with the aid of multipolar electrodes because many atrial electrograms have to be recorded simultaneously. However, in the animal laboratory and in the operation theatre multi electrode mapping of the atria offers a new method to study the effects of antiarrhythmics in atrial fibrillation by determination of 'refractoriness'. In the meantime, antiarrhythmic drugs prolonging the refractory period remain the drugs of choice to treat atrial fibrillation because the refractory period seems to be shorter than normal in patients with atrial fibrillation.

A THEORY TO EXPLAIN THE DIFFERENT CONVERSION RATE OF ATRIAL FIBRILLATION AND FLUTTER AFTER CLASS Ic ANTIARRHYTHMICS _____

Suttorp et al. recently demonstrated a higher conversion rate of atrial fibrillation than of atrial flutter following intravenous administration of flecainide or propafenone, two Class Ic antiarrhythmic agents[25]. On the basis of the wavelength theory for maintenance of circus movement reentry, the relatively poor conversion rate for atrial flutter may be explained by flecainide's actions to diminish conduction velocity (CV) while exerting little effect on refractoriness (RP) in the atria[26]. The resultant decrease in wavelength (CV x RP) would be expected to favor perpetuation of the reentrant mechanism responsible for the flutter. In the case of atrial fibrillation, flecainide-induced shortening of the wavelength through slowing of conduction might be expected to result in a greater number of wavelets and consequently more stable fibrillation. These facts notwithstanding, both flecainide and propafenone are clearly efficacious in converting atrial fibrillation, although relatively ineffective in converting atrial flutter.

This apparent paradox might be explained by differences in the response of endocardial and epicardial atrial tissues to sodium channel blockade as has been observed in ventricular tissues. Krishnan and Antzelevitch recently reported that strong sodium blockade produces different, sometimes opposite responses in canine ventricular epicardium when compared to endocardium [27]. Potent block of the sodium channels was found to depress excitability in epicardium to a much greater extent than in endocardium. As a result, measurements of the refractory period in epicardium were greatly dependent on the strength of the stimulus. In the example illustrated in Figure 2, potent blockade of the sodium channels with a high concentration of propanolol is shown to result in acceleration-induced marked prolongation of the effective refractory period (RP) in epicardium when a stimulus of 2,5 times diastolic threshold was employed. Postrepolarization refractoriness is evident in the epicardium (Figure 2B) but not the endocardium (Figure 2A) under these conditions. When the intensity of the stimulus was increased to 4 times diastolic threshold, postrepolarization refractoriness and RP prolongation at fast rates were no longer evident in the epicardium (Figure 2C).

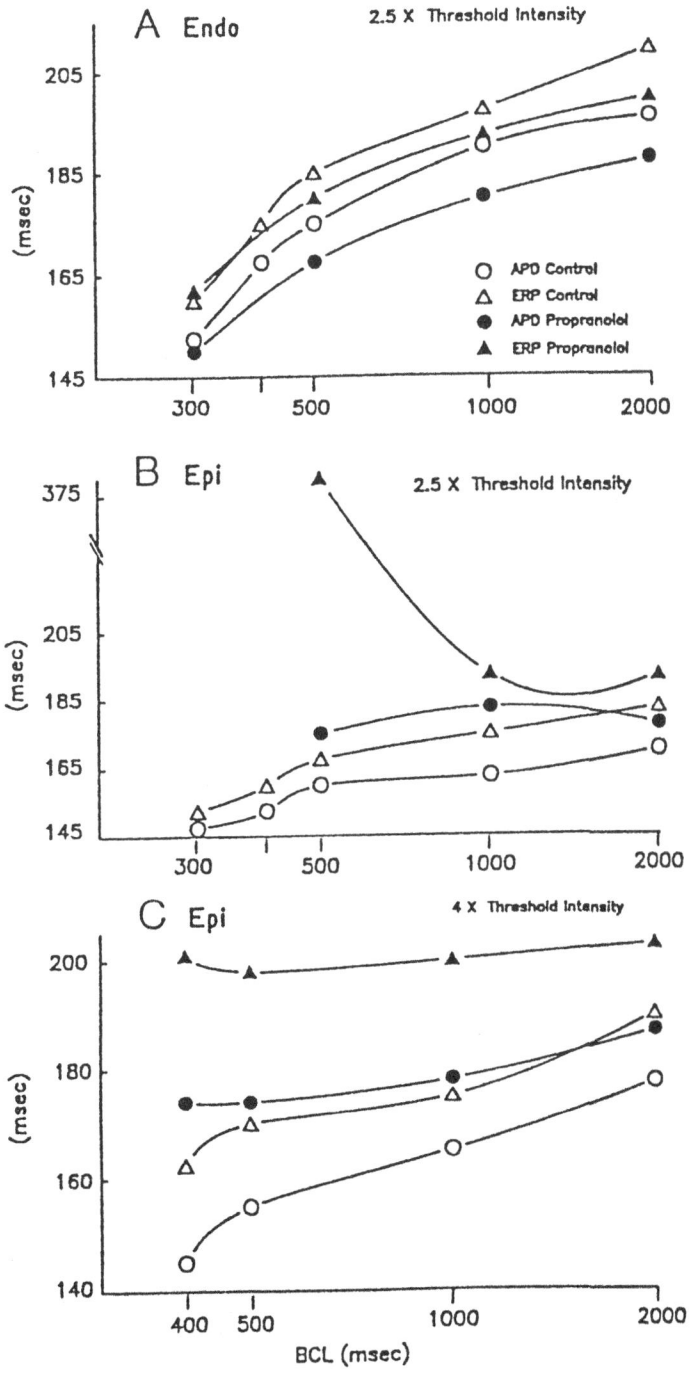

Figure 2.

Graphs showing rate dependence of action potential duration (APD) and effective refractory period (ERP) in endocardium (Endo) and epicardium (Epi) in the absence (open circle and triangle) and presence (closed circle and triangle) of 3 µg/ml propanolol (40 minutes in panels A and B, 45 minutes in panel C).
Panels A and B: protocols in which ERP was determined using test pulses 2,5 times diastolic threshold intensity.
Panel C: results obtained using test pulses 4 times diastolic threshold intensity (from Krishnan and Antzelevitch [27](with permission).

As a point of interest, most measurements of refractoriness following Class Ic agents have been performed using endocardial electrodes or in experiments employing endocardial atrial tissues exclusively. Although electrophysiologic differences between epicardium and endocardium have been reported in atria, a study of the differential effect of sodium blockers on these two atrial tissue subtypes has not been done[28]. If the data from canine ventricles apply to human atria, a reasonable hypothesis to explain the clinical results might be formulated based on the relative efficacy of flutter and fibrillation wave fronts to excite atrial epicardium exposed to potent sodium blockade. The greater source of current provided by organized flutter waves would be comparable to the situation in Figure 2C - the effect on epicardial refractoriness would be modest and termination of the reentry would be less likely. On the other hand, the smaller source of current provided by the fragmented fibrillation waves would be comparable to the situation graphically illustrated in Figure 2B - epicardial refractoriness would increase dramatically in response to potent sodium blockade, postrepolarization refractoriness would develop, and the likelihood of termination of fibrillation would be high. A test of this hypothesis clearly await experimental measurements of these parameter in atrial epicardial and endocardial tissues and cells.

A consequence of this theory, resulting from the experiments of the Antzelevitch group, might be that evaluation of antiarrhythmic drugs becomes still more complex. Apart from differences in response of the target cells to drugs, the electrical strength of the depolarization wave generated by the arrhythmia under study, should also be taken into account.

NONPHARMACOLOGIC TREATMENT
OF ATRIAL FLUTTER _____

Reentry is currently considered the arrhythmogenic mechanism of atrial flutter, as already suggested in 1920 by Lewis et al.[29] and later documented by Boineau et al. in dog studies[30]. Waldo et al. distinguish two different types of atrial flutter: the classical or type I (the sawtooth pattern of flutter waves in inferior ECG leads and a rate of 240 to 340 bpm), whereas type II is faster with a flutter rate of 340 to 430 bpm[31,32]. There is strong evidence that atrial flutter type I circulates around artificial or natural obstacles of the right atrium[29,30]. Fixed rapid atrial pacing close to the circuit can yield entrainment of atrial flutter type I which becomes manifest by constant fusion between the flutter and paced impulses except for the last beat, whereas the degree of fusion depends on the pacing rate. These findings are in agreement with the presence of an excitable gap in atrial flutter type I in contrast to type II where entrainment or resetting could never be achieved by atrial pacing. Furthermore, Waldo et al. have proposed criteria for the delineation of the site of ablation of atrial flutter type I based on the principles of entrainment[33].

Because of the stable pattern of atrial flutter, it is not surprising that attempts have been undertaken to eliminate atrial flutter with surgical or catheter ablation in case of drug refractoriness. During mapping of atrial flutter type I, several investigators have demonstrated fragmented deflections in the local bipolar atrial electrograms[34,35,36]. These multiphasic electrograms are usually interpreted as the recording of a pathway of excitation with a prolonged conduction time. These signals suggest the presence of a critical area of the reentry circuit[37]. This area is characterized by either a slow conduction of the activation front from entrance to exit or an anatomical barrier around which the activation wave travels in opposite directions[34]. To exclude standby pathways of excitation, fixed atrial pacing can be applied, and according to the criteria for entrainment, a dissociation of the fragmented signals from the tachycardia during entrainment unmasks standby pathways. However, in areas of critical slow conduction such a dissociation will not be encountered. DC shocks delivered in areas with multiphasic electrograms have been shown highly effective to ablate atrial flutter type I [34,35,36].

Concerning the anatomical position of the 'site of origin' of atrial flutter type I, Klein et al. have recently published preoperative endocardial and peroperative epicardial observations of 2 patients with atrial flutter type I [38]. The endocardial maps showed early potentials with reference to the flutter wave close to the coronary sinus orifice and epicardial maps demonstrated slow conduction in the right posteroseptal region; local cryosurgical ablation cured the arrhythmia. Chauvin and Brechenmacher and Saoudi et al. delivered DC catheter shocks in the posteroseptal area of the right atrium, which showed multiphasic local electrograms and could ablate atrial flutter in most cases [35,36].

Our group has performed peroperative mapping in patients with drug refractory atrial flutter type I, using unipolar 64 electrode grids and computer assisted analysis[39], or handhold tripolar probes. The endocardial maps showed 2 different patterns of activation: a reentry circuit travelling around the tricuspid valve ring or a reentry circuit with a region of slow conduction close to coronary sinus orifice, whereas the remaining right and left atrial muscular mass was passively activated from the reentry circuit (Figures 3 and 4).

Very recently, Ward et al. have demonstrated that a series of low energy DC shocks without precise catheter mapping is feasible to eliminate atrial flutter in patients[40]. These authors assumed that the 'site of origin' of atrial flutter type I was between the AV node area and coronary sinus orifice. The sites of ablation were localized by the anatomical landmarks of the triangle of Koch, visualized by the fluoroscopic position of catheters recording the His bundle and positioned in the coronary sinus orifice respectively. Although, third degree AV block was temporarily observed after the DC shocks, normal AV conduction resumed in all cases. More experience is needed for validation of this approach as a standard therapy in drug refractory atrial flutter type I.

In conclusion, the nonpharmacologic treatment of atrial flutter type I clearly illustrates the relationship between theories and therapeutical solution. However, final treatment of drug refractory atrial flutter type II still remains a challenge. His bundle ablation is today the only alternative treatment in case of drug refractoriness.

NONPHARMACOLOGIC TREATMENT OF ATRIAL FIBRILLATION

In the early 60-ties Moe et al. have reported theories on the mechanism of atrial fibrillation[41,42]. The arrhythmia is a condition in which multiple wavelets of excitation randomly wander through the atria. The perpetuation of atrial fibrillation depends on the number of wavelets, as was demonstrated by a computer model [41,42]. The multiple wavelet theory was further elaborated in canine hearts by Allessie et al., and later the concept of the leading circle with an unexcitable gap had been developed[43]. Allessie et al. confirmed the hypothesis of Moe, that a critical number of wavelets was required for perpetuation of the arrhythmia. The authors could determine that an average number

Figure 3.

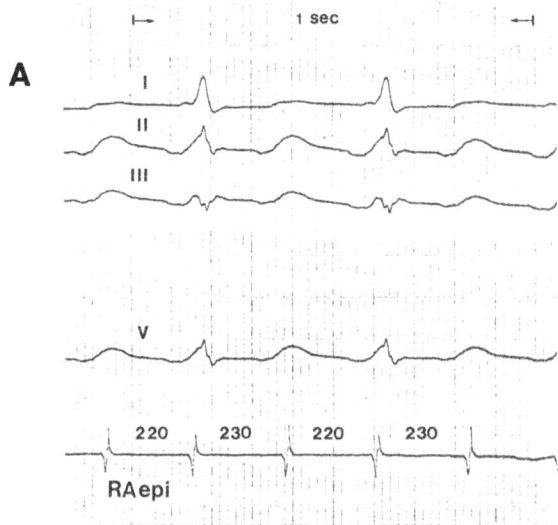

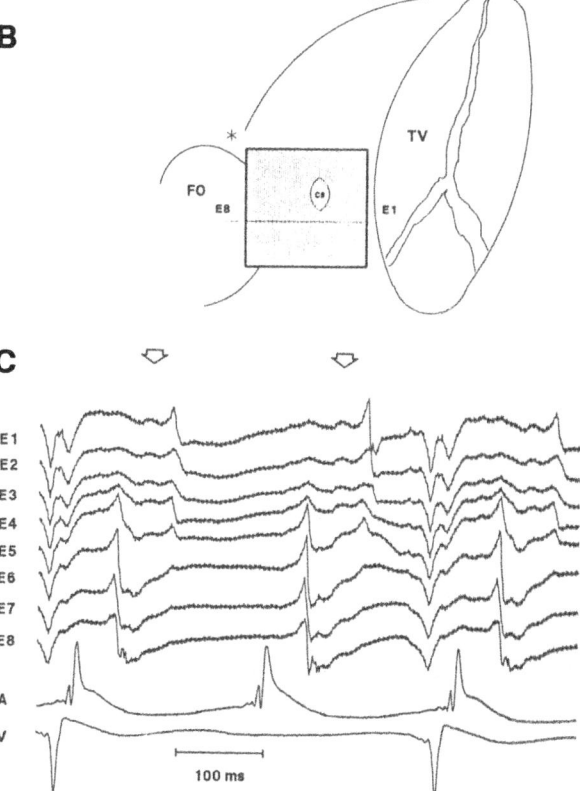

Figure 3.

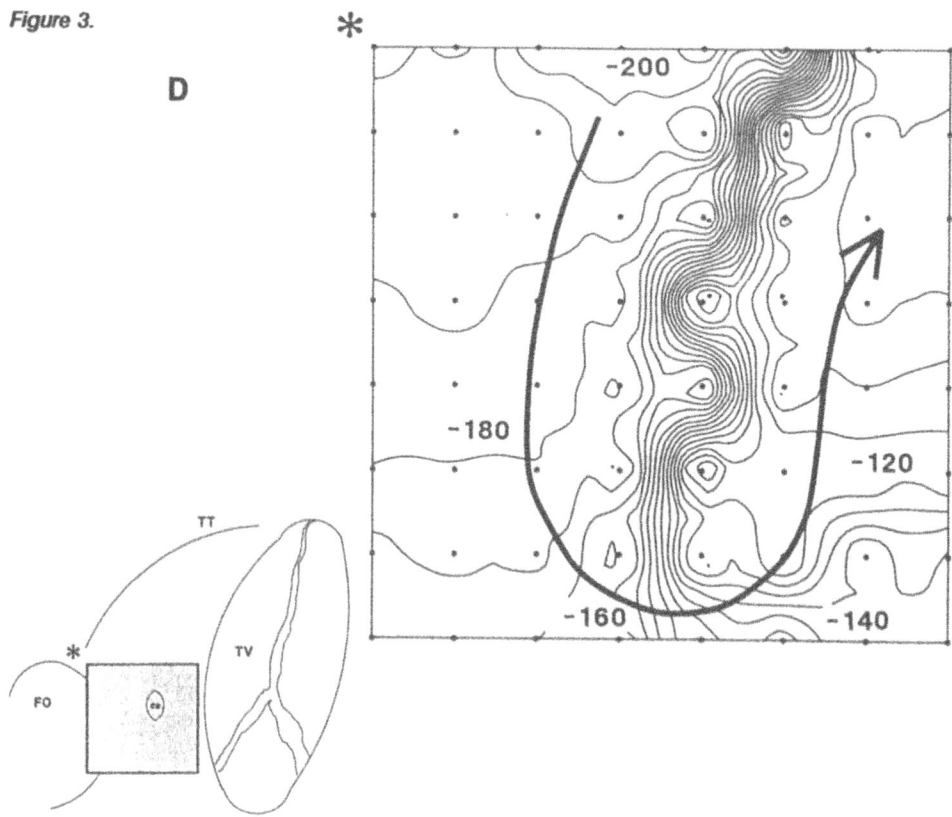

Figure 3. Results of peroperative endocardial mapping of atrial flutter type I. Panel A shows the peroperative EKG, leads I, II and III, and a precordial lead after thoracotomy. A stable atrial flutter type 1 with a cycle length of 220 msec is present. The local epicardial electrogram displays slight alterations of the cycle lengths. Panel B shows the position of the 64 unipolar multi-electrode grid with interspacing of 2 mm in the area between the fossa ovalis (FO) and the attachment of the septal slip of the tricuspid valve (TV) covering the coronary sinus (CS) orifice. Panel C displays the local unipolar electrograms half between top and bottom of the grid demonstrating a clear zone of difference in activation times of 90 msec between E1 to E3 and E4 to E8. Panel D displays the composite of isochrones showing a clear zone of slow conduction or block around which the activation wave of the flutter travels. Cryoablation of area around the coronary sinus orifice resulted in definitive elimination of the flutter.

Figure 4. Results of peroperative endocardial mapping of atrial flutter type 1. Panel A shows the peroperative EKG leads I, II and III, and a precordial lead after thoracotomy. From the epicardial recording an atrial cycle length of 240 msec is measured. Panel B shows the results of measurements of local activation times in the bipolar atrial electrograms using a handhold tripolar probe. A reentrant circuit is located around the tricuspid ring and shows a relatively slower conduction in the region of the coronary sinus orifice. Cryoablation of that region eliminated the atrial flutter.

Figure 4.

A

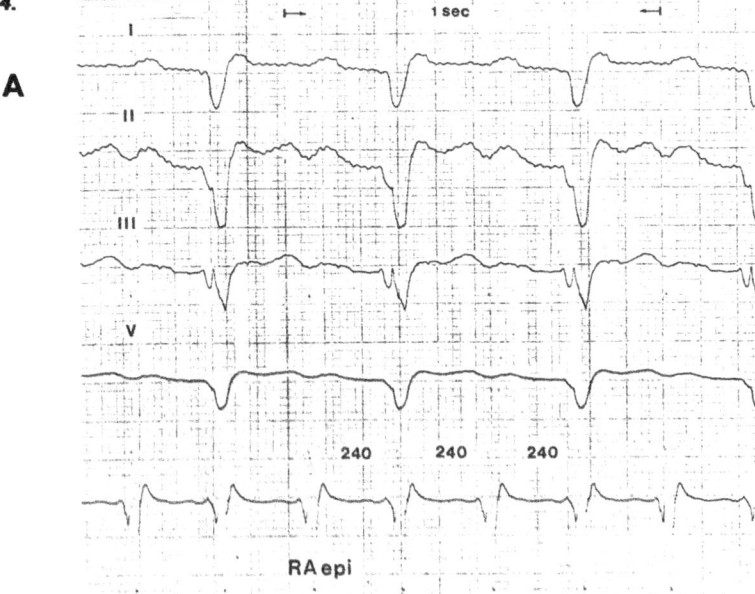

B

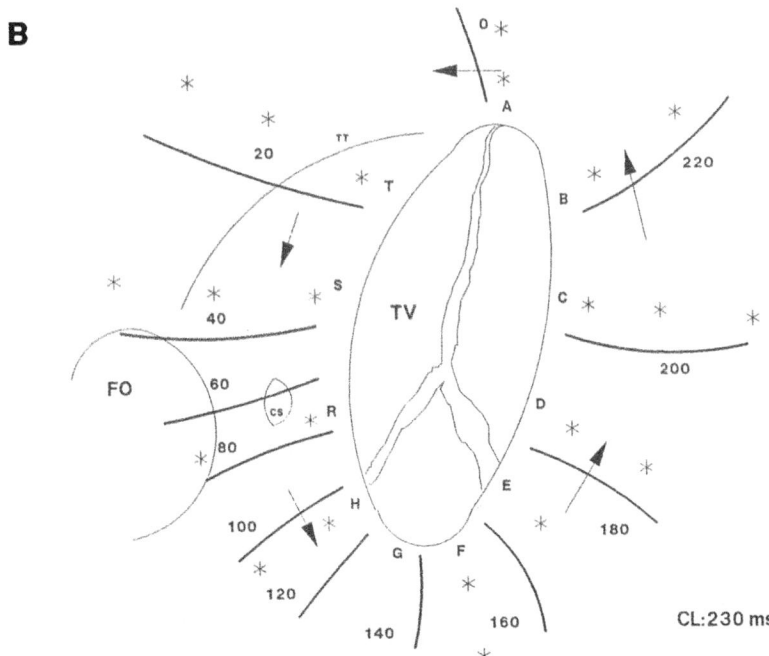

of at least 3 but not more than 6 simultaneously circulating wavelets in canine right and left atrium were required for the persistence of atrial fibrillation[24]. Very recently, Allessie et al. performed epicardial mapping of induced atrial fibrillation in patients who underwent surgical ablation of accessory AV pathways, and verified the hypothesis of multiple wavelets in human atrial fibrillation[44]. However, it was not possible to precisely define the smallest number of wavelets required in order to maintain atrial fibrillation in human atria. In addition, Rensma et al. have clearly demonstrated that inducibility of atrial fibrillation depends on the length of the excitation wave (defined by the product of refractory period and conduction velocity)[45]. Atrial fibrillation could only be initiated in animals by electrical stimuli if the wave length was shorter than 7.8 cm. Therefore, when the mean duration of the refractory period and/or mean conduction velocity cannot be prolonged sufficiently by antiarrhythmic drugs, manipulation of the atrial mass might be the next therapeutical step to eliminate drug refractory paroxysmal atrial fibrillation.

Because the atrial mass is constant, surgical methods to divide the atrial walls into segments, might yield an unfavorable condition for atrial fibrillation to emerge due to the diminished number of wavelets that can be harboured in the different atrial segments. Conceivably, the impulse formation of the sinus node and the transmission of sinus impulses to the ventricles to maintain chronotropy should be kept unaffected.

Based on these principles, Guiraudon et al. have designed the 'corridor' operation[46,7]. In their atrial surgery a right atrial conduit is constructed to isolate the sinus node and the atrioventricular node from the left and remaining right atrium in order to preserve physiologic drive of the ventricles. The excluded left and right atria can fibrillate without influence on the ventricular rhythm (Figure 5).

Our group has obtained experience with the 'corridor' operation in the surgical treatment of drug refractory *paroxysmal* atrial fibrillation[21,47]. Between 1987 and 1991, 24 patients with paroxysmal atrial fibrillation underwent surgical treatment. In 20 patients (83%) long-term successful isolation could be achieved, whereas in the remaining 4 patients an electrical leakage between left atrium and 'corridor' persisted after surgery, usually in the area adjacent to the coronary sinus. After a mean follow-up of 32 months all patients were alive

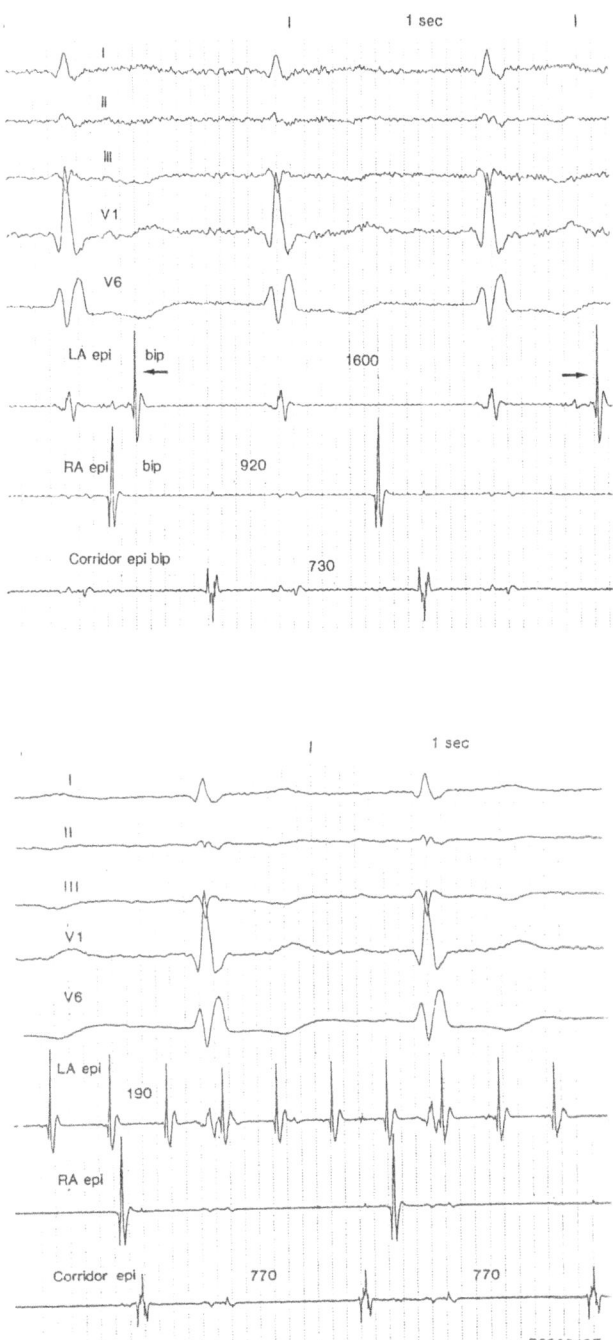

Figure 5.

Results of 'corridor' operation. Both panels show five electrocardiographic leads and the bipolar epicardial electrograms of left atrium (LA epi) and 'corridor' (Corridor epi) of the same patient (paper speed, 100 mm per min). In panel A the left atrium shows slow rhythm (cycle length, 1,600 msec) and the residual right atrium a faster rhythm (cycle length, 920 msec), whereas the 'corridor' has a sinus rhythm (cycle length, 730 msec) with 1:1 atrioventricular conduction and complete right bundle branch block. Panel B displays an atrium flutter (cycle length, 190 msec) in the left atrium. From both recordings it is evident that the sinus rhythm in the 'corridor' is not influenced by the impulses in other compartments[21] (with permission).

and 85% of the successfully operated patients were free of arrhythmia without drugs, whereas in only 1 patient paroxysmal atrial fibrillation reoccurred temporarily. The sinus node function remained undisturbed in 16 of 20 (80%) patients, whereas 4 patients needed pacemaker implantation for insufficient sinus rhythm at rest. Because the left atrium is allowed to fibrillate and lacks normal impulse formation after the 'corridor' operation, it is not surprising that active left atrial filling was always absent. However, Doppler echocardiography demonstrated preservation of right atrial contribution to right ventricular filling in 75% of the operated patients. All patients improved life style after surgery because of the absence of atrial fibrillation. A minor stroke occurred in 2 patients within 3 months after surgery and therefore anticoagulant therapy is still recommended. Our long-term experience has validated the concept and the clinical value of the 'corridor' operation when drug refractoriness of paroxysmal atrial fibrillation becomes clear[47].

To circumvent the disadvantage of possible left atrial thromboembolism after the 'corridor' operation, Cox et al. have developed the 'maze' procedure [48,49]. To describe the procedure in short, both atrial appendages are excised and the entrance of the pulmonary veins in the left atrium is isolated. On several appropriate sites of the left and right atrium incisions are made which divide the atria in several segments ('maze') in order to reduce the atrial mass. However, conduction of sinus impulses to activate both atria as well as the AV node are guaranteed by these atrial segments and thereby preserve atrial contribution to ventricular filling.

Between 1987 and 1991, 11 patients with paroxysmal atrial fibrillation, 9 patients with chronic atrial fibrillation and 2 patients with atrial flutter underwent the 'maze' operation[50]. There was no inhospital or late mortality. Atrial fibrillation was never seen beyond the 3 months postoperative period, but spontaneous atrial flutter was observed in 3 patients. In 9 of 22 (41%) patients a rate modulated dual chamber pacemaker was inserted postoperatively, but Cox et al. emphasized that 5 of 9 patients had preoperative sick-sinus syndrome and 2 patients did not need chronic stimulation during follow-up because of resumption of normal sinus node firing[51]. In only 2 cases (9%) the sinus node remained abnormal after the 'maze' operation. The surgical group of St Louis (U.S.A.) claims the preservation of atrial transport function after the 'maze' operation as documented by noninvasive techniques such as

Doppler examinations and dynamic magnetic resonance imaging scans. However, long-term follow-up is needed to define this presumed hemodynamic advantage because a deleterious effect of the multiple incisions inherent to the 'maze' operation on atrial contractility cannot be excluded.

In conclusion, the surgical approach of atrial fibrillation reflects clearly the benefits of experimental studies on atrial fibrillation. Although the selection criteria for surgery need further refinement, criteria for surgical therapy of atrial fibrillation are now well established.

CONCLUDING REMARKS _____

Although extensive clinical trials are needed to verify the theories resulting from experimental studies on atrial fibrillation and flutter, the first clinical applications favor the usefulness of these concepts. The introduction of the multiple circulating wavelets theory to explain atrial fibrillation, the wavelength concept and recent information on the characteristics of refractoriness in atrial fibrillation have set a new stage for therapeutic approach varying from new antiarrhythmic drugs to surgical techniques.

In our opinion, experimental investigators active in the area of arrhythmias will be challenged by new questions elicited by clinical trials. The resulting mutual interaction between laboratory and clinic might become a very fascinating area of cardiology.

References

[1]   Allessie MA, Lammers WJEP, Bonke FIM, Hollen J. Experimental evaluation of Moe's multiple wavelet hypothesis of atrial fibrillation. In: Zipes D, Jalife J (eds), Cardiac Electrophysiology and Arrhythmias, 1985, Grune & Stratton, pp 265-275.
[2]   Gilst WH van, Graeff PA de, Kingma JH, Wesseling H, Langen CDJ de. Capotpril reduces purine loss and reperfusion arrhythmias in the rat heart after coronary artery occlusion. Eur J Pharmacol 1984;100:113-117.
[3]   Six AJ, Louwerenburg JH, Kingma JH, Robles de Medina EO, van Hemel NM. Predicted value of ventricular arrhythmias for patency of the infarct-related coronary artery after thrombolytic therapy. Br Heart J 1991;66:143-146.
[4]   Rosenbaum MB, Lázzari JO, Elizari MV. The role of phase 3 and phase 4 block in clinical electrcardiography. In: Wellens HJJ, Lie KI, Janse MJ (eds), The conduction system of the heart. Martinus Nijhoff, The Hague, 1976, pp 126-142.
[5]   Janse MJ, Allessie MA. Experimental observations in atrial fibrillation. In: Falk RH,

Podrid PJ (eds), Atrial Fibrillation and Management. Raven Press Lts., New York, 1992, pp 41-57.

[6]   Amikam S, Riss E. The natural history of sick sinus syndrome following permanent pacemaker implantation. Abstracts Circulation 1977/1978;55 and 56:III-155.

[7]   Leitch JW, Klein G, Yee R, Guiraudon G. Sinus node-atrioventricular node isolation: Long-term results with the 'corridor' operation for atrial fibrillation. JACC 1991;17:970-975.

[8]   Coumel P. Neural aspects of paroxysmal atrial fibrillation. In: Falk RM, Podrid PJ (eds), Atrial fibrillation and management. Raven Press Ltd, New York, 1992, pp 109-125.

[9]   Han J, Millet D, Chizzonitti B, Moe GK. Temporal dispersion of recovery of excitability in atrium and ventricle as a function of heart rate. AM Heart J 1966;71:481-487.

[10]   Rosenqvist M, Brandt J, Schüller. Long-term pacing in sinus node disease: Effects of stimulation mode on cardiovascular morbidity and mortality. Am Heart J 1988;116:16-22.

[11]   Sutton R, Kenny RA. The natural history of sick sinus syndrome. PACE 1986;9:1110-1114.

[12]   Hemel NM van, Mast EG, Kingma JH, Bakema H, Ascoop CAPL. Factors interfering with stable chronic atrial pacing in the brady-tachycardia syndrome. (Abstract) PACE 1989;12:II,1237.

[13]   Task Forse of the Working Group on Arrhythmias of the European Society of Cardiology. The Sicilian Gambit: A new approach to the classification of antiarrhythmic drugs based on their actions on arrhythmogenic mechanisms. Circulation 1991;84:1831-1851.

[14]   Kühlkamp V, Haasis R, Seipel L. Atrial vulnerability and electrophysioly determined in patients with and without paroxysmal atrial fibrillation. PACE 1992;15:71-80.

[15]   Attuel P, Childers R, Cauchemer B, et al. Failure in rate adaptation of the atrial refractory period: its relationship to vulnerability. Int J Cardiol 1982;2:179-197.

[16]   Le Heuzey JY, Boutjdir M, Gagey S, Lavergne T, Guize L. Cellular aspects of atrial vulnerability. In: Attuel P, Coumel P, Janse MJ (eds), The atrium in health and disease. Mount Kisco, N.Y.: Futura, 1989, pp 81-94.

[17]   Cosio FG, Palacios J, Vidal JM, Cocina EG, Gómez-Sánchez MA, Tamargo L. Electrophysiologic studies in atrial fibrillation. Slow conduction of premature impluses: a possible manifestation of the background for reentry. Am J Cardiol 1983;51:122-130.

[18]   Lammers WJEP, Allessie MA, Rensma PL, Schalij MJ. The use of fibrillation cycle length to determine spatial dispersion in electrophysiological properties and to characterize the underlying mechanism of fibrillation. New Trends Arrhythmias 1986;2:109-112.

[19]   Opthof T, Ramdat Misier AR, Coronel R, Vermeulen JT, Verberne HJ, Frank RGJ, Moulijn AC, Capelle FJL van, Janse MJ. Dispersion of refractoriness in canine ventricular myocardium: effects of sympathetic stimulation. Circ Res 1991;68:1204-1215.

[20]   Ramdat Misier A, Opthof T, Hemel NM van, Defauw JJAM, Bakker JMT de, Janse MJ, Capelle FJL van. Increased dispersion of 'refractoriness' in patients with idiopathic paroxysmal atrial fibrillation. JACC 1992;19:1531-1535.

[21]   Defauw JJAMT, Guiraudon GM, Hemel NM van, Vermeulen FEE, Kingma JH, Bakker JMT de. Surgical therapy of paroxysmal atrial fibrillation with the 'corridor' operation. Ann Thorac Surg 1992;53:564-571.

[22]   Alessie R, Nusynowitz M, Abildskov JA, Moe GK. Nonuniform distribution of vagal effects on atrial refractory period. Am J Physiol 1958;194:406-410.

[23]   Zipes DP, Michalick MJ, Robbins GT. Effects of selective vagal and stellate ganglion stimulation on atrial refractoriness. Cardiovasc Res 1974;8:647-655.

[24]   Allessie MA, Lammers WJEP, Bonke FIM, Hollen J. Experimental evaluation of Moe's multiple wavelet hypothesis of atrial fibrillation. In: Zipes D and Jalife J (eds), Cardiac Electrophysiology and Arrhythmias. Grune & Stratton, 1985, pp 265-275.

[25]   Suttorp MJ, Kingma JH, Lie-A-Huen L, Mast EG. Intravenous flecained versus verapamil for acute conversion of paroxysmal atrial fibrillation or flutter to sinus rhythm. Am J Cardiol 1989;63:693-696.

[26]   Nathan AW, Camm AJ, Bexton RS, Hellestrand KJ. Intravenous flecainide acetate for the clinical management of paroxysmal tachycardias. Clin Cardiol 1987;10:317-322.

[27]   Krishnan SC, Antzelevitch C. Sodium channel block produces opposite electrophysiological effects in canine ventricular epicardium and endocardium. Circ Res 1991; 69:277-290.

[28]   Wang Z, Fermini B, Nattel S. Repolarization differences between guinea pig atrial endocardium and epicardium: evidence for the role of I_{to}. Am J Physiol 1991;260: H1501-H1506.

[29]   Lewis T, Feil HS, Strpud WD. Observations upon flutter and fibrillation: II. The nature of auricular flutter. Heart 1920;7:191-246.

[30]   Boineau JP, Schuessler RB, Mooney CR, Miller CB, Wylds AC, Hudson RD, Borremans JM, Brockus CW. Natural and evoked atrial flutter due to circus movement in dogs. Am J Cardiol 1980;45:1167-1181.

[31]   Wells JL, Karp RB, Kouchoukos NT, Maclean WAH, James TN, Waldo AL. Characterization of atrial fibrillation in man: Studies following open heart surgery. PACE 1978; 1:424-438.

[32]   Wells Jr JL , Maclean WAH, James TN, Waldo AL. Characterization of atrial flutter. Studies in man after open heart surgery using fixed atrial electrodes. Circulation 1979;60:665-673

[33]   Waldo AL, Okumura K, Olshansky B, Henthorn RW. Use of transient entrainment of tachycardias as an aid to the application of fulguration. In: Fontaine G, Scheinman MM (eds), Ablation in Cardiac Arrhythmias. Mount Kisco, NY, Futura Publishing, 1987, pp 277.

[34]   Cosio FG, Arribas F, Barbero JM, Wallmeyer C, Goicolea A. Validation of double spike electrograms as markers of conduction delay or block in atrial flutter. Am J Cardiol 1988;61:775-780.

[35]   Chauvin M, Brechenmacher C. Endocardial catheter fulguration for treatment of atrial flutter. Am J Cardiol 1988;61:471-473.

[36]   Saoudi N, Atallah G, Kirkorian G, Touboul P. Catheter ablation of the atrial myocardium in human type I atrial flutter. Circulation 1990;81:762-771.

[37]   Wit AL, Josephson ME. Fractionated electrograms and continuous electrical activity: Fact or artefact. In: Zipes DP and Jalife J (eds), Cardiac Electrophysiology and Arrhythmias. Grune and Stratton, Orlando, 1985, pp 343-351.

[38]   Klein GJ, Guiraudon GM, Sharma AD, Milstein S. Demonstration of macroreentry and feasibility of operative therapy in the common type of atrial flutter. Am J Cardiol 1986;57:587-591.

[39]   Bakker JMT de, Capelle FJL van, Janse MJ, Durrer D. An interactive computer system for guiding the surgical treatment of life-threatening ventricular tachycardias. IEEE Trans BME 1984;31:362-384.

[40]   O'Núnáin S, Linker NJ, Sneddon JF, Debbas NMG, Camm AJ, Ward DE. Catheter ablation by low energy DC shocks for successful management of atrial flutter. Br Heart J 1992;67:67-71.

[41]   Moe GK, Abildskov JA. Atrial fibrillation as self-sustaining arrhythmia independent of focal discharche. Am Heart J 1959;58:59-70.

[42]   Moe GK, Theinboldt WC, Abildskov JA. A computer model of atrial fibrillation. Am

Heart J 1964;67:200-220.
[43]   Allessie MA, Bonke FIM, Schopman FJG. Circus movement in rabbit atrial muscle as a mechanism of tachycardia III. The 'leading circle' concept: A new model of circus movement in cardiac tissue without the involvement of an anatomic obstacle. Circ Res 1979;41:9-18.
[44]   Allessie MA, Brugada J, Boersma L, Kirchhof C, Smeets J, Penn O, Wellens H. Mapping of atrial fibrillation in man. (Abstract) Eur Jeart J 1990;11:5.
[45]   Rensma PL, Allessie MA, Lammers WJEP, Bonke FIM, Schalij MJS. Length of excitation wave and susceptibility to reentrant atrial arrhythmias in normal conscious dogs. Circ Res 1988;62:395-410.
[46]   Guiraudon GM, Campbell CS, Jones DL, McLellan DG, MacDonald JL. Combined sino-atrial node atrio-ventricular isolation: a surgical alternative to His bundle ablation in patients with atrial fibrillation. (Abstract) Circulation 1985;72:III-220.
[47]   Hemel NM van, Defauw JAM, Kingma JH, Jessurun ER, Bakker J de, Guiraudon G. Longterm efficacy of surgical treatment for drug refractory paroxysmal atrial fibrillation using the 'corridor' procedure. (Abstract) Circulation 1991;84:II-194.
[48]   Cox JL. The surgical treatment of atrial fibrillation. IV. Surgical technique. J Thorac Cardiovasc Surg 1991;101:584-592.
[49]   Cox JL, Schuessler RB, D'Agostino HJ, Stone CM, Byung-Chul Ch, Cain ME, Corr PB, Boineau JP. The surgical treatment of atrial fibrillation. III. Development of a definitive surgical procedure. J Thorac Cardiovasc Surg 1991;101:569-583.
[50]   Cox JL, Boineau JP, Schuessler RB, Ferguson TB Jr, Cain ME, Lindsay BD, et al. Successful surgical treatment of atrial fibrillation. Review and clinical update. JAMA 1991;266:1976-1980.

Chapter 2

ATRIAL FUNCTIONAL ANATOMY

Gérard M. Guiraudon

Colette M. Guiraudon

Faculty of Medicine
Departments of Surgery and Pathology
University of Western Ontario
University Hospital
London, Ontario
Canada

23

J. H. Kingma et al. (eds.), Atrial fibrillation, a treatable disease?, 23–40.
© 1992 *Kluwer Academic Publishers.*

INTRODUCTION _____

Atrial anatomy plays a role in heart physiology by controlling, to an extent, heart rate, ventricular filling and myocardial contractility. Atrial fibrillation disrupts atrial functional anatomy by abolishing sinus node chronotropic function, atrial contraction, and by impairing AV nodal physiology.

We will describe the anatomical and physiological characteristics of the atria. Insights into atrial functional anatomy may identify therapeutic end-points, especially for surgical procedures aimed at atrial fibrillation.

GROSS ANATOMY _____

The atria are two pouches between the venous return and the atrioventricular orifice[1,2,3,4].

The *right atrium* is larger than the left (its capacity has been estimated about 57 ml). Its wall thickness, about 2 mm, is thinner than that of the left (3 mm). The right atrium, is constituted of 2 segments: the sinus venarum and the body. The *sinus venarum* is the smooth part of the RA located between the superior and inferior venae cavae. It has the shape of a cylinder with a large lateral opening into the body of the right atrium. That opening is well defined and circumscribed by a ridge constituted by the following structures: The terminalis muscle bundle, the precaval muscle bundle anterior to the superior vena cava orifice, the eustachian valve anterior to the inferior vena cava, and the tuber of lower. The septal part of the sinus venarum presents with the fossa ovalis.

The *body* of the right atrium is a saccular pouch between the orifice of the sinus venarum and the tricuspid valve orifice. It has three diverticuli: the right atrial appendage superiorly overlaying the aortic root, and two inferior appendages. The lateral wall presents with endocardial protracting transverse ridges: the pectinate muscles. The inferior wall presents with the opening of the coronary sinus and the two inferior appendages. The septal wall of the pouch lies anterior to the tuber of lower. It covers the posterior superior process of the left ventricle and the atrial membranous septum (triangle of Koch).

The venae cavae openings are at an angle directing the venous blood flow towards the tricuspid valve orifice.

The *left atrium* is a less complex cardiac chamber. It is smaller than the right but its wall is thicker (3 mm). Its organization is similar with venous inputs opening laterally and superiorly, and connected to the mitral valve orifice by a pouch (the body) which is oriented inferiorly (an inverted obliquely disposed earthen pot). The surface of the cavity is smooth without the many anatomical features of the right atrium. The left atrial appendage is a true diverticulum with a constricted orifice and a variable morphology.

The *atrial septum* comprises essentially the fossa ovalis, circumscribed by a ridge of myocardium (or limbus or anulus of Vieussens). The fossa ovalis is occluded by a membrane, the membranous portion of the atrial septum. The fossa ovalis is patent in 20% of subjects. The rest of the septal wall of the atria are in fact separated, anteriorly they can be easily dissociated by dissection and sandwich the AV node.

Atrial Wall Structure (Fig. 1, 2, 3)

The *atrial wall* is composed of three layers. The inner surface is covered by a connective tissue layer: the endocardium. The left endocardium is thicker. The cell layer that lines the endocardium is similar to endothelium. The outer surface is covered by the visceral epicardium. The atrial myocardium has the following characteristics:

1. Except for the interatrial bundle (Buchmann's bundle), each atrial myocardial bundle is confined to its chamber.
2. The atrial myocardium attaches onto the supra-valvular lamina of the mitral valve and tricuspid valve and on the right fibrous trigone, the atrial membranous septum and the intervalvular trigone.
3. The atrial myocardium is not homogeneous in thickness with thickens or ridges (pectinate muscles).
4. The atrial myocardium is not homogeneous within its thickness. It can be dissected into deep and superficial layers, and various bundles. There is a single interatrial bundle which connects the right and left atrium and is situated into the anterior wall of the left atrium, and the anterior medial wall of the right atrium.
5. There is very thin-walled areas of the atrial wall such as the "unprotected" area of the anterior wall of the LA, just behind the aortic root, and the thin supra-valvular lamina.

6. The atrial myocardium is a syncytium, making the entire atrial myocardium one anatomical and functional unit: On a thin histological slide, there is generally an orderly parallel arrangement of fibres, but there is "fibre disarray" if the entire wall thickness is considered.
7. The atrial myocardium is a complex disarrayed syncytium. The concept of the bundle is an illusion, and does not have the same meaning as bundle used in skeletal muscle organization.

The atrial myocardium has long been known to contain granules. These have been documented to contain a biologically active peptide, the atrial natriuric factor.

The atrial myocardium contains specialized myocardial structures: the sino-atrial node, and the atrio-ventricular node.

The *sinus node*. The sinus node was first described by Keith and Flack in 1907. In 1910, Lewis et al. documented the sinus node function as the heart pacemaker (Fig. 4-8).

The sinus node is a macroscopic structure easily identified by anatomical dissection on formalin fixed heart. Because of its height content in fibrotic tissue, it can be isolated as an oblong pit (node) of whitish tissue. It is situated in the crista-terminalis (precaval bundle) at the junction of the superior vena cava and the right atrium. Its position varies and it may be found in a large area, but is commonly located over the right lateral side of the sino-atrial junction[5]. There is a large artery coursing through the SA node. The sinus node artery arises from the proximal segment of the right coronary artery in 48% of cases, from the proximal segment of the circumflex coronary artery in 30% and from the posterior division of the right coronary artery in 22%[1]. The sinus node artery reaches the sinus node by coursing intramurally within the atrial wall. It circumscribes the superior vena cava either clockwise, or counter-clockwise. Histologically, the SA node is made of inter-connecting fasciculi of small cells set in a dense fibrous tissue matrix.

The *atrio-ventricular node* (Fig. 9). Specialized tissues of the junctional area can be divided into five zones: the atrial inputs, a transitional cell zone, the compact AV node, the penetrating AV bundle (His) and the branching AV bundles. The transitional AV node, and the compact node are atrial structures situated between the septal segment of the left and right atrial walls, posterior and inferior to the atrial membranous septum, within the triangle of Koch, who understood the importance of the tendon of Todaro: The Eustachian valve is prolonged into the septum by a tendinous structure which attaches into the "central fibrous body". The tendon of Todaro forms the posterior side of the triangle of Koch, of which the base is the coronary sinus ostium, and the anterior side   the muscular segment of the septal tricuspid valve leaflet. The apex of the triangle is at the atrial membranous septum. The following gross anatomy of the AV nodal area is consistent with the original description by Tawara[6], modern histological and reconstructive studies[7] and our dissections.

The penetrating bundle is within the membranous septum.

The compact AV node is continuous anteriorly with the penetrating bundle and cannot be distinguished from it. The compact node is a cluster of nodal tissue, with a half oval or triangular shape, which spans posteriorly and inferiorly within the interatrial septum from which it can be macroscopically dissected. The compact node is prolonged by the intermediate node: a fan-like bundle of pale myocardial fibres with fatty streaks, surrounding the compact node inferiorly and posteriorly. It merges with the atrial myocardium, where it can be distributed into three groups of nodal cells, corresponding to the three atrial inputs.

The atrial inputs are classified as deep, superficial and posterior (Fig. 10). The deep group is situated left to the Tendon of Todaro and is in close contact with the left atrial myocardium, near the apex of the AV node. The superficial group lies right to the tendon of Todaro and is in continuity with the septal right atrial myocardium. The "posterior" group, which should be labelled "inferior" is in continuity with a myocardial bundle which can be traced from the coronary sinus ostium.

The compact AV node as well as the intermediate node are surrounded by atrial myocardium and may communicate with the entire adjacent atrial myocardium. Because there is no discrete limits, and because the AV node is foremost a connecting structure, the anatomist is compelled to describe a larger AV nodal area which harbours the entire AV nodal functions (anatomical substrate) and extends beyond the anatomical landmarks (Fig. 11, 12, 13).

The AV nodal area is supplied by the AV node artery which arises either from the right coronary artery in the "posterior septal" region or from a dominant circumflex coronary artery.

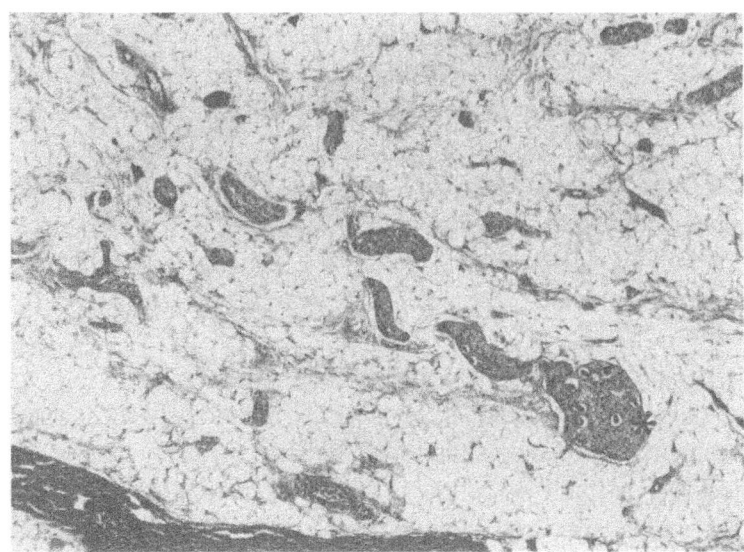

Figure 1.   Intra-atrial septum, Movat's Pentachrome x 22.5.   Adipose tissue with abundant neural structures, some with some with ganglion cells (✱) and small muscular fascicles.

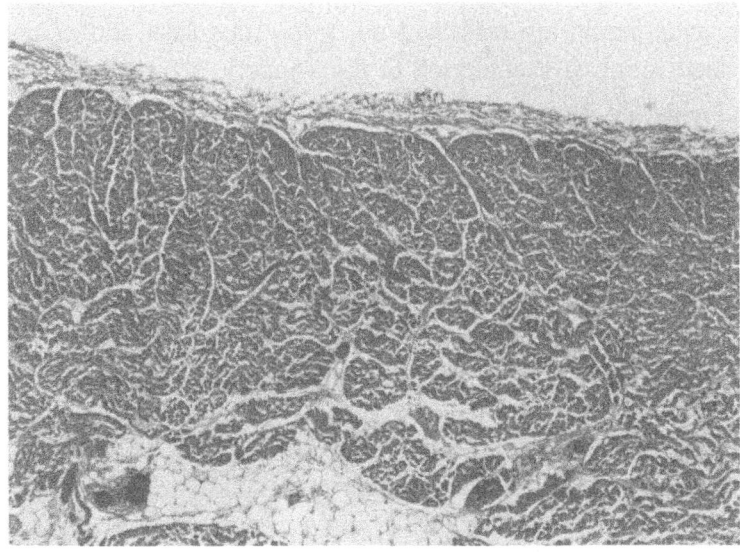

Figure 2.   Right atrial free wall, Movat's Pentachrome x 22.5.   Closely arranged fibres with variable orientation.

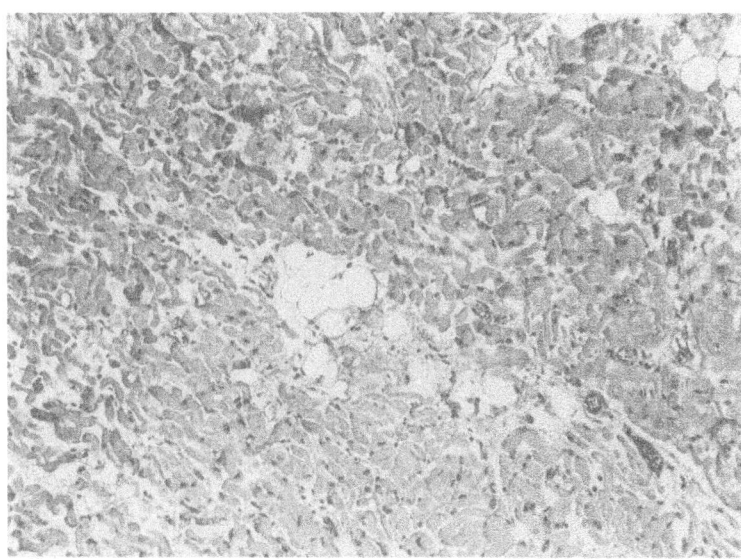

Figure 3.   Upper posterior right atrial free wall, Movat's Pentachrome x 56.25. Relatively large, zigzagging fibres, mixed with some fat and with variable orientation.

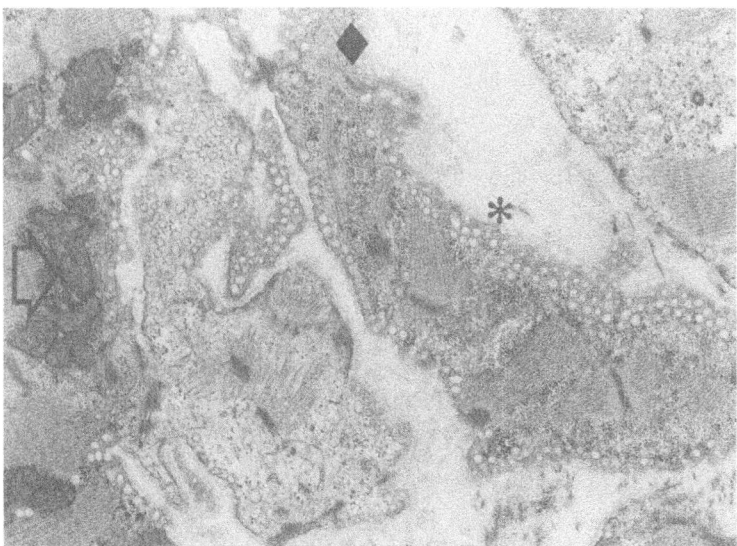

Figure 4.   Sinus node nodal cells. EM x 17500. Small cells with scant myofibrils, abundant pinocytic vesicles (✳) and basal lamina (♦), rare and small intercellular junctions (arrow).

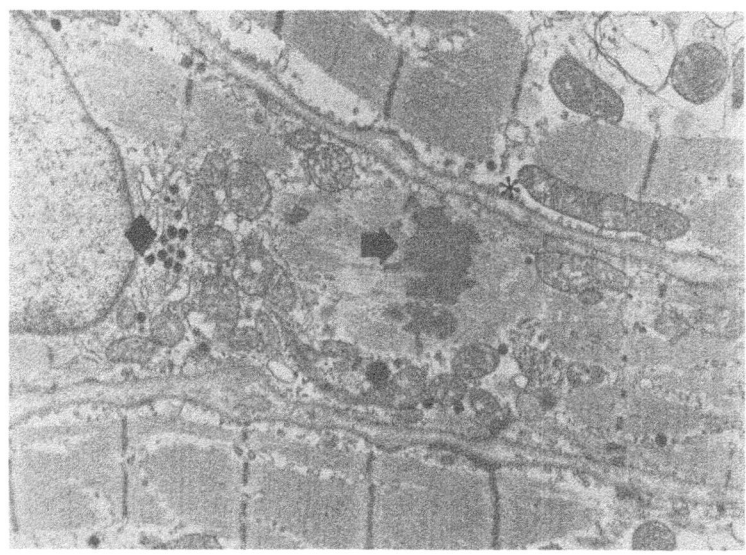

Figure 5.   Transitional sinus nodal cell (centre), in between two working atrial myocytes, EM
x 8400. Narrow cell with pinocytic vesicles (∗), atrial granules (♦) and marked
smearing of the Z bands (arrow).

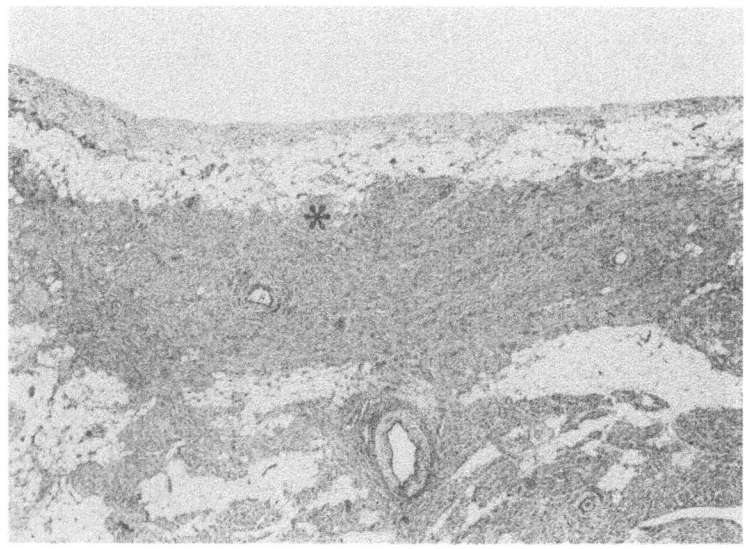

Figure 6.   Sinus node, Movat's Pentachrome x 11.25.   Dense oblong formation with central
artery, beneath the epicardial surface (∗).

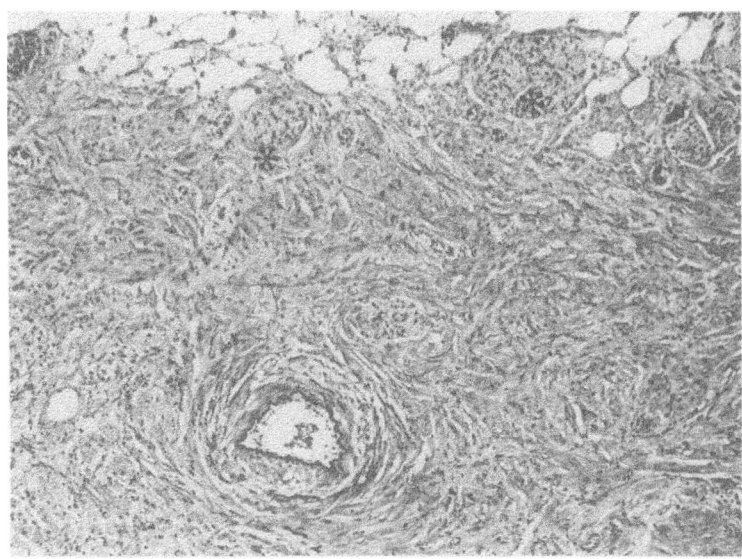

Figure 7.   Sinus node, Movat's Pentachrome x 45. Myocytes are wrapped within collagen and reticulin fibres, around the central artery, the wall of which blend with the nodal tissue. The epicardial fat is seen atop with several nerves (✻) in close contact with the node.

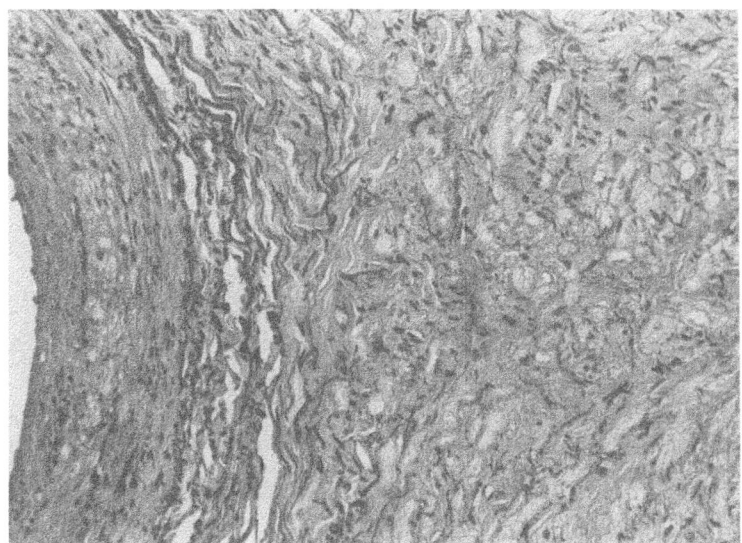

Figure 8.   Sinus node, Movat's Pentachrome x 140.6. Myocytes appear as clear, round cells, embedded in collagen and reticulin fibres.

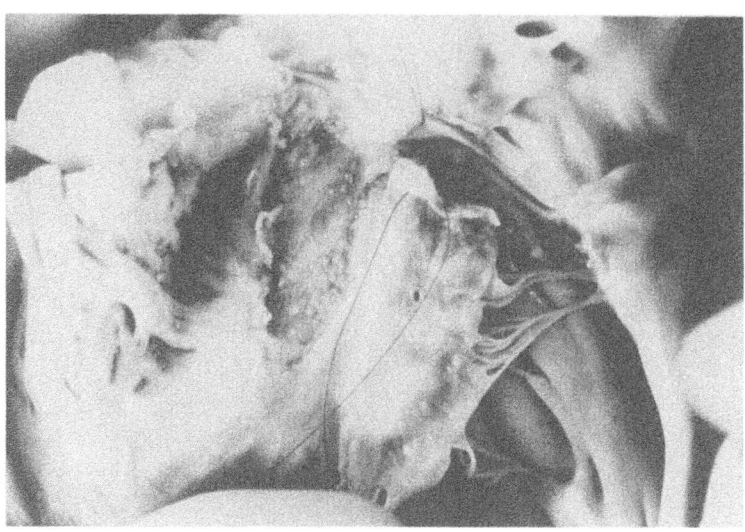

Figure 9. Dissection of Triangle of Koch. The right septal atrial wall has been resected and the intermedial node, compact node, and penetrating bundle are shown.

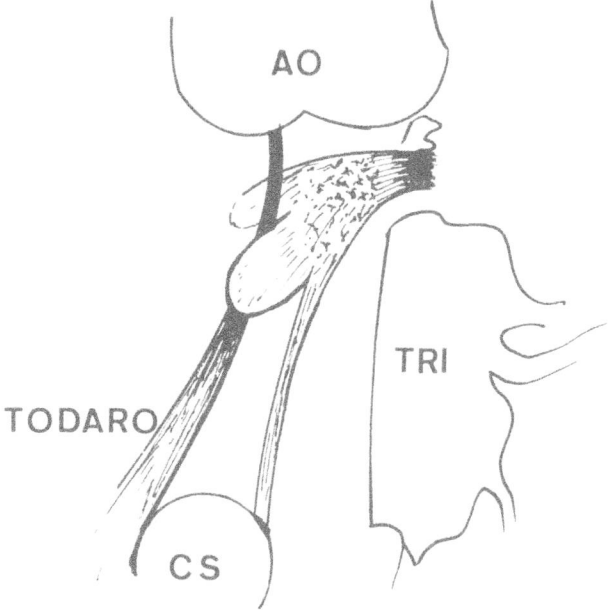

Figure 10. Schematic depiction of the heart specimen of Figure 9.

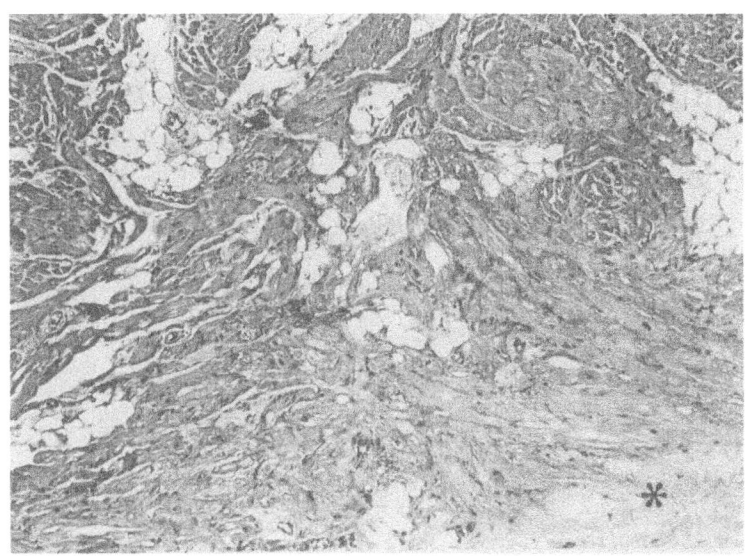

Figure 11. AVN, Movat's Pentachrome x 42. Large, clear fibres, mixed with some fat, seated on the tricuspid annulus (✳).

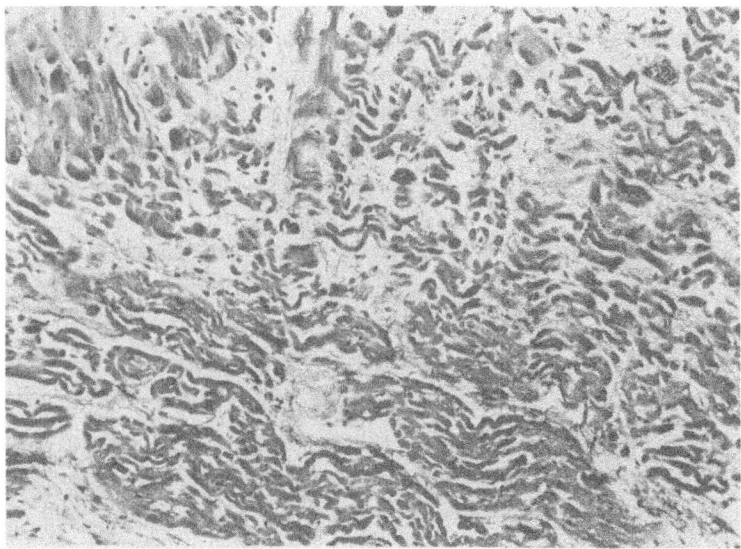

Figure 12. AVN, Movat's Pentachrome x 56.25. Dense, narrow, wavy, mostly transitional cells with conspicuous interstitial collagen and reticulin.

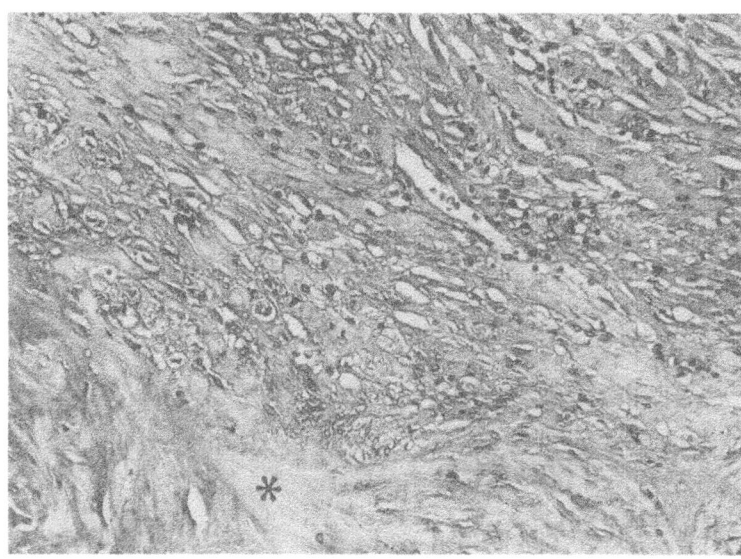

Figure 13. AVN, Movat's Pentachrome x 112.5. Penetration into the fibrous body (✱); cells
are large and clear and oriented at variable angle.

The ***internodal atrial myocardium.*** The presence of specialized conducting bundles between the SA node and the AV node has long been a contenti-
ous topic. Bundles have been described anatomically and histologically. There
is currently a consensus to deny the existence of specialized internodal
bundles and to explain the atrial activation patterns and preferential conduction
route on anatomical and functional grounds instead of hypothetical bundles.

Arterial blood supply. The atrial blood supply is supplied by the
coronary arteries and mediastinal arteries. The latter defines the non-coronary
artery flow. The atrial coronary artery branches are divided into three territorial
groups. The atrial coronary artery network is extensively anastomosed and
plays an important role in collateral blood supply. The coronary artery gives
rise, to arteries for the specialized conduction system (sinus node artery, AV
node artery). The non-coronary flow, most likely, provides a significant blood
flow to the atria. Major atrial arteries have been documented arising from a

large mediastinal artery, such as the sinus node artery arising from the right bronchial artery]1].

The lymphatic ducts parallel the coronary arteries and drain into mediastinal nodes.

Innervation. The atria, as well as the heart, are innervated by both sympathetic and parasympathetic fibres. The sympathetic fibres arise mainly from the forth and fifth segments of the thoracic spinal cord and via sympathetic connections in the cervical and thoracic cervical (stellate) ganglia and cardiac plexus. Post ganglionic sympathetic fibres are distributed to all regions of the heart. The sympathetic nerve that supplies the heart via the right stellate ganglion appear to play a major role in regulating myocardial contractility. The parasympathetic innervation originates in the dorsal efferent nuclei of the medulla oblongata and reaches the heart via the cardiac branches of the vagus nerve. The parasympathetic fibres supply essentially the SA node and the AV node.

Fractal anatomy. The mathematical concept of fractals, which provide order to the complex geometry of biological structures have been applied to the heart[8] several heart systems, including the conduction system, could be described in terms of fractal network.

FUNCTIONAL ANATOMY _____

Innervation. Cardiac, especially atrial denervation, is a difficult challenge. Most investigators, including ourselves, have failed to achieve complete surgical denervation in patients. This does not imply that imbalance in autonomic system is not an important factor in pathophysiology.

Blood supply. Atrial blood supply is the major source of non-coronary flow. Viability of atrial tissue is preserved even after suppression of coronary flow, as well documented by preservation of atria of heart transplant recipient. Normal atrial function, including sinus node function, may be present in recipients atria after heart transplant. Surgical experience shows as well that sinus node function[9], and/or AV nodal function persist after ligation of sinus node artery or AV nodal artery[10]. Acute ischemic myocardium is an exceptionally rare event. The rich arterial network of atrial blood supply plays a major role in collateral flow to the ventricles in ischemic heart disease.

Specialized Conduction System. Basic electrophysiology, as well as clinical electrophysiology and cardiac surgery have contributed to document that, 1) The function of sinus node, and AV node have an anatomical substrate which extends beyond the anatomically defined nodes; 2) The nodal functions are extremely resistant, and may be present even after extensive damage.

Electrophysiological studies by J. Boineau et al. have documented that the "pacemaker function" is present outside the actual node, and involves a large area of the superior caval atrial junction[11].

Recent developments in electrophysiological interventions to ablate AV nodal reentrant tachycardia have shown that the anatomical substrate of the AV nodal function is larger than the node of histologists and include a large segment of surrounding atrial tissue.

These considerations show that the sinus node function, and AV nodal function define an anatomical substrate, the limits of which extend far beyond the classic anatomical landmarks.

HEMODYNAMIC FUNCTION _____

The Frank Starling law[2] has dominated, and still dominates the concept of cardiac hemodynamics, in normal hearts, although the law has been described in a failing heart model, independently of any neurological and/or humeral control[12].

The relation between the volume of blood in ventricles at the moment they begin to contract (end diastolic volume) and the systolic pressure developed by the ventricle was first described in 1895 by Frank and later documented in the mammalian heart by Starling in 1914. The law is a manifestation of the length-tension relationship. It implies that increase in atrial pressure and or atrial systole is associated with increase in ventricular filling and end-diastolic volume and pressure which produce increased ventricular contractility, namely increase in ventricular systolic pressure and stroke volume. The Frank Starling law refers to a static model and does take into account, the interactions of systolic and diastolic dynamics, as well as gross motion of the heart and interaction of cardiac function with hemodynamics of preload and afterload and intrathoracic mechanics.

The Frank Starling law has three major shortcomings[12].

1. The law implies that cardiac output is uniquely determined by the right atrial pressure. Because right atrial pressure is very low in normal healthy individuals, it is difficult to conceptualize how a small change in atrial pressure (few millimetres of Mercury) may produce up to five fold increase in cardiac output.
2. The heart, according to the law of conservation of momentum moves within the chest. During the forward systolic acceleration of the blood, the heart moves backwards toward the atrium and engulfs the coming dynamics return blood flow.
3. The mammalian heart is a sucking pump as well. The excised mammalian heart empties and refills when placed in a dish of buffered solution. This suggests there is an active diastole, and that atrial pressure does not uniquely determine the magnitude of ventricular filling. It has been speculated that the ventricles are an elastic structure, with the energy of the elastic recoil stored during systole. The smaller the end systolic volume, the greater the recoil and consequently, the diastolic suction. The energy of the elastic recoil is stored within the sarcomere, and within the myocardial connective framework. In addition, diastolic compliance of the myocardium is controlled in part by calcium release and reuptake by the sacoplasmic reticulum.
4. The law does take into account the role of variation in heart rate (chronotropic function) in regulating cardiac output, as long as heart rate remains with physiological limits.

These considerations are just a few among many factors which determine and regulate cardiac output, not to mention neurological and humeral factors. Hemodynamic functions of the atria, should be reviewed with regards to these preceding considerations.

The atrium as a reservoir. The atria does not meet the criteria for a role as a reservoir, because the atrial capacity is too small, of the same order of magnitude as the stroke volume, and because the venous return flow is continuous except for a short time during atrial systole (reverse flow)[13]. The blood return flows through the atria as through a conduit. The atrial functional anatomy may be compared to that of the aortic root. The aortic root dilates to accommodate the stroke volume, while its elastic recoil returns the systolic energy and transforms intermittent flow in continuous flow. The atria are essentially a "compliant pouch" between a continuous input and intermittent output.

Atria as a Primer Pump.   The role of atrial contraction in filling the ventricle has been overestimated by the Frank Starling law. The loss of the atrial kick is essentially critical in failing heart[14-17]. In normal hearts, the atrial contraction allows the ventricle the "luxury" of a high end-diastolic pressure without the need for a "pricy" high atrial pressure. But we have stated, that in normal hearts the pressure increase is minimal with minimal effect on volume and pressure. Increase in stroke volume and myocardial contractility is mediated by other factors than atrial contraction and end diastolic volume. The atrium work that the atria contributes, is always a very small part of entire heart work (stroke work), in the order of magnitude of 5%]2-18]. Overall, the adjustment of cardiac output is essentially determined by heart rate and concomitant changes in myocardial contractility.

Atria as the Heart Pacemaker.   The chronotropic function is the critical factor in regulating cardiac output to body needs. This has been well documented in isolated heart, and human subjects. Chronotropic function is the unquestionable primary hemodynamic function of the atria. Atrioventricular synchrony has been extensively studied. The critical effects of the timing of atrial systole is a corollary of the role of atrial contraction. AV synchrony has a negligible role in normal heart, as well documented in patients with normal hearts and prolonged PR interval after electrophysiological intervention for AV nodal tachycardia. However, inappropriate timing of atrial contraction may impair venous return and induce symptoms.

To conclude, the hemodynamic function of the atria in the normal heart is essentially that of a compliant pouch between the venous return and ventricle to "buffer" the continuous high velocity venous inflow and intermittent ventricular flow. The systolic function appears, in the normal heart, more as part of a compliant pouch than a pump.

Atria and thrombosis

Thrombus formation does not occur in a normal heart, as in normal blood conduit. The blood is in continuous motion and endothelium layer is normal and fulfils its role. There is no stasis within the heart cavities, even within the appendages, which empty and refill at each cardiac cycle. In passing, it is interesting to note that there is no function attributed to atrial appendages, and that the dramatic differences in morphology of right and left appendages would suggest different role. Recent studies have suggested that the size of the atrium, not its contraction, may be the critical factor in thrombus formation[19], although most of them are thought to develop in the left atrial appendage, the constant wash-out of which is suppressed by atrial fibrillation.

COMMENTS

Normal functional anatomy may be instrumental in understanding pathophysiological anatomy, but is misleading in many instances. Pathophysiology is currently conceptualized as a different pathology, instead of modification or alteration of the normal physiology. However, the paramount function of the atria is the *chronotropic function*, whatever the circumstances.

References

[1]   McAlpine WA. Heart and coronary arteries. New York, New York, Springer-Verlag, 1975.
[2]   Katz AM. Physiology of the heart (second edition). New York, New York, Raven Press, 1992.
[3]   Gray H. Anatomy of the human body. Clemente CD (ed), Philadelphia, Lea & Febiger, 1985.
[4]   Rouviere H. Anatomie humaine - Descriptive et topographique. Cordier G, Delmas A (eds), Masson et Cie., Paris, France, 1962.
[5]   Anderson RH, Becker AE. Anatomy of conducting tissues revisited. Br Heart J 1978;40 (Supp):2-16.
[6]   Tawara S. Das Reizleitungssystem des Saugetierherzens. Jena: Verlag von Gustav Fischer, 1906.
[7]   Anderson RH, Becker AE, Brechenmacher C, et al. The human atrioventricular junctional area. A morphological study of the A-V node and bundle. Eur J Cardiol 1975;3:11-25.
[8]   West BJ, Goldberger AL. Physiology in fractal dimensions. Am Scientist 1987;75:354-365.
[9]   Guiraudon GM, Ofiesh JG, Kaushik R. Extended vertical trans-septal approach to the mitral valve. Ann Thorac Surg 1991;52:1058-1062.
[10]   Guiraudon GM, Klein GJ, Sharma AD, et al. Surgical ablation of posterior septal accessory pathways in the Wolff-Parkinson-White syndrome by a closed heart technique. J Thorac Cardiovas Surg 1986;92,3,1:406-413.
[11]   Boineau JP, Schuessler RB, Cain ME, et al. Activation mapping during normal atrial rhythms and atrial flutter. In: Zipes DP, Jalife J (eds.), Cardiac electrophysiology - From cell to bedside. 1990, Philadelphia, W.B. Saunders Co., pp. 537-548.

[12]   Robinson TF, Factor SM, Sonnenblick EH. The heart as a suction pump. Scientific American 1986;254,6:84-91.
[13]   Appleton CP, Hatle LK, Popp RL. Superior vena cava and hepatic vein Doppler echocardiograph in healthy adults. J Am Coll Cardiol 1987;10:1032-1039.
[14]   Baig MW, Perrins EJ. The hemodynamics of cardiac pacing: Clinical and physiological aspects. Progress in Cardiovascular Diseases XXXIII 1991;5:283-298.
[15]   Lamas GA. Physiological consequences of normal atrioventricular conduction: applicability to modern cardiac pacing. J Cardiac Surg 1989;4:89-98.
[16]   Samet P, Bernstein WH, Nathan DA, et al. Atrial contribution to cardiac output in complete heart block. Amer J Cardiol 1965;16:1-10.
[17]   Rydén L, Kruse I. Hemodynamic aspects of physiologic pacing. In: Barold SS (ed), Modern cardiac pacing. Mount Kisco, New York, Futura Publishing Co., 1985, pp. 19-32.
[18]   Atwood JE. Exercise hemodynamics of atrial fibrillation. In: Falk RH, Podrid PJ (eds), Atrial fibrillation - Mechanisms and management. New York, New York, Raven Press, 1992, pp. 145-163.
[19]   Kopecky SL, Gersh BJ, McGoon MD, et al. The natural history of lone atrial fibrillation. N Engl J Med 1987;317,11:669.

Chapter 3

THE PATHOLOGY OF DRUG RESISTANT

LONE ATRIAL FIBRILLATION IN

ELEVEN SURGICALLY TREATED PATIENTS

Colette M. Guiraudon

Nicolette M. Ernst

Gérard M. Guiraudon

Raymond Yee

George J. Klein

Departments of Pathology, Medicine & Surgery
University of Western Ontario
University Hospital
London, Ontario
Canada

and

University of Utrecht
Medical Faculty
Utrecht
The Netherlands

J. H. Kingma et al. (eds.), Atrial fibrillation, a treatable disease?, 41–58.

INTRODUCTION _____

Although atrial fibrillation (AF) is a common disease, there is relatively few publications on its associated pathology. Autopsy studies[1,2,3,4,5] report the lesions observed in a large variety of structural heart and systemic diseases causing multiple clinical presentations of AF (acute or chronic, permanent or paroxysmal). Others studies focuses on AF in rheumatic disease using autopsy examination[6] or biopsy studies[7,8] done during surgery for rheumatic mitral valve lesions. More recent works[9,10,11] address the problem of "lone" atrial fibrillation occurring in the absence of structural Heart Disease or of metabolic diseases. The pathological findings suggest that cardiomyopathic changes in the atria could be the anatomical substrate for the fibrillation. We report pathological findings in eleven cases of long-standing, drug-resistant AFs treated surgically with the *Corridor* operation[12-15].

MATERIAL AND METHODS _____

A. *Patient Selection.*   Eleven male patients, all males, age 24 to 67 (mean: 45), with drug resistant AF (Table 1), had a *Corridor* procedure. The duration of problematic AF was 2 to 20 years (mean: 8.7 years). Five patients had incessant AF (IAF) and six had paroxysmal AF (PAP).

Associated cardiac disease was found only in one patient: an underlying dilated cardiomyopathy, possibly related to a viral myocarditis in the past. One had a history of rheumatic fever, without cardiac involvement. Two patients (5 and 6) had non insulin dependent diabetes mellitus of recent onset.

Congestive heart failure was present only in the patient with the cardiomyopathy.

The atrial dimensions were determined by echocardiography. Three had mildly dilated right and left atria, one had more marked atrial dilatation and moderate biventricular dilatation.

Pre-operative sinus node (SN) function could be assessed in only seven patients, 5 of which had normal SN function.

None of these patients had significant coronary disease on the coronary angiogram (Table 1).

Table 1. Data on 11 patients with incessant/paroxysmal atrial fibrillation

Pt no.	Sex	Age (yrs)	Known cardiac disease	Duration (yrs)	Atrial enlargement	Sinus node function
1	M	53	IAF	9	0	n.a.
2	M	45	IAF	15	0	abnormal
3	M	40	PAF (*)	10	mildly dilated RA/LA	normal
4	M	24	IAF	5	mildly dilated RA/LA	n.a.[1]
5	M	50	IAF	4	0	n.a.[1]
6	M	67	PAF	13	0	normal
7	M	43	PAF	5	0	normal
8	M	51	PAF	4	0	normal
9	M	61	IAF	>20	moderately dilated RA/LA	n.a.
10	M	42	PAF (**)	2	mildly dilated RA/LA	normal
11	M	52	PAF	20	0	abnormal

NOTE: IAF   =   incessant atrial fibrillation
PAF   =   paroxysmal atrial fibrillation
0   =   not present; n.a. = not available
*   =   previous history of rheumatic fever (no mitral regurgitation)
**   =   underlying dilated cardiomyopathy, possibly related to a viral myocarditis in the past
1   =   due to the incessant atrial fibrillation, it was difficult to assess sinus node function

B. Available Biopsy Material. Excised right atrial tissue was obtained during the open heart surgery. In all cases, it was a segment of the right atrial lateral wall adjacent to the isolated sinus node region. Septal atrial fragments were also submitted in two and appendage in three patients. Tissue from the left atrium was obtained in three cases, right ventricular needle biopsies also in three and left ventricular in seven patients (Table 2).

C. Tissue Preparation. Tissue for light microscopy was fixed in 10% buffered formalin, processed as usual and stained with haematoxylin-eosin,

Movat's Pentachrome, congo red and perls.

Tissue for electron microscopy was fixed in the operating room in glutaraldehyde, rinsed in 0.1 cacodylate buffer and counterfixed in osmium tetroxide. Tissue was then embedded in epon araldite and semi-thin sections, 0.5 to 1 micron thick were done and stained with Toluidine Blue. Any of the blocks displaying longitudinal sections of cardiac myocytes were thin-sectioned and the 60 to 90 nm sections were stained with lead acetate and uranyl nitrate and put on 300 mesh grids.

D. *Tissue Evaluation for Light Microscopy.* Hypertrophy, fibrosis and fatty change were graded as absent, mild, moderate or severe. Presence or absence of abnormal deposits (iron, calcification, amyloidosis) and of an inflammatory infiltrate were assessed. The vasculature and nerve were examined.

E. *Tissue Evaluation for Electron Microscopy.* The criteria described by Maron[16,17] were used. For hypertrophy, they include enlarged fibres, wider than 12 microns for atrial fibres, and 15 for the left ventricular, increased number of mitochondria, excessive amount of glycogen, sarcoplasmic reticulum and Z bands material, large, ruffled nuclei with increased chromatin and widened intercalated discs. Degenerative myocyte changes include myofilament loss with replacement with mitochondria, glycogen, dilated sarcoplasmic reticulum, increased fat globules and lipofuchsin granules. In the interstitium, the presence of fibrosis, inflammation, amyloid fibrils and vascular abnormalities was assessed.

RESULTS _____

A. *Light Microscopy* (Table 2). No patients had evidence of amyloidosis, inflammation, iron deposits or diffuse vascular disease. In all patients, the number of nerves was dramatically decreased in the right atrial epicardium and particularly no ganglion cells were seen, although they are generally easily found in this location.

In the right atrium, fibrosis was seen in five, mild in three and moderate in two (Fig. 1). Fatty infiltration was present in five cases, mild in one, moderate in

Table 2.

LIGHT MICROSCOPY OF RIGHT ATRIUM

Pt	Fibrosis	Fat	Hypertrophy	Other findings	Other tissue available
1	0	0	+		
2	0	0	+ +		
3	0	0	+ +		LA: moderate hypertrophy LV: normal
4	+ +	0	+ + +		LV: mild hypertrophy
5	+ +	+ + +	+ +	Degenerated fibres	
6	+	+ +	+	Degenerated fibres SN tissue with fatty change	LV & RV: mild hypertrophy
7	0	0	0	Very thin wall	LV & RV: normal
8	+	0	+	SN tissue with fatty change and arterial dysplasia	LV: normal LA: moderate fibrosis and hypertrophy
9	+	+ +	+ +	Degenerated fibres SN tissue with fatty change and arterial dysplasia	LV: moderate hypertrophy and fat
10	0	+ +	+ +	SN tissue	RV & LV: normal LA: mild hypertrophy and fat
11	0	+	+ +	Degenerated fibres	

NOTE: 0 = none; + = mild; + + = moderate; + + + = severe

LA = left atrium; LV = left ventricle; RV = right ventricle

three and severe in one (Fig. 2). Hypertrophy was found in all cases but one, mild in three (Fig. 3), moderate in six and severe in one. Presence of degenerate fibres were generally associated with fatty infiltration and hypertrophy (Fig. 4). In four patients, tissue consistent with sinus node was found. In three cases, there was decreased cellularity (Fig. 5) with fat infiltration and, in one case, obliteration of the nodal cells with fibrosis. In two, the sinus node central artery showed mild to moderate mural thickening with intimal fibrosis and

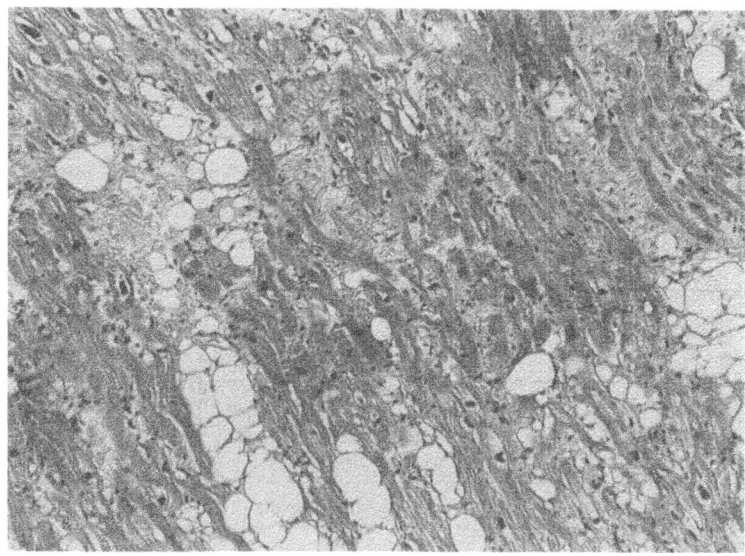

Figure 1. Patient 5, right atrium - Moderate fibrosis with fatty infiltration, hypertrophy and degenerated fibres. Movat's Pentachrome, magnification: x 127.

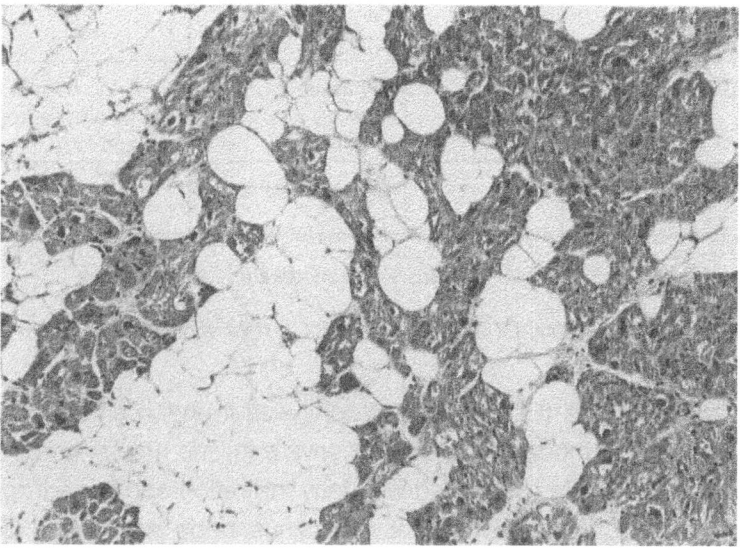

Figure 2. Patient 4, right atrium - Moderate hypertrophy and fatty infiltration. Movat's Pentachrome, magnification: x 127.

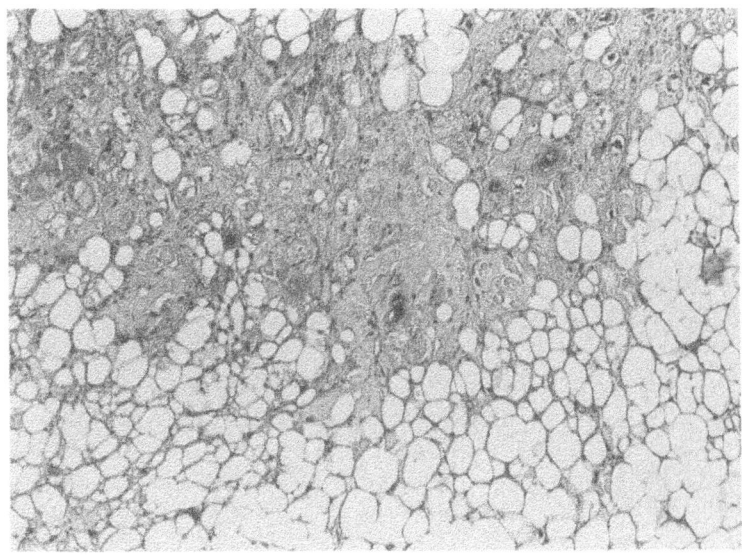

Figure 3.   Patient 5, right atrium - Severe fatty infiltration and degenerative changes. Movat's
Pentachrome, magnification: x 127.

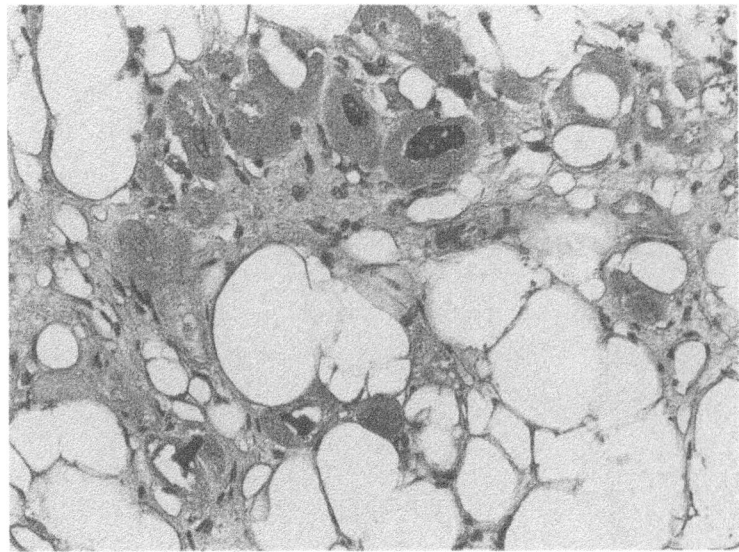

Figure 4.   Patient 5, right atrium - Marked degenerative changes, hyperchromatic nuclei and
fatty infiltration. Movat's Pentachrome, magnification: x 325.

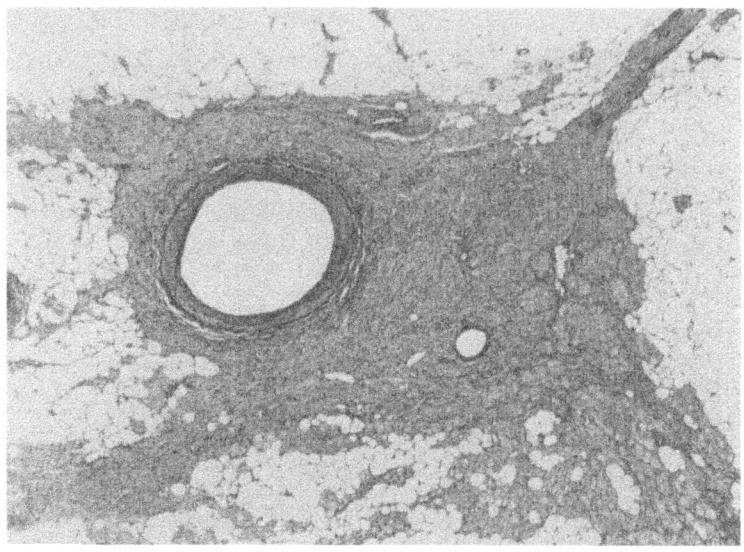

Figure 5. Patient 6, right atrium - Sinus node partially replaced with fat and hypocellular. Movat's Pentachrome, magnification: x 45.

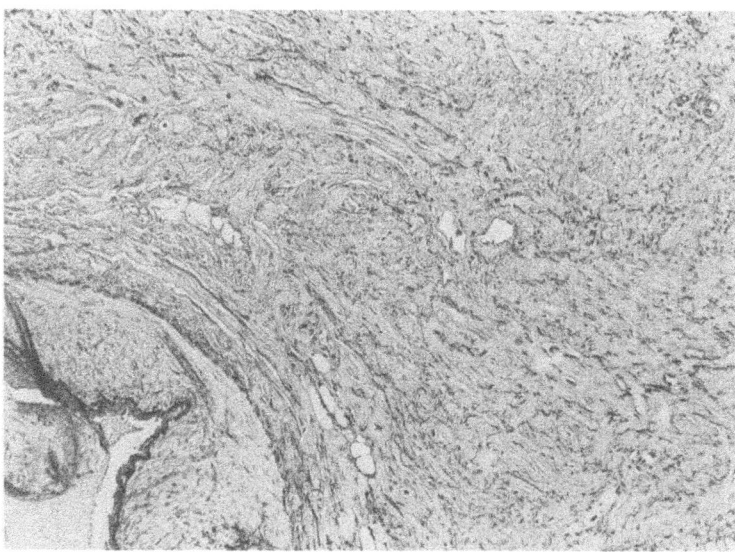

Figure 6. Patient 8, right atrium - Sinus node with fibromuscular dysplasia of the artery. Movat's Pentachrome, magnification: x 127.

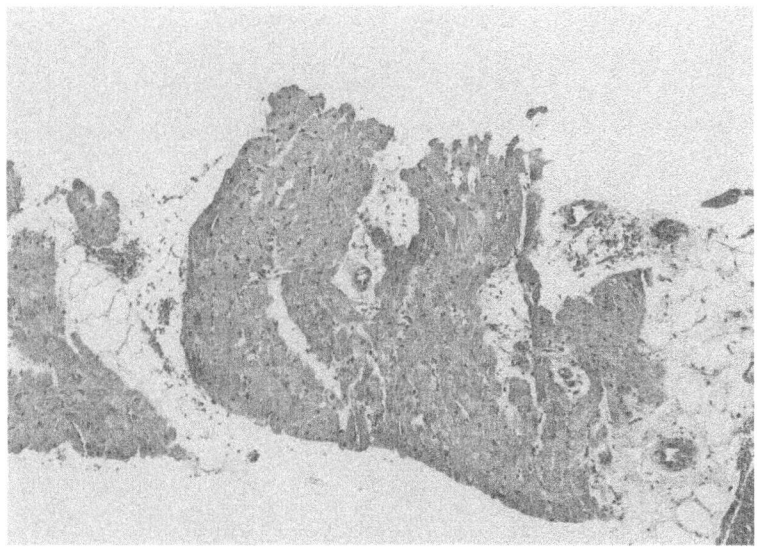

Figure 7. Patient 9, left ventricle - Moderate fatty infiltration. Movat's Pentachrome, magnification: x 32.

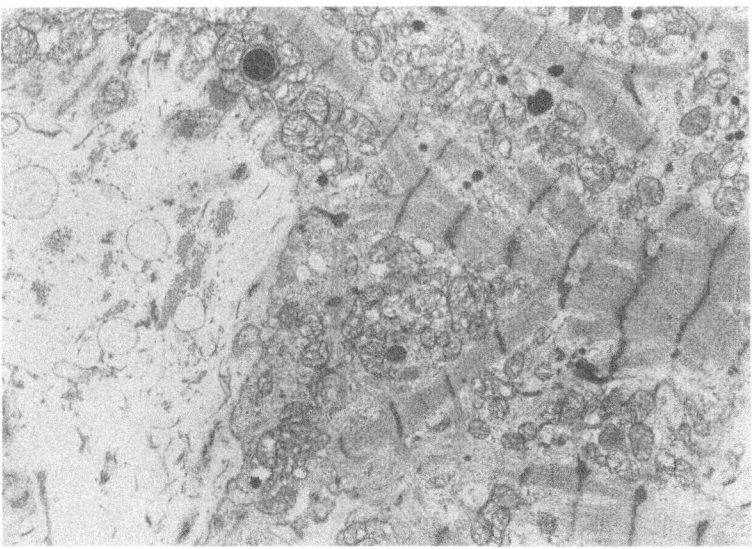

Figure 8. Patient 8, right atrium - Fibrillar loss and disorganization, increased mitochondria. Electron micrscopy, magnification: x 5280.

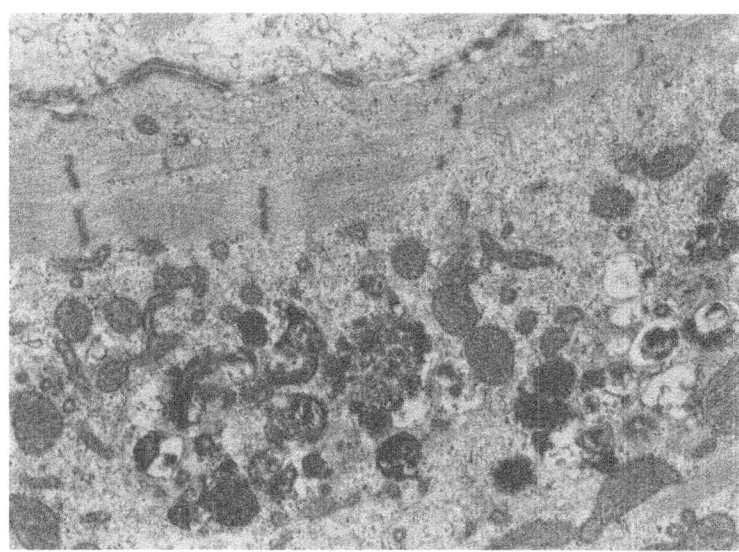

Figure 9. Patient 4, right atrium - Abundant lateral bodies, fibrillar loss and hypertrophic sarcoplasmic reticulum. Electron microcopy, magnification: x 14400.

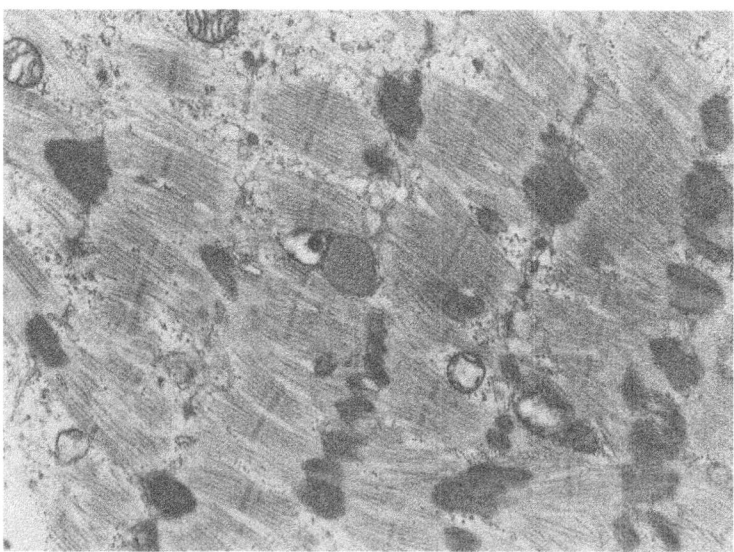

Figure 10. Patient 6, right atrium - Smearing of Z bands with pseudo-nemaline bodies. Electron microscopy, magnification: x 14400.

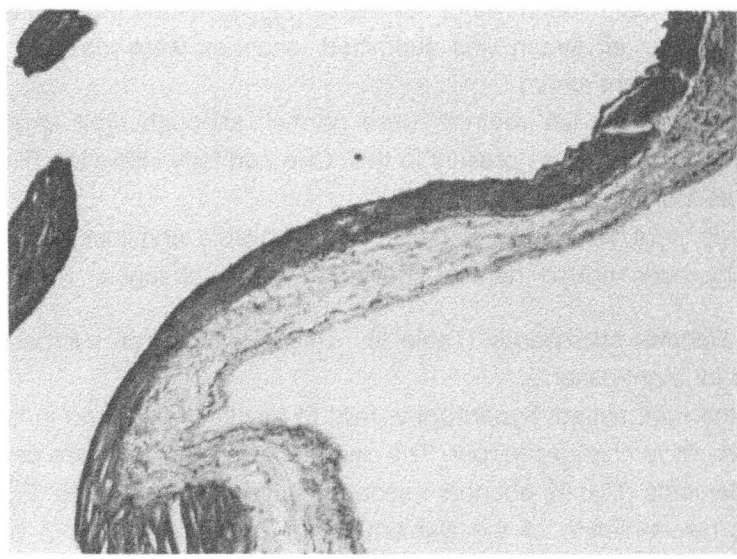

Figure 11. Patient 7, right atrium - Very thin atrial wall with well individualized epicardium, two to three rows of myocytes and a flat endocardium. Movat's Pentachrome, magnification: x 81.

Table 3.

ELECTRON MICROSCOPY OF THE RIGHT ATRIUM

Pt	Hypertrophy	Degenerative changes	Other findings	Other tissue available
3	0	0		LV & LA: mild hypertrophy
4	+ +	+ +	Transitional cells present Dilated RER Smearing of Z bands Disorganized fibrils	LV: mild hypertrophy
5	0	0	Smearing of Z bands	
6	+ + +	+ +		LV: moderate hypertrophy and degenerative changes RV: severe hypertrophy and mild degenerative changes
7	0	0	Nodal cells Smearing of Z bands	LV & RV: mild hypertrophy
8	+	+	Myelin figures Nodal cells Dilated RER Smearing of Z bands	LV: mild hypertrophy LA: mild hypertrophy and degeneration
9	+ +	+ +	Smearing of Z bands	
10	+	0		RV & LV: mild hypertrophy LA: mild hypertrophy and degeneration

NOTE: No EM samples were available for patients 1, 2 and 3.

0 = none; + = mild; + + = moderate; + + + = severe

smooth muscle cell hyperplasia of the media (Fig. 6). In the three cases where sample from the left atrium was submitted, changes were identical to those observed in the right atrium.

Four biopsies of the left ventricle were normal, although right atrial mild to moderate hypertrophy was present in two. One had fatty infiltration (Fig. 7). No fibrosis was found.

Three right ventricular biopsies were available and just one had mild hypertrophy, even though the atria showed moderate changes.

B. *Electron Microscopy* (Table 3). Tissue for electron microscopy was submitted for eight patients.

In the right atrium, hypertrophy, mild to severe, was found in five cases and degenerative changes in four. The degenerative changes were severe with few myofilaments (Fig. 8), abundant secondary lysosome granules (Fig. 9) and glycogen, disorientation of the filaments and disruption of the Z bands. In three cases, cells consistent with nodal or transitional cell morphology were present. Sarcoplasmic reticulum was markedly dilated in two and abundant in five. Z band smearing was prominent in four patients, reminiscent of nemaline bodies (Fig. 10). This feature has been described in transitional cells.

In the other chambers, the left atrium had similar lesions as the right atrium and mild hypertrophy was seen in the ventricles. In one case, severe hypertrophy and degenerative changes were present in both ventricles, associated with severe lesions of the atrium.

COMMENTS

There was a common finding in all cases, the dramatic decrease in nerves with no ganglion cell seen.

Classification:

The myocardial pathology can be classified in four groups:

1. Normal myocardium: Patient 7 had no myocyte or interstitial change. The only anomaly detectable, apart from the deficit in nerves, was a very thin atrial wall reduced to one to three layers of myocytes (Fig. 11) in between normal epicardium and endocardium.

2. Isolated hypertrophy: Patients 1,2,3 and 8 had only hypertrophy, mostly mild.

3. Cardiomyopathy, adiposis: Patients 5,6,9,10 and 11 had mostly markedly increased adipose tissue and extensive degenerative changes. Fibrosis was absent in two cases, mild in two and moderate in one. In one case, there was only mild hypertrophy and in the four others, moderate.

4. Case 4 had hypertrophy and fibrosis, with involvement of the left ventricle, and this suggests the possibility of a cardiomyopathy, possibly post-myocarditis.

Sinus node tissue was present in four 4 cases. Three sinus nodes had hypocellularity and fatty replacement. In two of these cases, the sinus node artery had fibro-muscular dysplasia.

DISCUSSION

Validation: Although the right atrial samples were small (1-2 cm^2), one may assume they were representative of diffuse lesions as suggested by identical changes observed in the 3 patients with concomitant right and left atrial biopsies.

Atrial fibrillation, characterized by its electrocardiographic pattern is associated with a reentry mechanism which requires a critical surface area to sustain [18]. G. Moe had speculated that atrial fibrillation was due to multiple wavelet activation, the perpetuation of which requires non-homogenous atrial conduction and refractoriness[19]. M. Allessie et al.[20,21] have confirmed that Moe's computer model hypothesis in animal models, and documented that the reentry mechanism was of the "leading circle" type and did not require an anatomical obstacle. Atrial anatomy plays an important role associated with its size (critical mass), its non homogeneous wall structure. Electrophysiological characteristics i.e. conduction velocity and refractoriness have a direct relationship to atrial size in perpetuation of atrial fibrillation. This was consistent with the evidence that atrial fibrillation is associated with structural heart disease, although the recent identification of "lone atrial fibrillation" suggested that atrial fibrillation may occur in the absence of anatomical substrate.

Our results document that lone atrial fibrillation is associated with significant cardiac pathology. A dramatic decrease in nerve and ganglion cells suggest that atrial myocardium electrophysiologic properties are altered by the lesions of the autonomous nervous system and are more likely instrumental in initiating and sustaining atrial fibrillation. This is consistent with the observation of James[2] on the selective cardio-neuropathy in atrial fibrillation[22], and more recent observations of P. Coumel[23,24,25] on vagal or adrenergic varieties of atrial fibrillation.

Associated myocardial pathology is consistent with current speculations that atrial myocardial pathology may be either primary or secondary or both. On the one hand, isolated mild myocardial hypertrophy suggests that atrial pathology may be secondary to atrial fibrillation (tachycardia induced cardio-myopathy). On the other hand, typical evidence of atrial cardiomyopathy suggests that inception and/or perpetuation of atrial fibrillation is enhanced by associated pathology.

Sinus node pathology. Sinus node tissue was observed in four patients, although the atrial fragment was excised away from the known location of the sinus node. The presence of sinus node tissue, in that area of the right atrial wall, may be due to either a more lateral location of the sinus node, ·or the presence of aberrant sinus nodal tissue away from the actual node as suggested by electrophysiological studies of J. Boineau[26] documenting scattered origins of sinus node activity. The high prevalence, in 3 nodes out of 4, of significant sinus node pathology is consistent with clinical evidence that sinus node dysfunction is associated with atrial fibrillation[27]. However, patients with sinus node pathology did not have evidence of sinus node dysfunction.

Pathological Diagnoses.

The patient with normal myocardium (Fig. 11) but with mural hypoplasia had cardiac pathology similar to the one we observed in two patients with sudden cardiac death[28]. The first patient had atrial flutter and fibrillation associated with myotonic dystrophy. At autopsy, the posterior right atrial wall was paper thin, with only scant atrophic myocytes embedded in fibrosis, and the second case was an apparently healthy young woman with the identical atrial lesions. In these two cases, there was atrophy and fibrosis, actually missing in patient 7, but the mechanism could be the same.

The isolated mild hypertrophy, observed in four patients is likely secondary to the fibrillation than primary. The fact that, when available, the ventricles were normal suggests that atrial fibrillation may induce atrial myocardial changes, while ventricular myocardium is protected.

Five patients had markedly increased adipose tissue with severe degenerative change. The morphology of the myocardium was similar to that of right ventricular dysplasia (RVD). Many authors recognize that RVD is not limited to the right ventricle[29-33]. Some cases of adiposis of the right atrium have been found in atrial tachycardias[34]. As there is yet no definite evidence as to the cause of the cardiac adiposis, it is difficult to elaborate if they are different entities. Case 9 also had moderate fatty infiltration of the left ventricle but, unfortunately, there was no tissue processed for electron microscopy to look for attenuation of the intercalated discs[35].

Case 4 (Fig. 9) had hypertrophy and fibrosis with involvement of the left ventricle, and this suggests the possibility of a cardiomyopathy, possibly post myocarditis. This patient had apparently normal cardiac function and anatomy preoperatively. Conversely, the patient suspicious of dilated cardiomyopathy secondary to a possible viral infection did not display the classical lesions of this condition.

CONCLUSION

There were several pathological patterns found in atrial fibrillation, some associated with cardiomyopathies, some others merely a result of the arrhythmia, but the constant decrease in autonomic nerves in this group of patients is the most striking feature.

Acknowledgements:
We thank Mrs Charlene M. Paquette for excellent manuscript editing and Mrs Elaine Hunter for quality photographic work.

References

[1]   Davies MJ, Pomerance A. Pathology of atrial fibrillation in man. Br Heart J 1972;34:520-525.

[2]   James TN. Diversity of histopathologic correlates of atrial fibrillation. In: Kulbertus HE, Olson SB, Schlepper M (eds), Atrial Fibrillation. Moludal, Sweden, Asta Publishers, 1982, pp 13-32.

[3]   Bharati S, Lev M. Histology of the normal and diseased atrium. In: Falk RH, Podrid PJ (eds), Atrial Fibrillation, Mechanisms and Management. New York, Raven Press, 1992, pp 15-39.

[4]   Hudson RE. The conducting system: anatomy, histology, pathology in acquired heart disease. In: Silver MD (ed), Cardiovascular Pathology. New York, Churchill Livingstone Inc., 1983, pp 633-682.

[5]   Ih S, Saitoh S. The histopathological substratum for atrial fibrillation in man. Acta Pathol Jpn 1982;32(2):183-191.

[6]   Fenoglio Jr JJ, Wagner BM. Studies in rheumatic fever; VI. Ultrastructure of chronic rheumatic heart disease. Am J Pathol 1973;73(3):623-640.

[7]   Unverferth DV, Fertel RH, Unverferth BJ, Leier CV. Atrial fibrillation in mitral stenosis: histologic, hemodynamic and metabolic factors. Int J Cardiol 1984;5(2):143-154.

[8]   Pham TD, Fenoglio Jr JJ. Right atrial ultrastructure in chronic rheumatic heart disease. Int J Cardiol 1982;1(3-4):289-304.

[9]   Frustaci A, Caldarulo M, Buffon A, Bellocci F, Fenici R, Melina D. Cardiac biopsy in patients with " primary " atrial fibrillation; histologic evidence of occult myocardial diseases. Chest 1991;100(2):303-306.

[10]   Sekiguchi M, Hiroe M, Kasanuki H, Ohnishi S, Hirosawa K. Experience of 100 atrial endomyocardial biopsies and the concept of atrial cardiomyopathy [abstract]. Circulation 1984;70 (suppl 2):118.

[11]   Kobayashi Y, Yazawa T, Baba T, Mukai H, Inoue S, Takeyama Y, Niitani H. Clinical, electrophysiological, and histopathological observations in supraventricular tachycardia. PACE 1988;11:1154-1167.

[12]   Guiraudon GM, Campbell CS, Jones DL, McLellan DG, MacDonald JL. Combined sino-atrial node atrio-ventricular isolation: a surgical alternative to His bundle ablation in patients with atrial fibrillation (abstract). Circulation 1985;72-II:III-220.

[13]   Guiraudon GM, Klein GJ, Sharma AD, Yee R. Use of old and new anatomic, electro-physiologic and technical knowledge to develop operative approaches to tachycardia. In: Brugada P, Wellens HJJ (eds), Cardiac arrhythmias: where to go from here? Futura Publishing Company, Inc., Mount Kisco, New York, 1987, pp 639-652.

[14]   Leitch JW, Klein G, Yee R, Guiraudon G. Sinus node-atrio-ventricular node insolation. Long-term results with the corridor operation for atrial fibrillation. JACC 1991;17:970-975.

[15].   Defauw JJAMT, Guiraudon GM, van Hemel NM, Vermeulen FEE, Kingma JH, de Bakker JMT. Surgical therapy of paroxysmal atrial fibrillation with the "corridor" operation. Ann Thorac Surg 1922;53:564-571.

[16]   Maron BJ, Ferrans VS. Ultrastructural features of hypertrophied human ventricular myocardium. Progress in Cardiovasc Dis 1978;3:207-238.

[17]   Maron BJ, Ferrans VJ, Roberts WC. Ultrastructural features of degenerated cardiac muscle cells in patients with cardiac hypertrophy. Am J Pathol 1975;79:387-434.

[18]   Garrey WE. Auricular fibrillation. Physiol Rev 1924;4:215.

[19]   Moe GK. On the multiple wavelet hypothesis of atrial fibrillation. Arch Int Pharmacodyn Ther 1962;140:183-188.

[20]   Allessie MA, Lammers WJEP, Rensma PL, et al. Flutter and fibrillation in experimental models: what has been learned that can be applied to human. In: Brugada P, Wellens HJJ (eds), Cardiac arrhythmias: where to go from here? New York, Futura Publishers, 1987, pp 67-82.

[21]   See chapter in this book.

[22]   Michelucci A, Padeletti L, Fradella GA, et al. Effects of pharmacologic autonomic blockade on atrial electrophysiologic properties in normal subjects and in patients with sinus node disease. Int J Cardiol 1985;8: 437-445.

[23]   Coumel P, Leenhardt A. Mental activity, adrenergic modulation and cardiac arrhythmias in patients with heart disease. In: Mental stress as a trigger of cardiovascular events. Circulation 1991;83-II:58-70.

[24]   Coumel P. Neural aspects of paroxysmal atrial fibrillation. In: Falk RH, Podrid PJ (eds), Atrial fibrillation: mechanisms and management. Raven Press Ltd., New York, 1992, pp 109-125.

[25]   Coumel P. Role of the autonomic nervous system in paroxysmal atrial fibrillation. In: Touboul P, Waldo AL (eds), Atrial arrhythmias. Current concepts and management. Mosby Year Book, 1991, pp 248-261.

[26]   Boineau JP, Canavan TE, Schuessler RB, et al. Demonstration of a widely distributed distributed atrial pacemaker complex in the human heart. Circulation 1988;77:1221-1237.

[27]   Atwood, J.E. Exercise hemodynamics of atrial fibrillation. In: Falk RH, Podrid PJ (eds), Atrial Fibrillation. Raven Press, New York, 1992, pp 145-163.

[28]   Pickering JG, Guiraudon CM, Klein GJ. Focal right atrial dysplasia and atrial flutter in a patient with myotonic dystrophy. PACE 1989;12:1317-1323.

[29]   Manyari DE, Klein GJ, Gulamhusein S, et al. Arrhythmogenic right ventricular dysplasia: a generalized cardiomyopathy? Circulation 1983; 68:251-257.

[30]   Guiraudon CM. Diagnostic of right ventricular dysplasia: a role for electron microscopy? Eur Heart J 1989;(Suppl D):82-83.

[31]   Ihiene G, Nava A, Corrado D, Rossi L, Penneli N. Right ventricular cardiomyopathy and sudden death in young people. N Eng J Med 1988;318:129-133.

[32]   Fontaine G, Fontaliran F, Martin de la Salle E, et al. Right ventricular dysplasias in ventricular tachycardias. In: Aliot E, Lazzara R (eds), Ventricular tachycardias: from mechanism to therapy. Boston, Martinus Nijhoff Publishers, 1987, pp 113-133.

[33]   Marcus FI, Fontaine GH, Guiraudon G, et al. Right ventricular dysplasia: a report of 24 adult cases. Circulation 1982;65:384-398.

[34]   Balsaver AM, Morales AR, Whitehouse FW. Fat infiltration of myocardium as a cause of cardiac conduction defect. Am J Cardiol 1967;19: 261-265.

[35]   Guiraudon CM, Guiraudon GM, Klein GJ. Arrhythmogenic right ventricular dysplasia: histological and electromicroscopy study of five cases (abstract). JACC 1988;2:181A.

Chapter 4

TERMINATION OF ATRIAL FIBRILLATION

BY CLASS IC ANTIARRHYTHMIC DRUGS, A PARADOX?

Maurits A. Allessie

Charles Kirchhof

Department of Physiology
Cardiovascular Research Institute Maastricht
University of Limburg
The Netherlands

J. H. Kingma et al. (eds.), Atrial fibrillation, a treatable disease?, 59–66.
© 1992 *Kluwer Academic Publishers.*

PATHOPHYSIOLOGIC MECHANISMS OF
ATRIAL FIBRILLATION _____

In 1962 Moe[1] proposed the so-called multiple wavelet hypothesis to explain the mechanisms of self perpetuating atrial fibrillation. According to this hypothesis fibrillation is maintained by the presence of a number of independent wavelets that travel randomly through the myocardium around multiple barriers of refractory tissue. The key element of this hypothesis is that the "wavefront becomes fractionated as it divides about islets or strands of refractory tissue, and each of the daughter wavelets may now be considered as independent offspring. Such a wavelet may accelerate or decelerate as it encounters tissue in a more or less advanced state of recovery. It may divide again or combine with a neighbor; it may be expected to fluctuate in size and change in direction. Its course, though determined by the excitability or refractoriness of surrounding tissue, would appear to be as random as Brownian motion"[2].

Maintenance of fibrillation will depend on the number of wavelets present. With only a small number of wavelets, they may at a certain moment die out or fuse into a single wavefront, leading to resumption of sinus rhythm or to atrial flutter. The average number, in turn, will depend on the atrial tissue mass and the average wavelength of the wavelets.

At the time this hypothesis was formulated, simultaneous recording from a sufficient number of sites in the atria to document the complex excitation pattern was impossible, and Moe wrote that "direct test of the hypothesis is difficult, if not impossible in living tissue"[1]. Progress in technology and electronics has made it possible to sample the electrical activity from several hundreds of cardiac sites enabling a direct test of Moe's hypothesis[3-5]. In the mapping study of Allessie et al. [3] atrial fibrillation was induced in isolated blood perfused canine hearts by a single premature stimulus. The refractory period was shortened by continuous administration of acetylcholine. During maintained fibrillation, the presence of multiple independent wavelets was demonstrated by two endocardial high density mapping electrodes. The width of the wavelets could be as small as a few mm, but broad wavefronts propagating uniformly over large segments of the atria were observed as well. Each individual wavelet existed only for a short time, no longer than a few hundred msec. Extinction of a wavelet could be caused by fusion or collision with another wavelet, by reaching the border of the atria, or by meeting refractory tissue. New wavelets could be formed by division of a wave at a local area of conduction block, or by an offspring of a wave travelling towards the other atrium. The critical number of wavelets required to maintain fibrillation was estimated to be between four and six.

In humans atrial fibrillation has been mapped during surgery in patients suffering from the WPW syndrome[4,5]. Atrial fibrillation was induced by programmed electrical stimulation and epicardial mapping was performed using high density multiple mapping electrodes. In essence the findings were the same as obtained in the canine heart.

Mapping both in animals and humans revealed the following characteristics of atrial fibrillation:

1) Although circulating excitation of the leading circle type[6] can occur, it is exceptional that an impulse follows the same circular route more than once. Rather, reentry as the basis for fibrillation means reexcitation of a given area that had already been excited shortly before by *another* wandering wavefront. This has been called "random reentry" by Hoffman and Rosen [7].
2) Wavelets can be as narrow as a few mm, but broad uniformly propagating wavefronts are very frequent.
3) There is a wide temporal and spatial variation in conduction velocity of the wandering waves between 15 cm/sec and more than 1 m/sec.
4) The life time of each wave is rather short, but "new" waves are constantly formed by division or offspring of the existing waves.
5) The critical number of wandering wavelets for perpetuation of fibrillation is between four and six.
6) In complex atrial fibrillation there are multiple macroreentrant circuits that continuously spin around the atrial myocardium in a rapidly changing pattern [8].

THE WAVELENGTH CONCEPT _____

For a reentrant arrhythmia to be sustained, all cells in the reentrant circuit must have recovered their excitability before being reexcited. This can only occur if the pathlength of the reentrant circuit is greater than the wavelength of the propagating impulse, which is given by the product of conduction velocity and refractory period. If the wavelength is short, either because of a short refractory period, slow conduction, or both, more reentrant wavelets can be present in a given tissue mass and therefore the likelihood for fibrillation will be increased. In normal myocardium, there is a close relationship between wavelength and the induction of atrial arrhythmias[9,10]. In conscious dogs in whom multiple electrodes for stimulation and recording had been sutured to both atria, refractory periods and conduction velocity were measured during programmed electrical stimulation. To change the wavelength, a variety of agents (acetylcholine, propafenone, lidocaine, ouabaine, quinidine, d-sotalol) were administered and refractory period duration, conduction velocity and their product were correlated with the induction of atrial arrhythmias by single early premature stimuli[10]. In all dogs (n=19), atrial arrhythmias (n=549) could be induced including atrial fibrillation (n=208). Although at shorter refractory periods a relatively high incidence of atrial fibrillation was observed, prolongation of the refractory period did not always prevent atrial fibrillation.

In fact, the predictive value of refractory period duration alone, or conduction velocity alone, for induction of arrhythmias was poor. Because of the variety of drugs administered, values for conduction velocity and refractory period varied widely. Atrial fibrillation could be induced over a wide range of refractory periods (50 to 150 msec) and conduction velocities (50 to 140 cm/sec). For each of these parameters there was an overlap between the population of "no arrhythmias" and atrial fibrillation. When however the wavelength was used as a criterion, there was a clear separation between both populations. The critical wavelength for atrial fibrillation was 8 cm. It must be emphasized however that these results were obtained in normal atria in which the electrophysiological characteristics are fairly homogeneous throughout the atrial tissue.

THE SUBSTRATE OF ATRIAL FIBRILLATION _____

In diseased atria with a more inhomogeneous distribution of conduction velocities and refractory periods, certainly there does not exist such a thing as a *single* wavelength. Rather different wavelengths will exist at different sites which in addition will vary with changes in heart rate and direction of propagation. In such atria it may not be easy to demonstrate a similar relationship between wavelength and vulnerability to arrhythmias. Abnormalities in atrial electrophysiology and structure are probably important for the clinical development of atrial fibrillation. Shortened atrial refractoriness and diminution of the rate dependent change in refractoriness have been associated with a higher vulnerability to fibrillation[11-13]. Furthermore, membrane potential abnormalities which will lead to impaired conduction have been found in atrial fibers of patients with chronic atrial fibrillation[14,15]. Also extensive degenerative changes are present in atria of such patients[16]. With increasing age, electrical uncoupling of side to side fiber connections and development of collageneous septa have been reported[17]. From the above described multiple wavelet theory and the wavelength concept it is clear that all these factors will promote the occurrence of fibrillation in the human atria. Chronic atrial fibrillation is often preceded by episodes of paroxysmal atrial fibrillation [18]. The transition from paroxysmal to chronic fibrillation may be due to a further progression of an underlying etiological process, or fibrillation itself may cause changes in the myocardium which favor its irreversibility[19]. Pathological studies showed significantly more degenerative atrial changes in long-term than in short-term fibrillation[16]. The reported high oxygen consumption by the atria during fibrillation may explain this phenomenon by creating relative ischemia and resulting progressive fibrosis[20]. Prevention and treatment of atrial fibrillation should be focused on modification of the above mentioned factors. Mapping of atrial excitation in patients during cardiac surgery could open new ways to study the relative importance of wavelength and structural inhomogeneities in the occurrence of clinical atrial fibrillation[4,5,8].

THE ANTIFIBRILLATORY ACTION
OF CLASS IC DRUGS

The concept of a critical wavelength for reentrant arrhythmias suggests to describe the anti-arrhythmic properties of cardiac drugs in terms of wavelength. Drugs which shorten the wavelength must be regarded as pro-arrhythmic, whereas agents prolonging the wavelength possess anti-arrhythmic properties. An increase in wavelength is most effectively accomplished by a combined increase in refractory period and conduction velocity. Compounds whose action on one variable is totally or partially counteracted by an opposite effect on the other are less effective. When the wavelength is long, a large area of unidirectional conduction block is required for reentry. On the other hand, when the impulse is short -either by depressed conduction or by short refractoriness- small arcs of conduction block may already set up reentrant circuits. Since conduction block is more likely to occur in a small than in a large part of the myocardium, the *inducibility* of reentrant arrhythmias will be directly related to the length of the cardiac impulse[9,10].

For the perpetuation of reentrant rhythms the wavelength is also of crucial importance. Interventions which prolong the wavelength will increase the minimal size of intra-myocardial circuits. If an excitable gap is present in the reentrant loop, prolongation of the wavelength will first reduce and finally close the excitable gap, leading to instability and a higher chance of block of the circulating impulse. In the case of *multiple* reentering wavelets as during fibrillation, a prolongation of the wavelength will result in an increase in average circuit size. Since the tissue mass in a given heart is constant, the total number of wandering impulses will thus diminish and the likelihood of fusion and dying out of the wavelets will increase. As a consequence the prolongation of the wavelength during fibrillation may diminish the number of wavelets below the critical number for perpetuation and spontaneous termination may result. On the other hand, interventions which shorten the wavelength might either stabilize the reentrant process by creating or enlarging an excitable gap or it may lead to degeneration into multiple smaller circuits (fibrillation). In the study of Rensma et al.[10] class III drugs have been shown to be the most powerful agents to prolong the wavelength. However it should be kept in mind that many class III drugs show a reverse use dependency. This means that at higher heart rates the effect on the duration of the refractory period becomes less compared to slow heart rates.

Class Ic drugs have been shown to posses strong anti-fibrillatory properties[21,22]. In Langendorff perfused pig hearts the induction of multiple premature beats during acute regional ischemia always resulted in ventricular fibrillation. In the presence of Org 7797 (2-10 microMol) in no instance ventricular fibrillation could be induced[21]. In chronically instrumented conscious dogs, Org 7797 (3 mg/kg/h) reduced the inducibility of atrial fibrillation to 25% and the duration of fibrillation to 10%[22]. However both in the ventricles and the atria the wavelength of the activation wave was not lengthened by class Ic drugs and at higher concentrations the wavelength actually was found to become shorter[21,22]. This paradoxical finding that, despite the marked effects on conduction velocity and refractory period, administration of Org 7797 did not affect the wavelength appeared to invalidate the concept that the wavelength is a crucial parameter for both inducibility and stability of atrial fibrillation. However it should be kept in mind that the effects of a drug during pacing are not necessarily the same as during fibrillation. To prevent or terminate fibrillation, a drug should exert its effects at very short cycle lengths. If one looks at the effects on the maximal pacing rate, it was found that Org 7797 markedly prolonged the shortest attainable wavelength during incremental pacing[22]. While in the normal canine atria a progressive rate dependent shortening of the wavelength was found from 16 cm to 10 cm, administration of Org 7797 at 1, 2, and 3 mg/kg/h, limited the rate dependent shortening of wavelength to 10.6, 11.3, and 13.7 cm respectively. Thus the anti-fibrillatory action of class Ic drugs seems to be primarily based on a limitation of the physiological rate-dependent shortening of the wavelength. At higher concentrations the physiologic adaptation of the refractory period to higher heart rates was completely abolished and in some cases was even changed into a slight rate dependent lengthening of the refractory period. Thus Org 7797 may not affect or even shorten the algebraic product of conduction velocity and refractory period at slow heart rates, but it markedly prolonged the wavelength of the highest possible heart rate as found during fibrillation. As a result the average number of wandering wavelets will diminish which will lead to a higher statistical chance of spontaneous termination of atrial fibrillation.

References

[1]   Moe GK. On the multiple wavelet hypothesis of atrial fibrillation. Arch Int Pharmacodyn Ther 1962;140:183-188.
[2]   Moe GK, Abildskov JA. Atrial fibrillation as a self-sustaining arrhythmia independent of focal discharge. Am Heart J 1959;58:59-70.
[3]   Allessie MA, Lammers WJEP, Bonke FIM, Hollen J. Experimental evaluation of Moe's multiple wavelet hypothesis of atrial fibrillation. In: Zipes DP, Jalife J (eds), Cardiac Arrhythmias. Grune & Stratton, New York, 1985, pp 265-276.
[4]   Cox JL, Canavan TE, Schuessler RB, et al. The surgical treatment of atrial fibrillation. II. Intraoperative electrophysiologic mapping and description of the electrophysiological basis of atrial flutter and atrial fibrillation. J Thorac Cardiovasc Surg 1991;101:406-426.
[5]   Konings KTS, Allessie MA. Mapping of atrial fibrillation in man. New trends in arrhytmias 1991;7:81-84.
[6]   Allessie MA, Bonke FIM, Schopman FJG. Circus movement in rabbit atrial muscle as a mechanism of tachycardia. III. The "leading circle" concept: a new model of circus

movement in cardiac tissue without the involvement of an anatomic obstacle. Circ Res 1977;41:9-18.

[7]   Hoffman BF, Rosen MR. Cellular mechanisms for cardiac arrhythmias. Circ Res 1981; 49:1-15.

[8]   Cox JL, Boineau JP, Schuessler RB, Ferguson TB, Lindsay BD, Cain ME, Corr PB, Kater KM, Lappas DG. A review of surgery for atrial fibrillation. J Cardiovasc Electrophysiol 1991;2:541-561.

[9]   Smeets JL, Allessie MA, Lammers WJEP, Bonke FIM, Hollen J. The wavelength of the cardiac impulse and reentrant arrhythmias in isolated rabbit atrium. Circ Res 1986;58: 96-108.

[10]   Rensma PL, Allessie MA, Lammers WJEP, Bonke FIM, Schalij MJ. The length of the excitation wave as an index for the susceptibility to reentrant atrial arrhythmias. Circ Res 1988;62:395-410.

[11]   Michelucci A, Padeletti L, Fradella GA. Atrial refractoriness and spontaneous or induced atrial fibrillation. Acta Cardiol 1982;5:333-344.

[12]   Attuel P, Childers R, Cauchemez B, Poveda J, Mugica J, Coumel P. Failure in the rate adaptation of the atrial refractory period: its relationship to vulnerability. Int J Cardiol 1982;2:179-197.

[13]   Olsson SB, Brorson L, Varnauskas E. Monophasic action potential studies of atrial fibrillation. In: Kulbertus HE, Olsson SB, Schlepper M (eds), Atrial Fibrillation. Molndal, Sweden, 1982, pp 83-91.

[14]   Hordof AJ, Edie R, Malm JR, Hoffman BF, Rosen MR. Electrophysiologic properties and response to pharmacologic agents of fibers from diseased human atria. Circulation 1976;54:774-779.

[15]   Rosen MR, Bowman FO, Mary-Rabine L. Atrial fibrillation: the relationship between cellular electrophysiologic and clinical data. In: Kulbertus HE, Olsson SB, Schlepper M (eds), Atrial Fibrillation. Molndal, Sweden, 1982, pp 62-69.

[16]   Davies MJ, Pomerance A. Pathology of atrial fibrillation in man. Br Heart J 1972;34:520-525.

[17]   Spach MS, Miller WT, Geselowitz DB, Barr RC, Kootsey JM, Johnson EA. The discontinuous nature of propagation in normal canine cardiac muscle. Circ Res 1981;48: 39-54.

[18]   Godtfredsen J. Atrial fibrillation: course and prognosis - a follow-up study of 1212 cases. In: Kulbertus HE, Olsson SB, Schlepper M (eds), Atrial Fibrillation. Molndal, Sweden, 1982, pp 134-145.

[19]   Salmon DR, McPherson DD, Augustine DE, Holida MD, White CW. A canine model of chronic atrial fibrillation: echocardiographic and electrocardiographic validation. Circulation 1985;72:III-250.

[20]   White CW, Kerber RE, Weiss HR, Marcus ML. The effects of atrial fibrillation on atrial pressure-volume and flow relationships. Circ Res 1982;51:205-215.

[21]   Janse MJ, Wilms-Schopman F, Opthof, T. Mechanism of antifibrillatory action of Org 7797 in regionally ischemic pig heart. J Cardiovasc Pharmacol 1990;15:633-643.

[22]   Kirchhof C, Wijffels M, Brugada J, Planellas J, Allessie M. Mode of action of a new class Ic drug (Org 7797) against atrial fibrillation in conscious dogs. J Cardiovasc Pharmacol 1991;17:116-124.

Chapter 5

CHARACTERISTICS OF PATIENTS WITH CHRONIC ATRIAL

FIBRILLATION AND THE PREDICTION OF SUCCESSFUL

DC ELECTRICAL CARDIOVERSION

Isabelle C. van Gelder

Harry J.G.M. Crijns

Kong I. Lie

Department of Cardiology
Thoraxcenter
University Hospital Groningen
The Netherlands

67

J. H. Kingma et al. (eds.), Atrial fibrillation, a treatable disease?, 67–86.
© 1992 *Kluwer Academic Publishers.*

INTRODUCTION _____

Chronic atrial fibrillation is a common arrhythmia found in about 0.4% of the adult population. The prevalence increases with age, being 2-4% after 60 years of age. In cardiac patients the prevalence is about 4%, and up to 40% in patients with overt congestive heart failure[1-3]. In the Framingham study the overall incidence in both sexes of developing atrial fibrillation was two per thousand in each biennium, rising sharply with age[4]. Rheumatic heart disease and cardiac failure were the most powerful predictive precursors, with at least a sixfold excess risk. Men with coronary artery disease had a statistically significant doubled risk of developing chronic atrial fibrillation, whereas women did not have an increased risk[5].

Chronic atrial fibrillation can be distinguished from paroxysmal atrial fibrillation. Unfortunately a clear division between these two forms of atrial fibrillation is not always made in different studies. Chronic atrial fibrillation was defined by our group as documented atrial fibrillation with a duration of >24 hours. *In addition*, sequential precardioversion electrocardiograms must show the arrhythmia, i.e. must show absence of intercurrent sinus rhythm. This definition is based on clinical practice, since mostly 24 hour Holter monitoring is the only readily available tool to document the continuous nature of the arrhythmia. Therefore our group used Holter monitoring to validate the 24 hour criterion[6]. It must be realized that this definition includes *paroxysmal long-standing* (lasting between 24 hours and 6 months) atrial fibrillation and as such it is different from the definition of chronic atrial fibrillation used by Suttorp et al. (see Chapter 6).

In order to prevent or reverse adverse effects caused by chronic atrial fibrillation the general goal of the clinician is to restore and maintain sinus rhythm in these patients.

DC electrical cardioversion is an effective method of terminating atrial fibrillation[7], introduced in 1962 by Lown et al.[8]. The indications for electrical cardioversion as well as its efficacy in restoring sinus rhythm depends on the patient's clinical profile. Since the introduction of the electrical cardioversion this profile has changed. Although a systematic study into the magnitude of this change has never been undertaken, it can be supposed that the lower incidence of rheumatic heart disease and the higher age in the population both play a role. In addition it is well known that congestive heart failure is an increasing problem. Also, the introduction of new diagnostic and therapeutic modalities for conditions predisposing to atrial fibrillation may relate to this change. The clinical profile of atrial fibrillation patients may also have changed due to the fact that the detection of the underlying heart disease improved, especially through echocardiography, thus changing the composition of the 'lone' atrial fibrillation group. The increased interest in atrial tachyarrhythmias in the last years has led to new studies into the treatment of chronic atrial fibrillation. In this chapter we discuss the present characteristics of patients with chronic atrial fibrillation and try to determine the probability of successful DC electrical cardioversion on the basis of the patient's clinical profile. In addition, clinically useful guidelines for the management of these patients are presented.

CHARACTERISTICS OF PATIENTS WITH CHRONIC ATRIAL FIBRILLATION _____

Table 1 shows an overview of the clinical characteristics of chronic atrial fibrillation patients between 1966 and 1991. It suggests that the clinical profile changed in course of time. Unfortunately, no data on the clinical characteristics of *all* patients with chronic atrial fibrillation can be given, since the clinical profiles reported in different studies depend heavily on the entry criteria. At best, patients referred for cardioversion or selected for prevention trials with oral anticoagulation may be studied from the literature[9-18]. Thus only selected patient groups of atrial fibrillation are available. In these studies restrictions were often used for duration of the arrhythmia, left atrial size and number of previous episodes at entry into the study.

Age of the patients referred for the respective studies tends to increase, although not drastically, despite an ageing population nowadays. This may be caused by the fact that older patients are often not treated by cardiologists but other physicians who tend to be more conservative and who accept atrial fibrillation as predominant rhythm. The AFASAK trial was not conducted to convert atrial fibrillation but to prevent thromboembolic events. This can explain the higher age in this study. As is shown in Table 1 only few patients suffer from rheumatic heart disease nowadays. In the AFASAK trial rheumatic heart disease was one of the exclusion criteria. In contrast, at present patients suffer more frequently from coronary artery disease and arterial hypertension. Due to improved diagnostics in the last decades, the composition of the 'lone' atrial fibrillation group may have altered. However, it has not resulted in a relative

Table 1. Characteristics of patients with chronic atrial fibrillation. Differences between older and more recent studies.

First author	Szek	Lown	Cram	Resn	Bjer	Söd*	Lund	AFA#	Bro*	Juul@	VanG
year	1966	1967	1968	1968	1969	1975	1988	1989	1989	1990	1991
reference	(9)	(10)	(11)	(12)	(13)	(14)	(15)	(16)	(17)	(18)	(6)
age (mean, years)	45	-	55	-	53	58	63	74	58	59	60
patients	145	350	237	180	437	117	100	1007	43	183	246
male (%)	-	-	53	58	58	68	57	54	58	81	56
AFL(%)	0	0	0	0	-	6	0	0	0	0	22
Underlying disease											
CAD (%)	10	12	8	9	-	32	10	25	19	16	24
RhHD (%)	81	70	56	56	63	26##	22##	0	35##	5##	24
HYT (%)	-	-	14	1	-	9	22	32	12	26	11
CHD (%)	3	-	-	4	-	-	2	-	-	-	6
CM (%)	-	-	-	9	-	-	4	-	16	-	10
NonRh VD (%)	-	-	-	-	-	-	-	-	-	-	8
HThyr,corr (%)	4	-	1	3	-	6	4	5	-	-	2
'Lone' (%)	2	10	16	18	-	-	21	-	-	-	15
Miscellaneous	-	8	5	-	-	8	15	-	19	-	0
Previous duration (months)											
0-6 (%)	-	-	-	34	31	76	-	-	33	-	30
7-12 (%)	-	-	-	20	14	15	-	-	4	-	10
13-36 (%)	-	-	-	20	15	9	-	-	63**	-	21
37-60 (%)	-	-	-	9	9	0	-	-	-	-	14
> 60 (%)	-	-	-	17	31	0	-	-	-	-	25
mean (years)	2.5	-	-	-	-	-	-	-	2.9	0.4	4.3
median (years)	-	-	-	-	-	-	-	-	-	0.3	2
Left atrial size long axis, mean (mm)	-	-	-	-	-	-	-	-	>45	42	46
NYHA III+IV (%)	-	-	48	-	29	6	-	-	-	-	27

-: not available; *: patiens with a duration > 36 months were excluded in this study; #: rheumatic heart disease was exclusion criterion; @: patients with a duration of atrial fibrillation > 1 year were excluded; **: duration > 1 year was not further specified; ##: including non rheumatic valvular disease. AFA= AFASAK trial(16); AFL= atrial flutter; Bjer= Bjerkelund(13); Bro=Brodsky(17); CAD= coronary artery disease; CHD= congenital heart disease; CM= cardiomyopathy; corr= corrected; Cram= Cramer(11); HThyr= hyperthyroidism; Hyt= arterial hypertension; Juul= Juul-Möller(18); Lund= Lundström(15); Non Rh VD= nonrheumatic valvular disease; Resn= Resnekow(12); RhHD= rheumatic heart disease; Söd=Södermark(14); Szek=Szekely(9); VanG= Van Gelder(6)

decline of patients suffering from atrial fibrillation without underlying detectable heart disease. This is difficult to explain but may be related to a change in referral pattern. Another important characteristic in relation to outcome of treatment is the previous duration of the arrhythmia. As far as data are available, there are only small differences between the earlier and present studies. However, many have not given this information, which precludes the study of the changes between older and more recent investigations at this point. This also applies for the presence or absence of heart failure and for the left atrial size.

In our study almost all referred patients were included. Previous arrhythmia duration, left atrial size and röntgenographic heart size were not used as exclusion criteria. Therefore, our population may reflect closely the clinical profile of the patients referred for cardioversion at present (Table 2). A total of 302 patients were referred for DC electrical cardioversion to our department between 1986 and 1989. Fifty-six patients were excluded: twenty-three (8% of the total referred population) due to the presence of sinus rhythm at admission, the other 33 for unstable heart failure, cardiogenic shock or the presence of severe

Table 2. **Characteristics of 246 patients undergoing DC cardioversion between 1986 and 1989 at the University Hospital Groningen**

Age (range, years)*		60 ± 12 (25-86)
Male/female (n)		137/109
Atrial fibrillation/atrial flutter (n)		191/ 55
Underlying heart disease:		
Coronary artery disease	(%)	24
Rheumatic heart disease	(%)	24
Hypertension	(%)	11
Congenital heart disease	(%)	6
Cardiomyopathy	(%)	10
Non rheumatic valvular disease	(%)	8
Hyperthyroidism, corrected	(%)	2
'Lone' arrhythmia	(%)	15
Previous cardiac surgery		
CABG/valvular surgery		25/49
Previous duration: mean (months)		28 ± 45
median (range, months)		8 (0.04-300)
Previous episodes of fibrillation/flutter (n)*		1.8 ± 2.0
Total duration arrhythmia (months)*		52 ± 66
median (range, months)		24 (0.04-400)
NYHA class I/II/III/IV:		84/97/62/3
Cardiac thoracic ratio (%)*		53 ± 7
Left atrial size, long axis (mm)*		46 ± 8
apical view (mm)*		68 ± 10
Right atrial size, apical view (mm)*		60 ± 8
Left ventricular end diastolic diameter (mm)*		52 ± 9
Left ventricular end systolic diameter (mm)*		37 ± 9
Height of fibrillation wave in lead V1 (mm)*		1.3 ± 0.7
Plasma potassium concentration (mmol/L) *,**		4.3 ± 0.5
Treated with diuretics / ACE inhibitors (n)		110 / 44

*mean±standard deviation, **at the cardioversion. ACE= angiotensin converting enzyme; bpm= beats per minute; CABG= coronary artery bypass grafting; NYHA = New York Heart Association.

systemic disease. Thus almost 10% of the patients were excluded because of spontaneous restoration of sinus rhythm at the day of cardioversion. This was often at least 4 weeks after the initial appointment, due to the start of oral anticoagulation (see below). By definition, these patients did not have chronic atrial fibrillation.

THERAPEUTIC STRATEGY OF
CHRONIC ATRIAL FIBRILLATION _____

Atrial fibrillation is associated with subjective complaints[10], deterioration of the left ventricular function[19,20], increased risk of thromboembolic complications[21,22], increase of atrial sizes[23,24] and an increased mortality [1,3,4]. In order to prevent or reverse these effects, restoration of sinus rhythm is the general goal of the clinician in patients with atrial fibrillation. There are two possible approaches: chemical cardioversion and Direct Current (DC) electrical cardioversion. For recent onset paroxysmal atrial fibrillation chemical cardioversion is very effective, especially with new class IC and class III antiarrhythmic drugs. However, lower cardioversion rates are observed if the duration of the arrhythmia exceeds 24 hours[11,25-29]. Moreover, chemical conversions remain more time consuming than DC cardioversions. The chance on proarrhythmic effects related to the use of antiarrhythmic drugs for cardioversion of atrial fibrillation obliges the patient to be in hospital under close electrocardiographic monitoring. Up to now cost-effectiveness of chemical and DC cardioversion have not been compared. It seems reasonable to assume that DC cardioversion is more cost-effective in patients with atrial fibrillation with a duration > 24 hours since the procedure is more effective, and the duration of the procedure is shorter, and it may be performed on an outpatient basis. On the other hand, the need for general anaesthesia remains a disadvantage and a considerable cost factor.

DIRECT CURRENT ELECTRICAL CARDIOVERSION _____

Prior to the cardioversion the potassium level should be checked and the procedure should be cancelled when the potassium concentration is < 3.5 mmol/l in order to avoid the induction of arrhythmias. Also, the success rate may be decreased in the presence of hypokalemia as arrhythmogenic responses may occur not only at the ventricular but also at the atrial level. Conceivably, the latter leads to reinduction of atrial fibrillation.

Electrocardioversion may be arrhythmogenic by itself but especially in the setting of digitalis toxicity sustained ventricular arrhythmias may be found[10,30-32]. In addition, toxic doses of digitalis have been shown to reduce the energy requirement for inducing ventricular ectopy after cardioversion[30]. Therefore, since the introduction of DC electrical cardioversion it has been recommended to withhold digitalis at least 24 hours prior to the shock[10]. However, Ditchey and Karliner[33] showed that digitalis had no significant arrhythmogenic potential during cardioversion if there is no evidence of digitalis toxicity. Therefore, cardioversion during digitalis treatment is no longer contraindicated. Only in case of suspected digitalis toxicity cardioversion should be postponed, if possible, or caution should be exercised. In such cases it is recommended to start with a low dose of energy.

Patients with previous hyperthyroidism should only be cardioverted at least 3 months after achievement of the euthyroid state, since a high recurrence rate has been documented in case of earlier restoration of sinus rhythm[34]. After a period of at least 3 months of euthyroidism there may be an excellent cardioversion and maintenance rate. This implies that an attempt to restoration of sinus rhythm should be done in all these patients.

During the procedure facilities for resuscitation must be available. A continuous drip infusion with glucose 5% is introduced before the cardioversion and allows for emergency infusion of atropine 0.5 mg or isoprenaline 0.4 mg%. An anesthesiologist should be present not only for a professional induction of anaesthesia but also to prevent complications associated with e.g. apnea necessitating endotracheal intubation.

Anticoagulation to prevent thromboembolic events during and after the electrical cardioversion is clearly indicated[13,35]. Although no randomized trials have been performed, one large comparative study showed that the frequency of thromboembolic events without anticoagulants was 5.3% and with anticoagulants 0.8%[13]. Arbitrarily therapy should start at least 4 weeks before cardioversion in all patients with atrial fibrillation > 24 hours to allow time for adherence of a preexisting thrombus. Thromboembolic complication have been described up to 10 days after the cardioversion since atrial activity may not resume for 1-4 weeks[36-38]. Therefore, and for protection in case of a recurrence of atrial fibrillation soon after cardioversion, it is reasonable to continue anticoagulation at least 1 month after the shock. In our institution anticoagulation is considered effective if the prothrombin time is between 2.4 and 4.8 INR. In case of a prothrombin time > 4.8 INR at the day of DC electrical cardioversion we postpone the procedure, since it suggests that anticoagulation was inadequate during the last weeks.

DC electrical cardioversion must be performed in the post absorptive state during light general anaesthesia. Anaesthesia using short-acting drugs is preferred. Drugs with a shorter half-life may enhance cardioversion on an outpatient basis[39,40]. From this approach significant savings can be expected and for the patients it is less apprehensive compared to hospitalization. A drawback is, however, that patients may suffer late anesthesiological sequelae of the procedure. Therefore, this approach should not be followed unless specific postanesthetic care out of the hospital is provided and guaranteed.

For all cardioversions, except for very rapid ventricular tachyarrhythmias (ventricular fibrillation/flutter), synchronization to the QRS complex is important to avoid the vulnerable period of the cardiac cycle. Therefore, the lead with the highest R-wave amplitude should be selected for synchronization. Electrocardiographic tracings derived from the paddle electrodes may give motion artifacts and errors in R-wave sensing.

The paddle electrodes can be positioned at two sites. Firstly, the anterolateral position, with one paddle placed right parasternally at the level of the first or second rib and the other one in the midaxillary line at the fourth or fifth intercostal place. Secondly the anteroposterior position, with one paddle placed in the left infraclavicular region and the other one along the right sternal border. Although Lown[10] stated that the anteroposterior position reduces the energy requirement with about 50% and thus lowers the complication rate, this could not be confirmed by others[12]. Kerber et al.[41] showed that there was no clear advantage for any position. Position of the paddles on bone should be avoided as much as possible since this impedes the flow of current through the heart [42]. To prevent burns defibrillator pads or gel should be used adequately. Firm pressure must be applied to the paddle electrodes (size at least 11 x 11 cm) in order to reduce transthoracic impedance. Larger defibrillator pads lower the transthoracic impedance[42-44]. In patients with atrial flutter the initial dose may be set at 50 Joules of stored energy, whereas in atrial fibrillation this initial dose should be at least 100 to 200 Joules. Thereafter, as part of routine we follow a protocol with a stepwise increase of the energy till the highest energy setting.

Delivering the shock with the maximum energy level twice will not improve outcome[36]. The procedure is ended after restoration of sinus rhythm or 1 attempt at the highest level of stored energy. Time between consequent shocks should be between 1 and 1.5 minute in order to prevent myocardial damage[43]. Care must be taken that the rhythm can be recorded quickly and accurately after each cardioversion attempt. In many cases this will prevent unnecessary shocks.

Electrical cardioversion may succeed only if the electrical current through the myocardium is strong enough to depolarize a critical mass of atrial myocardium. The actual current flow is determined not only by the actual delivered energy but also by the transthoracic impedance. If the transthoracic impedance is high, low energy may generate inadequate current to achieve cardioversion. Therefore, it has been suggested that determining the transthoracic impedance before the shock may improve outcome, may shorten the procedure and decrease toxic effects to the myocardium. Up to now Dalzell et al.[44] and Kerber et al.[45] reported on the precardioversion measurements of the transthoracic impedance. It was concluded, that a high impedance and low energy output generated too low current to successfully cardiovert patients with atrial fibrillation[44]. Kerber et al.[45] used an impedance-based energy adjustment technique, by which the operator-selected energy was automatically increased if the preshock impedance exceeded 70 Ω. This resulted in a significant improvement in shock success-rate in patients with a high transthoracic impedance.

IMMEDIATE OUTCOME OF
DC ELECTRICAL CARDIOVERSION _____

Immediate outcome of DC electrical cardioversion in chronic atrial fibrillation patients in older and more recent studies is shown in Table 3 [6,9-14,46]. The success percentages of the newer studies are lower compared to the earlier studies. Especially our study shows a low success percentage: 70% in atrial fibrillation patients. The latter may be explained by three factors. Firstly, we used maintenance of sinus rhythm for at least 24 hours after the cardioversion as criterion for successful electrical cardioversion. In contrast, in previous studies establishment of sinus rhythm immediately after the shock was considered a successful cardioversion. If we had used that definition the success percentage would have been 74%. Secondly, considering the previous duration of the

Table 3. Immediate success percentage of older and more recent studies of electrical cardioversion of chronic atrial fibrillation.

First author	[ref]	year	success %	pretreatment with AAD
Szekely	[9]	1966	87	+
Lown	[10]	1967	94	+
Resnekow	[12]	1968	86	+/−
Bjerkelund	[13]	1969	80	?
Södermark	[14]	1975	85	+
Dittrich	[15]	1989	76	+/−
Van Gelder	[6]	1991	70	−

+/− = part of the patients; ? = unknown. AAD = antiarrhythmic drugs.

arrhythmia, the number of previous episodes and the New York Heart Association classification for exercise tolerance, these parameters indicate that the study patients should be characterized as difficult-to-treat. Finally, patients were not pretreated with antiarrhythmic drugs. Whether this indeed lowered the efficacy of electrical cardioversion is debatable, since the benefit of precardioversion institution of antiarrhythmics has been questioned[12,14,47,48, see below).

Similar to our study, the lower success rate in the report of Bjerkelund and coworkers[13] may relate to the inclusion of difficult-to-treat patients, as indicated by the previous duration, underlying heart disease and New York Heart Association classification for exercise tolerance (Table 1). Dittrich et al.[46] also reported a low success percentage. Detailed information about baseline characteristics of their patients is however not available, but significantly lower cardioversion rates are reported in patients with congestive cardiomyopathy and pulmonary disease.

Parameters related to success of the cardioversion differ among studies. However, most have shown that a long previous duration significantly reduces success of the cardioversion. Similarly, using multivariate analysis, we found that a shorter previous duration of the arrhythmia ($p < 0.001$) favoured success of the cardioversion. Other independent parameters significantly related to successful cardioversion were the presence of atrial flutter instead of fibrillation ($p < 0.02$) and a lower age ($p < 0.05$)[6]. In contrast to earlier studies parameters like left atrial size[10,12], underlying disease[48] and heart size[12,13] were not related to success of the cardioversion. Several explanations may be offered for these discrepancies. The most important is that almost all earlier studies did not use multivariate analysis, thereby potentially overestimating some predicting factors. In addition, only relatively small patient groups were investigated.

Up to now no clinically useful decision algorithms, allowing for prediction of cardioversion outcome, have been established. Estimations of probability of conversion may guide the clinician in the management of patients with chronic atrial fibrillation. With the formula of the logistic regression analysis used in our study the chance on a successful cardioversion can be determined[6].

$$P \text{ (failure cardioversion)} =$$

$$\frac{\exp(-3.7 + 0.023 \times prev\ dur - 2.3 \times (AF=0/FL=1) + 0.03 \times age)}{1 + \exp(-3.7 + 0.023 \times prev\ dur - 2.3 \times (AF=0/FL=1) + 0.03 \times age)}$$

AF = atrial fibrillation; dur = duration; FL = atrial flutter; prev = previous.
Previous duration in months, age in years.

For example, a 40 year old patient with atrial fibrillation since 1 month has a chance of a successful cardioversion of 91%, whereas a 80 year old patient with atrial fibrillation since 12 months only has a probability of success of 67%. Using these easy to obtain clinical characteristics decisions to perform cardioversion may depend on the calculated probability of conversion[6]. In this way highly unsuccessful cardioversions may be avoided, improving the cost-benefit ratio.

Cardioversion threshold.

The cardioversion threshold for atrial fibrillation has been defined as the amount of stored energy delivered at the successful attempt. As is shown in Table 4 our study showed the highest mean cardioversion threshold, whereas Lown [10] found a lower cardioversion threshold. In the study of Lown a longer duration of atrial fibrillation and smaller fibrillatory waves increased the energy requirement for cardioversion. Using multivariate analysis we found that parameters significantly related to a lower cardioversion threshold were (a) the presence of atrial flutter in stead of atrial fibrillation (p=0.00001) (affirming earlier studies[10,12]), and (b) female sex (p<0.005). The lower cardioversion threshold in women may be explained by assuming that they have a lower mean chest

I. C. van Gelder et al.

Table 4. Comparison of cardioversion thresholds

First author	[ref]	year	CVT	% success with >200 J
Lown	[10]	1967	100	18
Resnekow	[12]	1968	210	55
Van Gelder	[6]	1991	240	74

CVT = cardioversion threshold

circumference and therefore may have a lower transthoracic impedance. In addition, atrial muscle mass presumably is lower. A longer duration of the arrhythmia influenced the cardioversion threshold unfavourably although this difference was not significantly different ($p = 0.06$). This has also been found by Lown[10].

From the threshold data it was possible to generate an algorithm which allows for precardioversion calculation of the probability of successful cardioversion at a certain setting of stored energy. Multivariate analysis gives an algorithm of the following form[36]:

279-134 x (AF=0/FL=1) - 41 x (M=0/F=1) + 0.1 x (prev dur, months)

(AF = atrial fibrillation; FL = atrial flutter; F = female; M = male; prev dur = previous duration)

This means for example that for a woman suffering from atrial fibrillation since 12 months, an energy level of at least 239 Joules is required to achieve a 95% probability of cardioversion with a single shock.

The clinical relevance may be obvious. A maximum cardioversion rate may be achieved, without the need for administering multiple shocks. Multiple shocks may be potentially hazardous, since it extends the cardioversion procedure and prolongs the duration of the anaesthesia with its associated risks. In addition, administration of multiple shocks increases the chance of producing myocardial damage. The precardioversion calculation of the cardioversion threshold simultaneously with the determination of the actual transthoracic impedance may further optimize the procedure.

The cardioversion threshold was 200 Joules or higher in 74% of our patients. Delivering the highest dose of energy twice resulted in cardioversion in only an additional 3% of patients, and such a second full energy attempt may therefore be omitted[36].

Effects of antiarrhythmic drugs on the cardioversion threshold.

Little is known about the effects of antiarrhythmic drugs on the atrial defibrillation threshold in humans. Pretreatment with quinidine has been reported to facilitate cardioversion[49], but this has been questioned in other studies [12,14,48]. Echt et al.[50] performed a study in dogs evaluating the ventricular defibrillation threshold with differently acting antiarrhythmic drugs. From that study it was concluded that antiarrhythmics which act as sodium channel blocker increase the defibrillation threshold whereas antiarrhythmics which prolong the action potential duration decrease the defibrillation threshold. We found that patients pretreated with flecainide (2 mg/kg body weight in 30 minutes intravenously followed by 100 mg orally) showed an increased energy requirement for cardioversion of chronic atrial fibrillation to sinus rhythm[47]. The number of patients eventually converting to sinus rhythm did not differ from that in patients not pretreated. In view of the above mentioned it is reasonable to assume that all drugs with class I action may hamper cardioversion. In future studies the value of pure class III antiarrhythmic drugs in increasing the cardioversion rate while decreasing energy requirements, should be studied. One disadvantage of loading with antiarrhythmic drugs before electrical cardioversion is however that it is time consuming and necessitates a longer hospital admission for safety reasons[51-53].

COMPLICATIONS _____

Complications are listed in Table 5 and occur in 5-27%[6,31,32,54]. Below the most commonly seen complications are discussed. Minor complications due to superficial skin burns or chest muscle or skeleton pains are not considered.

Myocardial damage. Myocardial damage, accompanied with myocardial necrosis has been reported after large doses of energy in animals[43,55]. Except for the total delivered energy dose, myocardial damage seemed to be related to the size of the paddle electrodes and time between subsequent shocks[43]. The smaller the paddle electrodes and the shorter time between subsequent shocks, the larger the extent of myocardial damage. However, a wide safety margin was demonstrated between the effective dose of energy used for cardioversion and the dose required to produce significant myocardial damage in dogs[56,57]. In earlier years it has been recognized that myocardial damage was considerably less when DC cardioversion was used compared to Alternating Current cardioversions[10] and nowadays only DC shocks are used.

Creatine kinase (CK) release has been reported to occur after cardioversion in humans[55,58], but only small concomitant increases of creatine kinase MB isoenzyme (CK-MB) have been reported. In one study this increase of CK-MB was significantly lower compared to a control group of patients with a myocardial infarction 24 hours after onset of symptoms[58]. This almost rules out the occurrence of myocardial damage in patients undergoing DC electrical cardioversion for chronic atrial fibrillation using the commonly used ranges of delivered energy. However, a limitation may be that this method is too insensitive to detect local damage[56] which may also hold for myocardial scintigraphy [59,60].

ST segment elevations have been reported to occur in about 20% of cardioversions[58,61,62], especially in patients with a previous pericardiotomy [58], but have not been associated with CK-MB release or necrosis. The mechanism of the ST segment elevations remains unclear but it may be associated with a lower cardioversion rate and a lower maintenance rate of sinus rhythm after the shock[58].

Cardiac arrhythmias and conduction disturbances. Arrhythmias are the most common complications reported after DC cardioversion. Ventricular arrhythmias have been related to the use of digitalis and quinidine[10,31,32] and were difficult to terminate, sometimes leading to death. In one recent study all ventricular tachycardias, occurring immediately after the shock were self terminating within 30 seconds[36]. Obviously, improper synchronisation can lead to ventricular fibrillation[10,36] but is easy to terminate. Atrial arrhythmias such as supraventricular premature beats, couplets and nonsustained supraventricular tachycardias occur very frequently after cardioversion and may be related to recurrence of the arrhythmia[36]. These arrhythmias are not mentioned in Table 5. Other, new, atrial arrhythmias may be related to unmasking underlying tachycardia circuits after conversion to sinus rhythm, which may have been suppressed during the arrhythmia[36].

The occurrence of conduction disturbances due to unmasking of a sick sinus syndrome with or without AV nodal disease occur often after cardioversion and are related to the previous duration of atrial fibrillation: up to 45% in patients with atrial fibrillation of several years duration[10,36]. This may necessitate pacemaker therapy after successful cardioversion in some cases[36].

Table 5. Complications due to DC electrical cardioversion alone

First author Reference Year	Van Gelder [36] 1991	Åberg [32] 1968	Resnekow [54] 1967	Rabbino [31] 1964
Number of patients	246	207	204	35
AF	191	176	180	35
AFL	55	31	24	0
Total Complications (%)	8.8	8.5	5	27
Myocardial damage (%)				
Increase CK-MB	0	–	–	–
Arrhythmias (%)				
Ventricular arrhythmias				
Non sustained ventricular tachycardia	1.6	–	–	–
Ventricular fibrillation	0.4	2.5	0	9#
Atrial arrhythmias				
Sustained AT	0.4	–	–	–
Sustained CMT	0.4	–	–	–
Sustained AVNT	1.2	–	–	–
Parox AT with block	0.4	–	–	6
Underlying sick sinus syndrome				
Asystole	1.2	0.5	0.5	3
needed pacemaker	0.4	0	0	–
Sympt AVN rhythm	0.8	–	–	–
Sympt A rhythm	0.8	3	0.5	–
2nd degree SA block	0.4	–	–	3
C. Thromboembolic events (%)	0.4	1	1.5*	6*
D. Acute Congestive Heart Failure (%)	0.4	1.5	2.5	–
E. Hypotension (%)	0	–	3.5	–
F. Mortality (%)	0	0	0.5@	6#

– = not available; * = no anticoagulants; @ = during treatment with Q-36 hrs after the shock; # = probably cardioversion during digitalis toxicity.
AF = atrial fibrillation; AFL = atrial flutter; AVN = atrioventricular nodal; CM = circus movement; CV = cardioversion; Parox = paroxysmal; SA = sinoatrial; Sympt = symptomatic; T = Tachycardia.

SUMMARY and GUIDELINE _____

Selection of patients with chronic atrial fibrillation for DC electrical cardioversion: relation with clinical characteristics

There are two possible approaches to restore sinus rhythm in patients with chronic atrial fibrillation: chemical cardioversion and DC electrical cadioversion. For the effects of chemical cardioversion in paroxysmal longstanding atrial fibrillation the reader is referred to Chapter 6 (Suttorp et al.). In the present chapter DC electrical cardioversion is described. However, before treating patients with chronic atrial fibrillation the probability of success of the therapy should be evaluated. Firstly the probability of a successful electrical cardioversion has to be determined. Secondly, the chance of maintenance of sinus rhythm after cardioversion must be estimated. Whether patients will maintain sinus rhythm after the cardioversion is described in the Chapters 6 (Suttorp et al.) and 7 (Crijns et al.). To improve the cost-effectiveness of the procedure the probability of successful DC electrical cardioversion may be assessed beforehand using several clinical variables. In previous studies acute cardioversion outcome was related to the duration of the arrhythmia, the underlying heart disease, atrial size and the degree of congestive heart failure. Atrial size and underlying heart disease were of no importance in the later studies. If this depends on a time-dependent difference in clinical profile, e.g. underlying disease is uncertain. However, at present most of the patients with chronic atrial fibrillation suffer from coronary artery disease and arterial hypertension instead of rheumatic heart disease. 'Lone' atrial fibrillation has also been associated with intractability, but occasionally with a favourable outcome. The discrepancies between these studies may reflect differences in characterization of 'lone' arrhythmia as well as in the diagnostic effort put into identifying a specific underlying cause, rather than a true difference in outcome. Congestive heart failure is not necessarily a significant negative predictive parameter. Therefore, at present the only clinical parameters of importance determining success of the cardioversion in patients with chronic atrial fibrillation are the patient's age and the duration of the arrhythmia. Using the formula mentioned above the chance of a successful cardioversion can be determined. Decisions to perform cardioversion might depend on a probability of cardioversion of e.g. 75%.

In atrial fibrillation the initial dose of stored energy may be set at at least 100 Joules. In a more sophisticated approach, and in an attempt to avoid unnecessary shocks, the threshold may also be calculated, as is shown above.

All patients should be anticoagulated effectively for > 1 month and the protrombin time should be ascertained at the day of the electrical cardioversion. The role of echocardiography in determining the risk of pericardioversion embolization still needs to be established (see also chapter on anticoagulation).

Drugs given to control the ventricular response (digitalis, verapamil and beta-blockers) can be continued during the procedure and eventually be stopped after sinus rhythm has been restored. Only if digitalis toxicity is suspected, the procedure is better postponed. The potassium concentration should always be verified before the shock. Obviously, overt congestive heart failure and hyperthyroidism should be well controlled before cardioversion is performed.

Cardioversion can be performed on an outpatient basis if postanaesthetic care out of hospital is provided.

As long as the usefulness of antiarrhythmic drugs during the shock has not been affirmed, drug pretreatment before DC electrical cardioversion should be avoided.

Whether patients with paroxysmal longstanding atrial fibrillation should be treated chemically or by DC electrical cardioversion remains a point of discussion at this moment. Due to the excellent success rates using DC electrical cardioversion in this patient group and the more time consuming procedure when using antiarrhythmic drugs one may prefer DC electrical cardioversion.

References

[1] Godtfredsen J. Atrial fibrillation. Etiology, course and prognosis. A follow-up study of 1212 cases. Copenhagen: University of Copenhagen, 1975 (Thesis).
[2] Petersen P, Godtfredsen J. Atrial fibrillation-a review of course and prognosis. Acta Med Scand 1984;216:3-9.
[3] Onundarson PT, Thorgeirsson G, Jonmundsson E, Hardarson Th. Chronic atrial fibrillation-epidemiologic features and 14 years follow-up: a case control study. Eur Heart J 1987;8:521-527.
[4] Kannel WB, Abbott RD, Savage DD, McNamara PM. Epidemiologic features of chronic atrial fibrillation. N Engl J Med 1982;306:1018-1022.
[5] Kannel WB, Abbott RD, Savage DD, McNamara PM. Coronary heart disease and atrial fibrillation: the Framingham study. Am Heart J 1983;106:389-396.
[6] Van Gelder IC, Crijns HJ, Van Gilst WH, Verwer R, Lie KI. Prediction of uneventful cardioversion and maintenance of sinus rhythm from Direct-Current electrical cardioversion of chronic atrial fibrillation and flutter. Am J Cardiol 1991;68:41-46.

[7] DeSilva RA, Lown B. Cardioversion and defibrillation. Am Heart J 1980;100:881-895.
[8] Lown B, Neuman J. New method for terminating cardiac arrhythmias. JAMA 1962;182:548-555.
[9] Szekely P, Batson GA, Stark DCC. Direct current shock therapy of cardiac arrhythmias. Br Heart J 1966;28:366-373.
[10] Lown B. Electrical cardioversion of cardiac arrhythmias. Br Heart J 1967;29:469-487.
[11] Cramer G. Early and late results of conversion of atrial fibrillation with quinidine. Acta Med Scand 1968;490:1-102.
[12] Resnekov L, McDonald L. Appraisal of electroconversion in treatment of cardiac dysrhythmias. Br Heart J 1968;30:786-811.
[13] Bjerkelund C, Orning OM. The efficacy of anticoagulant therapy in preventing embolism related to DC electrical cardioversion of atrial fibrillation. Am J Cardiol 1969;23:209-215.
[14] Södermark T, Edhag O, Sjögren A, Jonsson B, Olsson A, Orö L, Danielsson M, Rosenhamer G, Wallin H. Effect of quinidine on maintaining sinus rhythm after conversion of atrial fibrillation or flutter. A multicenter study from Stockholm. Br Heart J 1975;37:486-492.
[15] Lundstrom T, Ryden L. Chronic atrial fibrillation. Long term results of direct current cardioversion. Acta Med Scand 1988;223:53-59.
[16] Petersen P, Godtfredsen J, Boysen G, Andersen ED, Andersen B. Placebo-controlled, randomized trial of warfarin and aspirin for prevention of thromboembolic complications in chronic atrial fibrillation. Lancet 1989;i:175-178.
[17] Brodsky MA, Allen BJ, Capparelli EV, Luckett CR, Morton R, Henry WL. Factors determining maintenance of sinus rhythm after chronic atrial fibrillation with left atrial dilatation. Am J Cardiol 1989;63:1065-1068.
[18] Juul-Möller S, Edvardsson N, Rehnquist-Ahlberg N. Sotalol versus quinidine for the maintenance of sinus rhythm after direct current conversion of atrial fibrillation. Circulation 1990;82:1932-1939.
[19] Braunwald E. Symposium on cardiac arrhythmias: introduction with comments on the hemodynamic significance of atrial systole. Am J Med 1964;37:665-669.
[20] Morris Jr JJ, Entman M, North WC, Kong Y, McIntosh H. The changes in cardiac output with reversion of atrial fibrillation to sinus rhythm. Circulation 1965;31:670-678.
[21] Wolf PA, Dawber TR, Thomas, Jr HE, Kannel WB. Epidemiologic assessment of chronic atrial fibrillation and risk of stroke: The Framingham study. Neurology 1978; 28:973-77.
[22] Wolf PA, Kannel WB, McGee DL, Meeks SL, Bharucha NE, McNamara PM. Duration of atrial fibrillation and imminence of stroke: The Framingham study. Stroke 1983;14:664-667.
[23] Petersen P, Kastrup J, Brinch K, Godtfredsen J, Boysen G. Relation between left atrial size and duration of atrial fibrillation. Am J Cardiol 1987;60:382-384.
[24] Sanfilippo AJ, Abascal VM, Sheehan M, Oertel LB, Harrigan P, Hughes RA, Weyman AE. Atrial enlargement as a consequence of atrial fibrillation. Circulation 1990;82:792-797.
[25] Teo KK, Harte M, Horgan JH. Sotalol infusion in the treatment of supraventricular tachyarrhythmias. Chest 1985;87:113-118.
[26] Crijns HJGM, Van Wijk LM, Van Gilst WH, Kingma JH, Van Gelder IC, Lie KI. Acute conversion of atrial fibrillation to sinus rhythm: clinical efficacy of flecainide acetate. Comparison of two regimens. Eur Heart J 1988;9:634-638.
[27] Suttorp MJ, Kingma HJ, Jessurun ER, Lie-A-Huen L, Van Hemel NM, Lie KI. The value of class IC antiarrhythmic drugs for acute conversion of paroxysmal atrial fibrillation or flutter to sinus rhythm. J Am Coll Cardiol 1990;16:1722-1727.
[28] Suttorp MJ, Polak PE, Van 't Hof A, Rasmussen HS, Lacante P, Dunselman PH, Kingma JH. Efficacy and safety of a new selective class III antiarrhythmic agent dofetilide in paroxysmal atrial fibrillation or atrial flutter. Am J Cardiol 1992;69:417-419.
[29] Di Marco JP. Cardioversion of atrial flutter by intravenous ibutilide, a new class III antiarrhythmic agent (abstr). J Am Col Cardiol 1991;17:324A.

[30] Lown B, Kleiger R, Williams J. Cardioversion and digitalis drugs: changed threshold to electric shock in digitalized animals. Circulation Research 1965;17:519-531.
[31] Rabbino MD, Likoff W, Dreifus LS. Complications and limitations of direct-currrent countershock. JAMA 1964;190:417-420.
[32] Åberg H, Cullhed I. Direct current countershock complications. Acta Med Scand 1968;183:415-421.
[33] Ditchey RV, Karliner JS. Safety of electrical cardioversion in patients without digitalis toxicity. Ann of Int Med 1981;95:676-679.
[34] Nakazawa HK, Handa S, Nakamura Y, Oyanagi H, Hasegawa M, Ishikawa N, Ozaki O, Ito K. High maintenance rate of sinus rhythm after cardioversion in post-thyrotoxic chronic atrial fibrillation. Int J Cardiol 1987;16:47-55.
[35] Dunn M, Alexander J, De Silva R, Hildner F. Antithrombotic therapy in atrial fibrillation. Chest 1989;95:118S-127S.
[36] Van Gelder IC. Management of chronic atrial fibrillation in the nineties. Thesis, University of Groningen, The Netherlands, 1991.
[37] Lipkin DP, Frenneaux M, Stewart R, Joshi J, Lowe T, McKenna WJ. Delayed improvement in exercise capacity after cardioversion of atrial fibrillation to sinus rhythm. Br Heart J 1988; 59:572-77.
[38] Manning WJ, Leeman DE, Gotch PJ, Come PC. Pulsed doppler evaluation of atrial mechanical function after electrical cardioversion of atrial fibrillation. J Am Coll Cardiol 1989;13:617-623.
[39] Edvardsson N, Olsson SB. Outpatient electroconversion of chronic atrial fibrillation. In: Kulbertus HE, Olsson SB, Schlepper M. Atrial fibrillation. Kiruna, Sweden. Mölndal: AB Hässle 1981:242-249.
[40] Lesser MF. Safety and efficacy of in-office cardioversion for treatment of supraventricular arrhythmias. Am J Cardiol 1990;66:1267-1268.
[41] Kerber RE, Jensen SR, Grayzel J, Kennedy J, Hoyt R. Elective cardioversion: influence of paddle-electrode location and size on success rates and energy requirements. N Engl J Med 1981;305:658-662.
[42] Crampton R. Accepted, controversial and speculative aspects of ventricular defibrillation. Progr in Cardiovasc Dis 1980;23:167-186.
[43] Dahl CF, Ewy GA, Warner ED, Thomas, ED. Myocardial necrosis from direct current countershock. Circulation 1974;50:956-961.
[44] Dalzell GWN, Cunningham SR, Anderson J, Adgey J. Electrode pad size, transthoracic impedance and success of external ventricular defibrillation. Am J Cardiol 1989;64:741-744.
[45] Kerber RE, Martins JB, Kienzle MG, Constantin L, Olshansky B, Hopson R, Charbonnier F. Energy, current and succes in defibrillation and cardioversion: clinical study using an automated impedance-based method of energy adjustment. Circulation 1988;77:1038-1046.
[46] Dittrich HC, Erickson JS, Schneiderman T, Blacky R, Savides T, Nicod PH. Echocardiographic and clinical predictors for outcome of elective cardioversion of atrial fibrillation. Am J Cardiol 1989;63:193-197.
[47] Van Gelder IC, Crijns HJGM, Van Gilst WH, De Langen CDJ, Van Wijk LM, Lie KI. Effects of flecainide on the atrial defibrillation threshold. Am J Cardiol 1989;63:112-114.
[48] Waris E, Kreus KE, Salokannel J. Factors influencing persistence of sinus rhythm after DC shock treatment of atrial fibrillation. Acta Med Scand 1971;189:161-166.
[49] Rossi M, Lown B. The use of quinidine in cardioversion. Am J Cardiol 1967;19:234-238.
[50] Echt DS, Black JN, Barbey JT, Robertson Coxe D, Cato E. Evaluation of antiarrhythmic drugs on defibrillation energy requirements in dogs. Circulation 1989;79:1106-1117.
[51] Selzer A, Wray HW. Quinidine syncope. Paroxysmal ventricular fibrillation occurring during treatment of chronic atrial arrhythmias. Circulation 1964;30:17-26.

[52] Crijns HJ, Van Gelder IC, Lie KI. Supraventricular tachycardia mimicking ventricular tachycardia during flecainide treatment. Am J Cardiol 1988;62:1303-1306.
[53] Falk RH. Flecainide-induced ventricular tachycardia and fibrillation in patients treated for atrial fibrillation. Ann Int Med 1989;111:107-111.
[54] Resnekov L, McDonald L. Complications in 220 patients with cardiac dysrhythmias treated by phased direct current shock and indications for electroconversion. Br Heart J 1967;29:926.
[55] Ehsani A, Ewy GA, Sobel BE. Effects of electrical countershock on serum creatinine phosphokinase isoenzyme activity. Am J Cardiol 1976;37:12-18.
[56] Tacker Jr. WA, Van Vleet JF, Geddes LA. Electrocardiopgraphic and serum enzymic alterations associated with cardiac alterations induced in dogs by single transthoracic damped sinusoidal defibrillator shocks of various strengths. Am Heart J 1979;98:185-193.
[57] Patton JN, Allen JD, Pantridge JF. The effects of shock energy, propanolol and verapamil on cardiac damage caused by transthoracic countershock. Circulation 1984;69:357-368.
[58] Van Gelder IC, Crijns HJ, Van Der Laarse A, Van Gilst WH, Lie KI. Incidence and clinical significance of ST segment elevation after electrical cardioversion of atrial fibrillation and atrial flutter. Am Heart J 1991;121:51-56.
[59] Doherty PW, McLaughlin PR, Billingham M, Kernoff R, Goris ML, Harrison DC. Cardiac damage produced by direct current counter shock applied to the heart. Am J Cardiol 1979;43:225-232.
[60] Metcalfe MJ, Smith F, Jennings K. Does cardioversion of atrial fibrillation result in myocardial damage? Br Med J 1988;296:1364-1365.
[61] Chun PKC, Davia JE, Donohue DJ. ST segment elevation with elective DC cardioversion. Circulation 1981;63:220-224.
[62] Zelinger AB, Falk RH, Hood WB. Electrical-induced sustained myocardial depolarization as a possible cause for transient ST elevation post-DC elective cardioversion. Am Heart J 1982;103:1073-1074.
[63] Gajewski J, Singer RB. Mortality in an insured population with atrial fibrillation. JAMA 1981;245:1540-1544.
[64] Ewy GA, Ulfers L, Hager D, Rosenfeld AR, Roeske WR, Goldman S. Response of atrial fibrillation to therapy: role of etiology and left atrial diameter. J Electrocardiol 1980;13:119-124.

Chapter 6

PHARMACOLOGICAL CARDIOVERSION OF

PAROXYSMAL ATRIAL FIBRILLATION OR

ATRIAL FLUTTER TO SINUS RHYTHM

Maarten J. Suttorp

Emile R. Jessurun

J. Herre Kingma

Department of Cardiology
St Antonius Hospital
Nieuwegein
The Netherlands

J. H. Kingma et al. (eds.), Atrial fibrillation, a treatable disease?, 87–103.

INTRODUCTION _____

Next to premature atrial and ventricular extrasystoles, atrial fibrillation and atrial flutter are probably the most frequently occurring arrhythmias in man. Atrial fibrillation, "the grandfather of cardiac arrhythmias", is prevalent in 0.4% of the general population and is estimated to effect 2% to 4% of adults >60 years of age. Depending on the degree of congestive heart failure the prevalence of atrial fibrillation in the cardiac population may rise to approximately 40%[1-3]. The prevalence of atrial flutter is estimated to be less than 0.1% in the general population. The paroxysmal form of atrial fibrillation seems present in up to 40% of the patients[4].

We define paroxysmal atrial fibrillation or atrial flutter as arrhythmias with sporadic, recurrent or frequent episodes of atrial fibrillation or atrial flutter that may last a few seconds to several months. However, this type of arrhythmia has to convert spontaneously or be restored to sinus rhythm by using pharmacological therapy or direct-current countershock. Furthermore, incessant paroxysmal atrial fibrillation or atrial flutter has been defined as frequent daily attacks covering more than 12 hours per day. Paroxysmal atrial fibrillation or atrial flutter should be subdivided into recent onset or long-standing atrial arrhythmias. Recent onset atrial fibrillation or atrial flutter is defined by our group as a rhythm disturbance lasting less than 24 hours, and as long-standing if the arrhythmia last more than 24 hours but less than six months[5].

Paroxysmal atrial fibrillation or atrial flutter can be considerably more disabling than the chronic form. These atrial arrhythmias can present themselves in various ways, requiring specific treatment according to the nature of its presentation, and if possible to correct the underlying disorder. In addition to the role of an electrophysiological substrate, these arrhythmias can also depend on either vagal or adrenergic stimulation of atrial myocardium by the autonomic nervous system[6]. Furthermore, atrial fibrillation, especially its chronic form, is frequently associated with an increased risk for development of thromboembolic events[7].

The initial treatment, directed at adequate control or regulation of ventricular rate during a paroxysm of atrial fibrillation or atrial flutter, can usually be achieved by various drugs like digoxin, verapamil, and ß-adrenergic blocking agents. However, one should be aware that this mode of therapy is often inappropriate, because of the possible long-term pathophysiologic consequences for patients with persisting atrial fibrillation or atrial flutter. Therefore, most patients deserve an attempt to restore sinus rhythm by using pharmacological or electrical cardioversion, or both. This can only be obtained safely after a careful stratification of the thromboembolic risk in the individual patient and when the underlying cause of the disease, if detectable, has been treated.

In this chapter, starting with a brief overview of the possible mechanisms of antiarrhythmic drug effects, we will review the various modes of pharmacological therapy for acute control of the ventricular rate and the immediate conversion of paroxysmal atrial fibrillation and atrial flutter to sinus rhythm.

POSSIBLE MECHANISMS OF ANTIARRHYTHMIC DRUG EFFECTS

Atrial fibrillation and atrial flutter are both considered to be based on some form of atrial reentry[8]. On the basis of the leading circle concept of atrial reentry it has been shown that, both theoretically and experimentally, prolongation of the wavelength, i.e. the product of conduction velocity and refractory period, leads to termination and prevention of atrial tachyarrhytmias by increasing the minimal circuit size[9-11]. According to this wavelength theory, either a critical increase in conduction velocity or refractory period, or both, seems necessary to terminate the reentrant circuit.

The precise electrophysiologic mechanisms by which the various antiarrhythmic agents exert their beneficial effects for conversion of atrial fibrillation or atrial flutter remains speculative. The effect of class IC antiarrhythmic agents for terminating or suppressing atrial fibrillation remains difficult to explain in comparison to class III antiarrhythmic drugs, which prolong the refractory period with less effect on conduction. Class IC antiarrhythmic agents primarily decrease conduction velocity and have a less pronounced effect on atrial refractoriness. Thus, the mechanism of block by a critical increase in wavelength does not seem to function, but possibly due to the loss of conduction and subsequent extinction of the wave fronts. Perhaps the rate-dependent decrease in conduction velocity by class I agents might explain this action [12]. However, the antifibrillatory effect of class IC agents might also be explained by prolongation of the wavelength by increasing the atrial refractory period at very short cycles[13].

The concept of a critical wavelength for reentrant tachyarrhythmias suggests that antiarrhythmic agents that shorten the wavelength should be regarded as potentially arrhythmogenic, while drugs that prolong the wavelength possess ideal antiarrhythmic properties. Furthermore, class I antiarrhythmic drugs, except perhaps propafenone (due to its weak ß-blocking properties), seem more effective if a vagal mechanism is predominant. In contrast, class II antiarrhythmic drugs seem more effective when an adrenergic mechanism is involved[14].

ACUTE PHARMACOLOGICAL INTERVENTION OF ATRIAL FIBRILLATION OR FLUTTER

Control of ventricular heart rate during atrial fibrillation or atrial flutter.

Control and regulation of ventricular response during atrial fibrillation or atrial flutter can be achieved pharmacologically. The ventricular rate can be reduced by using antiarrhythmic agents which can decrease atrioventricular conduction, thereby improve ventricular filling by increasing the diastolic filling period, resulting in an augmentation of stroke volume[15].

Currently, a variety of antiarrhythmic agents are used for this purpose such as: digoxin, calcium channel blockers, ß-adrenoceptor blocking agents, amiodarone, or a combination of these antiarrhythmic agents. However, class I antiarrhythmic agents are less suitable for control of ventricular heart rate, because of its potency to sustain or even facilitate atrioventricular conduction in certain circumstances, causing various adverse cardiac effects[16,17]. Quinidine and disopyramide may facilitate atrioventricular conduction by their anticholinergic effect. Some reports have shown that class IC antiarrhythmic drugs effect a decrease and regularization of the atrial rate making 1:1 atrioventricular conduction possible. Furthermore, if the ventricular response is sufficiently high a rate-dependent widening of the QRS complex can occur [17].

Digoxin. Digitalis glycosides have been in clinical use for over more than 200 years and are widely used for decreasing the rapid ventricular rate during atrial fibrillation. It is assumed that the vagotonic effect of digoxin is considered to play a predominant role in the ability to control heart rate in patients with atrial fibrillation or atrial flutter[18,19]. Conduction of the atrioventricular node is slowed. The prolongation of atrioventricular nodal refractoriness by digoxin is largely responsible for the slowed ventricular response at rest[18]. Furthermore, digitalis decreases atrial refractoriness.

Digoxin fails to control exercise-induced tachycardia in patients with atrial fibrillation or atrial flutter as it has little direct effect on atrioventricular nodal conduction[20,21]. However, up to now, digoxin has not shown any effect in converting atrial fibrillation to sinus rhythm[22]. One should be aware that if digitalization promotes restoration of sinus rhythm, it does so as result of slowing of the ventricular rate which leads to an overall hemodynamic improvement.

Calcium channel blockers. The calcium channel blockers verapamil and diltiazem increase refractoriness and prolong conduction time in the atrioventricular node. Therefore, these agents can effectively decrease ventricular rate in atrial fibrillation or atrial flutter both at rest and during exercise[23,24] and improve exercise performance[25]. However, intravenous verapamil may be more likely than diltiazem to cause or exacerbate heart failure due to a greater negative inotropic effect[26]. The addition of digoxin to calcium channel blocker therapy improves control of heart rate during exercise[27]. The effective conversion rate of atrial fibrillation or atrial flutter to sinus rhythm with verapamil is as high as 15%[28-31], however in a recent study from our group, we observed a conversion rate of only 6%[32]. This low conversion rate reflects only spontaneous conversion. Calcium antagonists may even impair conversion to sinus rhythm and prolong the duration of these arrhythmias [33,34]. It is conceivable, that there may be a critical shortening of atrial refractoriness which sustains atrial fibrillation due to reflex sympathetic activity mediated by the vasodilatory action of verapamil. However, despite the ineffectiveness for acute restoration of sinus rhythm, verapamil and perhaps diltiazem remains the standard therapy for acute control of the ventricular response during atrial fibrillation or atrial flutter, because of its specific and rapid onset of action[24,28,35].

ß-adrenoceptor blocking agents. In general, ß-adrenoceptor antagonists (ß-blockers) can be used to improve control of exercise-induced atrial fibrillation or atrial flutter[36,37]. Decreasing ventricular response is probably due to the direct depressant effect on conduction in the atrioventricular node. However, ß-blockers have negative inotropic effects and may precipitate heart failure in some patients. In addition, treatment with ß-blockers may be associated with a range of side effects, including cold extremities, fatigue, impotence, bronchospasm in patients with bronchial asthma and glucose intolerance in diabetic subjects. Certain central nervous symptoms are associated with the use of lipophilic ß-blockers[38]. Combination of the treatment with digoxin may be important to prevent the need for high doses of ß-blockers and thereby reducing the risk of adverse effects[37].

Sotalol. Sotalol, a relative new ß-adrenoceptor blocking agent with additional class III antiarrhythmic properties, acts by blocking ß-receptors as well as lengthening the action potential duration and the effective refractory period in atria, ventricle, atrioventricular node and bypass tracts[39]. In various studies both intravenous and oral sotalol showed a significant decrease of ventricular rate during atrial fibrillation or atrial flutter[40,41]. In postoperative studies performed by our group, the antiarrhythmic effect of both low- and high-dose sotalol was demonstrated by a significant decrease in mean heart rate during sinus rhythm[42,43]. Furthermore, the maximal heart rates during supraventricular tachyarrhythmia in patients treated with sotalol, were significantly lower than those in the group given a placebo[43].

Esmolol. Intravenous esmolol, an ultrashort-acting ß-blocker with an elimination half-life of 9.2 minutes, compares favorably with intravenous verapamil in the acute management of patients with atrial fibrillation or atrial flutter and a rapid ventricular rate. Platia and co-workers reported that 50% of esmolol-treated patients with recent onset atrial fibrillation converted to sinus rhythm. Reduction of blood pressure has been reported in 8% to 12% of patients receiving intravenous esmolol[31].

Amiodarone. In 1967, amiodarone, a benzofurane derivate, was first introduced as an anti-anginal drug because of its coronary and systemic vasodilatory properties and was later recognized as an effective class III anti-arrhythmic agent[44]. Amiodarone prolongs the action potential duration and slows conduction velocity[45]. This agent has a heart rate limiting action and will help to control the ventricular response during atrial fibrillation or atrial flutter. A major limitation to the use of amiodarone is its toxicity, which can affect many organ systems. During long-term administration this agent can cause a number of serious adverse effects, such as: pulmonary toxicity, hyper- and hypothyroidism, corneal microdeposits and photosensitivity. Most of these adverse effects are reversible upon dose reduction or discontinuation although one should be aware that the elimination of amiodarone from the body is very slow.

Pharmacological cardioversion of atrial fibrillation or atrial flutter to sinus rhythm.

Many therapeutic regimens aimed at establishing and maintaining sinus rhythm have been studied, including digoxin, calcium antagonists, quinidine, procainamide, disopyramide, flecainide, propafenone, various ß-blocking agents, amiodarone and just recently the experimental highly selective class III antiarrhythmic agent dofetilide (UK-68,798).

Previous reports have shown that both digoxin and calcium antagonists are not effective in this respect[22,46,47]. In fact, a combination of digoxin with verapamil has sometimes been used to attempt to perpetuate the patient into atrial fibrillation in cases of intractable paroxysmal atrial fibrillation[14].

Class IA antiarrhythmic agents.

Quinidine. Quinidine, a class IA antiarrhythmic agent, is the oldest and most widely used agent for early conversion of atrial fibrillation or atrial flutter to sinus rhythm. This agent decreases atrial conduction and enhances atrioventricular nodal conduction by its vagolytic action, but increases the action potential duration. Quinidine should be administrated orally at a dose of 0.5 to 2 g daily. For patients with atrial fibrillation the conversion rate varies between 40-80%, depending on underlying disease and duration of the arrhythmia[48]. However, adverse effects are observed in more than 20% of treated patients and frequently causes intolerable noncardiac (diarrhea, pyrexia, rash) and cardiac (e.g. torsades de pointes) adverse effects.

Procainamide. Intravenous procainamide, a class IA antiarrhythmic agent, appears to be an effective agent for rapidly converting paroxysmal atrial fibrillation to sinus rhythm. It slows conduction velocity and increases the action potential duration and thus the refractory period. Administration of procainamide at a rate of up to 30 mg/min (maximum dose 20 mg/kg body weight) is effective in 43% to 90% of patients for terminating atrial fibrillation, with an overall conversion success rate of 58%[49-51]. However, the small size of these studies precludes more definitive conclusions. The responders had a shorter mean duration of the atrial arrhythmia or normal left atrial dimensions, or both, as compared to the non-responders. In patients with uncompromised left ventricular function the infusion with procainamide was generally safe and well tolerated.

Disopyramide. Disopyramide phosphate, a class IA antiarrhythmic agent, seemed to be only moderately effective in converting atrial fibrillation or atrial flutter to sinus rhythm. The antiarrhythmic actions of disopyramide resemble those of quinidine and procainamide. Furthermore, disopyramide has anticholinergic effects. The reported conversion rate varies from 20 to 71% for patients with atrial fibrillation and 38% to 43% for patients with atrial flutter [52,53]. After coronary artery bypass graft operation intravenous disopyramide at a dose of 2 mg/kg body weight, followed by infusion or oral therapy, caused conversion of atrial arrhythmia to sinus rhythm in 48% of the patients within 12 hours, but at the expense of urinary retention in 11.5% and an alarming incidence (30%) of 1:1 conduction in atrial flutter[54]. Intravenous disopyramide proved to be a moderately effective agent for restoring sinus rhythm, but the occurrence of adverse effects related to its use, especially the anticholinergic effects, demands caution and even may preclude its wide spread use[53].

Class IC antiarrhythmic agents.

Flecainide. Flecainide acetate is a class IC antiarrhythmic agent currently used in the management of ventricular and supraventricular tachy-arrhythmias. It slows intracardiac conduction and prolongs the refractory period to a lesser degree[55-57].

Intravenous flecainide, at a dose of up to 2 mg/kg bodyweight administrated in 10 minutes, showed an overall efficacy for restoring sinus rhythm of between 65% to 90% in patients with paroxysmal atrial fibrillation [32,58]. In patients with atrial flutter the overall conversion rate varies between 0% and 40%[32,58]. Besides underlying heart disease, the successful conversion to sinus rhythm depends on the duration of the arrhythmia. If atrial fibrillation lasted ≤ 24 hours a conversion rate of up to 90% has been reported

(Table 1). However, in patients with paroxysmal atrial fibrillation lasting >24 hours the conversion rate for restoring sinus rhythm decreases and varies between 40% and 83%. Interestingly, conversion to sinus rhythm was achieved very rapidly in the majority of patients, and usually within 30 minutes[32,58]. As contrasted to class IA antiarrhythmic drugs, flecainide decreased ventricular response in patients whose arrhythmia was not converted. It has been noted that during flecainide infusion the QRS interval widens due to slowing of intraventricular conduction[58]. Atrial flutter cycle length showed an increase after flecainide infusion[58]. Mild transient adverse effects during and shortly

Table 1. **Rate of Conversion to Sinus Rhythm with Intravenous Flecainide Acetate**

		AF		AF <24 hrs		AFI	
Study		Pts (n)	SR (%)	Pts (n)	SR (%)	Pts (n)	SR (%)
Goy	1985	39	74	—	—	6	33
Borgeat	1986	30	67	—	—	—	—
Nathan	1987	10	90	—	—	10	20
Crozier	1987	25	76	25	76	10	40
Crijns	1988	20	65	13	77	—	—
Suttorp	1989	32	72	22	86	7	0
Suttorp	1990	20	90	14	93	5	20

AF = atrial fibrillation; AFI = atrial flutter; SR = sinus rhythm.

after flecainide infusion are frequently noted. These adverse effects are dizziness, paresthesia, dryness of mouth, short-lasting hypotension and transient conduction disturbances[32,58].

In conclusion, intravenous administration of flecainide is highly effective and very useful for immediate conversion of paroxysmal atrial fibrillation but exerts almost no effect for acute conversion of atrial flutter. However, pharmacological conversion with flecainide should be used in patients with uncompromised left ventricular function and only during close electrocardio-graphic cardiographic monitoring, because of its transient effects on cardiac conduction.

Propafenone. Propafenone hydrochloride has been classified as a class IC antiarrhythmic agent with weak beta-adrenoceptor antagonist activity [62]. It primarily slows intra-atrial and atrioventricular node conduction[63]. Clinically, no substantial increase in atrial refractoriness has been observed.

Propafenone hydrochloride, administrated intravenously at a dose of up to 2 mg/kg bodyweight in 10 minutes, showed an overall conversion rate of between 9% and 62% in patients with paroxysmal atrial fibrillation. Recent studies have demonstrated that intravenous propafenone is potentially effective with only mild side effects, in terminating paroxysmal atrial fibrillation and in controlling ventricular response during atrial fibrillation or atrial flutter[64-66]. Propafenone seems less effective for restoration of sinus rhythm in patients with atrial flutter with an overall success rate reported of only 33% and 40% [58]. The success rate for conversion depends on the duration of the arrhythmia as shown in Table 2. Intravenous propafenone achieved successful cardioversion to sinus rhythm in 50% to 71% if atrial fibrillation lasted less than 48 hours, but only 26% to 50% of those with longstanding atrial fibrillation. Conversion to sinus rhythm was achieved in most of the patients within 30 minutes after starting the propafenone infusion[58].

Table 2. **Rate of Conversion to Sinus Rhythm with Intravenous Propafenone Hydrochloride.**

		AF		AF < 48 hrs		AFI	
Study		Pts (n)	SR (%)	Pts (n)	SR (%)	Pts (n)	SR (%)
Connolly	1987	12	50	12	50	2	0
Vita	1989	23	9	5	?	–	–
Bianconi	1989	68	62	56	71	15	33
Suttorp	1990	20	55	14	57	5	40

AF = atrial fibrillation; AFI = atrial flutter; SR = sinus rhythm;
? = unknown.

Contrary to class IA antiarrhythmic agents, propafenone decreases the ventricular rate before conversion and in refractory patients[58]. In patients with atrial flutter, a significant slowing of the atrial flutter rate has been observed. A remarkably low incidence of adverse effects is reported during and after infusion of propafenone at a dose of 2 mg/kg body weight in 10 minutes, especially in patients with an uncompromised left ventricular function [58]. Furthermore, the plasma levels at 20 minutes after start of the infusion with propafenone in patients with conversion to sinus rhythm were almost twice as high as the plasma levels of the patients without arrhythmia conversion. This suggests that either a higher dosage or a faster rate of administration that leads to sufficiently high tissue levels is probably necessary for greater efficacy.

Thus, propafenone is a moderate effective agent for conversion of recent onset atrial fibrillation to sinus rhythm with almost no adverse effects, but is less effective for converting atrial flutter. Its use seems to be safe, except in patients with severe congestive heart failure.

Class II antiarrhythmic agents.

Esmolol. Intravenous esmolol is a relative new ß-blocking agent with an ultra-short duration of action. At a dose ranging from 8 to 16 mg/minute, 50% of patients with recent onset atrial fibrillation or atrial flutter converted to sinus rhythm[31]. Conversion to sinus rhythm occurred at a mean time of 29 minutes. One advantage of this short-acting titratable drug, is the facility with which drug effects can be controlled, especially in a critical care setting. The mechanism of conversion remains unknown. It could be explained, by a significant slowing of the ventricular heart rate and thereby leading to an overall hemodynamic improvement which facilitates conversion to sinus rhythm. In addition, the depression of high adrenergic states by esmolol could also be of influence in restoring sinus rhythm. Only a few adverse effects were noted, such as hypotension that immediately disappears after discontinuation of the esmolol infusion.

Sotalol. The efficacy and safety of this class II antiarrhythmic drug with additional class III properties will be discussed below.

Class III antiarrhythmic agents.

Amiodarone. This class III antiarrhythmic agent, at an intravenous dose of up to 7.5 mg/kg body weight in 30 minutes, is reported to achieve rapid conversion of paroxysmal atrial fibrillation or atrial flutter to sinus rhythm in between 48 to 81% of the patients with a relative lack of acute toxicity in contrast to its long term usage[67-69]. Amiodarone has a rate limiting action and will help to control the ventricular rate even if atrial fibrillation or atrial flutter persists. Intravenous amiodarone can depress left ventricular function and therefore should be used with caution in patients with cardiac failure.

Sotalol. Sotalol, a relative new ß-blocking agent with additional class III antiarrhythmic properties, appears to be effective in suppressing both supraventricular and ventricular arrhythmias[39].

Intravenous sotalol, as a bolus of up to 1.5 mg/kg body weight, has been found moderately effective for conversion of atrial fibrillation or atrial flutter to sinus rhythm. Sotalol may achieve restoration of sinus rhythm in between 25 and 60% of the patients with paroxysmal atrial fibrillation[40,41]. However, none of the patients with atrial flutter reverted to sinus rhythm. The mean ventricular rate decreased in all of the patients. However, it should be emphasized that the sotalol dosages used and the small number of patients preclude definite conclusions.

Dofetilide. Dofetilide (UK-68,798) is a new highly selective class III antiarrhythmic agent that has undergone extensive preclinical evaluation[70]. Dofetilide selectively prolongs refractoriness by blocking the potassium outward channels without any effects on conduction[71].

In a recent dose-ranging study, dofetilide showed an overall efficacy rate of 53% for converting atrial fibrillation to sinus rhythm, whereas the overall conversion rate in patients with atrial flutter was as high as 80%[72]. Interestingly, 71% of all the patients had longstanding atrial fibrillation or flutter (Table 3).

The QTc intervals showed a significant increase after infusion of dofetilide, representing an increase in the refractory period. No significant QRS widening was noted, indicating that the drug does not influence cardiac conduction. Furthermore, blood pressure also remained stable and not a single adverse experience was noted in these patients. In conclusion, dofetilide seems an effective and well-tolerated new antiarrhythmic agent for converting paroxysmal atrial fibrillation or atrial flutter. In particular, its successful outcome in usually drug resistant atrial flutter, frequently requiring direct-current cardioversion, is very promising and underscores the importance of selective class III antiarrhythmic action for the termination of reentry tachycardias.

Table 3. **Rate of Conversion to Sinus Rhythm with Intravenous Dofetilide**

	AF (%)	AFI (%)
Dose		
Low-dose group	3/ 6[*]	1/ 2[*]
High-dose group/15 min	3/ 6	2/ 2
High-dose group/10 min	4/ 7	1/ 1
All treated patients	10/19 (53)	4/5 (80)
Duration of arrhythmia		
≤24 hours	4/ 6[#]	0/ 1[#]
>24 hours	6/13	4/ 4

[*] difference not significant compared with high-dose groups,
[#] difference not significant compared with >24 hours.
   AF = atrial fibrillation; AFI = atrial flutter.

CONCLUSIONS

Atrial fibrillation and atrial flutter remains the most common sustained arrhythmias in man and constitute a clinical problem for almost every practising physician at some point of time. Better understanding of the mechanisms involved in the occurrence and termination of the arrhythmia has opened new therapeutic approaches. Nowadays it seems of paramount importance to start antiarrhythmic treatment as soon as possible for appropriate control of heart rate and to restore sinus rhythm, with the expectation to reduce the risk of various complications, such as tachycardia-induced cardiomyopathy, increasing left atrial size and systemic thromboembolism.

During the last decade a major leap forward has been made in the approach to these atrial arrhythmias, such as the development and use of new class IC antiarrhythmic agents flecainide and propafenone, the class III and ß-blocking agent sotalol, but also very selective class III agents like dofetilide. At present, there is increasing evidence that class IC antiarrhythmic agents, especially flecainide when used intravenously, are extremely effective for acute conversion of paroxysmal atrial fibrillation to sinus rhythm. However, one should use these class IC antiarrhythmic drugs cautiously and only during close ECG monitoring, because of its transient adverse effects on cardiac conduction. Further insights into alternative antiarrhythmic therapy, such as direct-current and radio-frequency ablation techniques, modern pacing devices and also new promising surgical procedures (Corridor and Maze operation) will refine management even further. These new prospects may have important implications for the practising physician. In future, the new generation of class III antiarrhythmic drugs, with very few adverse effects, may prove able to convert atrial flutter rapidly to sinus rhythm. The historical use of the two oldest and most popular cardiac drugs for the acute management of paroxysmal atrial fibrillation or atrial flutter, digitalis and quinidine, seem to have passed their prime.

References

[1]   Ostrander LD, Brandt RL, Kjelsberg MO, Epstein FH. Electrocardiographic findings among the adult population of a total natural community. Tecumseh, Michigan. Circulation 1965;31:888-897.

[2]   Selzer A. Atrial fibrillation revisited. N Engl J Med 1982;306:1044-1045.

[3]   Godtfredsen J. Atrial fibrillation. Etiology, course, and prognosis: a follow-up study of 1212 cases. Copenhagen, Munksgaard, 1975.

[4]   Takahashi N, Seki A, Imataka K, Fujh J. Clinical features of paroxysmal atrial fibrillation. An observation of 94 patients. Jpn Heart J 1981;22:143-149.

[5]   Suttorp MJ. Paroxysmal atrial fibrillation and atrial flutter: current concepts and new strategies. Thesis. University of Groningen, The Netherlands, 1992.

[6]   Coumel P. Atrial fibrillation. In: Tachycardias. Surawicz B, Pratap Reddy C and Prystowsky EN (eds), Boston, Martinus Nijhoff, 1984:231-244.

[7]   Stroke Prevention in Atrial Fibrillation Study Group Investigators. Preliminary report of the stroke prevention in atrial fibrillation study. N Engl J Med 1990;322:863-868.

[8]   Waldo AL. Mechanisms of atrial fibrillation, atrial flutter, and ectopic atrial tachycardia: a brief review. Circulation 1987;75(Supp III):37-40.

[9]   Allessie MA, Bonke FIM, Schopman FJG. Circus movement in rabbit atrial muscle as a mechanism of tachycardia. III. The "leading circle" concept: A new model of circus movement in cardiac tissue without the involvement of an anatomic obstacle. Circ Res 1977;41:9-18.

[10]   Smeets JLRM, Allessie MA, Lammers WJEP, Bonke FIM, Hollen J. The wavelength of the cardiac impulse and reentrant arrhythmias in isolated rabbit atrium. Circ Res 1986;58:96-108.

[11]   Rensma PL, Allessie MA, Lammers WJEP, Bonke FIM, Schalij MJ. The length of the excitation wave as an index for the susceptibility to reentrant atrial arrhythmias. Circ Res 1988;62:395-410.

[12]   Buchanan JW Jr, Saito T, Gettes LS. The effects of antiarrhythmic drugs, stimulation

frequency, and potassium-induced resting membrane potential changes on conduction velocity and dV/dt_{max} in guinea pig myocardium. Circ Res 1985;56:696-703.

[13]   Janse MJ, Wilms-Schopman F, Opthof T. Mechanism of antifibrillatory action of org 7797 in regionally ischemic pig heart. J Cardiovasc Pharmacol 1990;15:633-643.

[14]   Coumel P. Clinical approach to paroxysmal atrial fibrillation. Clin Cardiol 1990;13:209-212.

[15]   Rawles JM. What is meant by a "controlled" ventricular rate in atrial fibrillation? Br Med J 1990;63:157-161.

[16]   Falk RH. Flecainide-induced ventricular tachycardia and fibrillation in patients treated for atrial fibrillation. Ann Int Med 1989;111:107-111.

[17]   Marcus FL. The hazards of using type IC antiarrhythmic drugs for the treatment of paroxysmal atrial fibrillation. Am J Cardiol 1990;66:366-367.

[18]   Rosen MR, Wit AL, Hoffman BF. Electrophysiologic and pharmocology of cardiac arrhythmias. IV. Cardiac antiarrhythmic and toxic effects of digitalis. Am Heart J 1975;89:391-399.

[19]   Klein HO, Kaplinski E. Digitalis and verapamil in atrial fibrillation and flutter. Drugs 1986;31:185-197.

[20]   Beasly R, Smith DA, McHaffie DJ. Exercise heart rates at different serum digoxin concentrations in patients with atrial fibrillation. Be Med J 1985;290:9-11.

[21]   Lewis R, Lakhani M, Moreland TA, McDevitt DG. A comparison of verapamil and digoxin in the treatment of atrial fibrillation. Eur Heart J 1987;8:148-153.

[22]   Falk RH, Knowlton AA, Bernard SA, Gotlieb NE, Battinelli RN. Digoxin for converting recent-onset atrial fibrillation to sinus rhythm. Ann Int Med 1987;106:503-506.

[23]   Klein HO, Pauzner H, Di Segni E, David D, Kaplinsky E. The beneficial effects of verapamil in chronic effects of verapamil in chronic atrial fibrillation. Arch Intern Med 1979;139:747-749.

[24]   Ellenbogen KA, Dias VC, Plumb VJ, Heywood JT, Mirvis DM. A placebo-controlled trial of continuous intravenous diltiazem infusion for 24-hour heart rate control during atrial fibrillation and atrial flutter: A multicenter study. J Am Coll Cardiol 1991;18:891-897.

[25]   Lundström T, Rydèn L. Ventricular rate control and exercise performance in chronic atrial fibrillation: Effects of diltiazem and verapamil. J Am Coll Cardiol 1990;16:86-90.

[26]   Böhm M, Schwinger RHG, Erdmann E. Different cardiodepressant potency of various calcium channel antagonists in human myocardium. Am J Cardiol 1990;1039-1041.

[27]   Roth A, Harrison E, Mitani G, Cohen J, Rahimtoola SH, Elkayam U. Efficacy and safety of medium- and high-dose diltiazem alone and in combination with digoxin for control of heart rate at rest and during exercise in patients with chronic atrial fibrillation. Circulation 1986;73:316-324.

[28]   Waxman HL, Myerburg RJ, Appel R, Sung RJ. Verapamil for control of ventricular rate in paroxysmal supraventricular tachycardia and atrial fibrillation and atrial flutter. Ann Intern Med 1981;94:1-6.

[29]   Singh BN, Nademanee K, Baky SH. Calcium antagonists, clinical use in the treatment of arrhytmias. Drugs 1983;25:125-153.

[30]   Schwartz JB. Verapamil in atrial fibrillation: The expected, the unexpected, and the unknown. Am Heart J 1983;106:173-176.

[31]   Platia EV, Michelson EL, Porterfield JK, Das G. Esmolol versus verapamil in the acute treatment of atrial fibrillation or atrial flutter. Am J Cardiol 1989;63:925-929.

[32]   Suttorp MJ, Kingma JH, Lie-A-Huen L, Mast EG. Intravenous flecainide versus verapamil for acute conversion of paroxysmal atrial fibrillation or flutter to sinus rhythm. Am J Cardiol 1989;63:693-696.

[33]   Shenasa M, Kus T, Fromer M, LeBlanc RA, Dubuc M, Nadeau R. Effect of intravenous and oral calcium antagonists (diltiazem and verapamil) on sustenance of atrial fibril-

lation. Am J Cardiol 1988;62:403-407.

[34] Falk RH, Knowlton AA, Manaker S. Verapamil-induced atrial fibrillation. N Engl J Med 1988;318:640-641.

[35] Zipes DP. Management of cardiac arrhythmias. In: Braunwald E, ed. Heart Disease: a Textbook of Cardiovascular Medicin. Philadelphia: WB Saunders, 1988:665-669.

[36] Yahalom J, Klein HO, Kaplinsky E. Beta-adrenergic blockade as adjunctive oral therapy in patients with chronic atrial fibrillation. Chest 1977;71:592-596.

[37] David D, Di Segni E, Klein HO, Kaplinsky E. Inefficacy of digitalis in the control of heart rate in patients with chronic atrial fibrillation: Beneficial effect of an added beta adrenergic blocking agent. Am J Cardiol 1979;44:1378-1382.

[38] Lewis RV, McDevitt DG. Adverse reactions and interactions with beta-adrenoceptor blocking drugs. Medical Toxicology 1986;1:343-361.

[39] Singh BN, Phil D. Sotalol: A beta blocker with unique antiarrhytmic properties. Am Heart J 1987;114:121-139.

[40] Fogelman F, Lightman SL, Sillett RW, McNicol MW. The treatment of cardiac arrhythmias with sotalol. Eur J Clin Pharmacol 1972;5:72-76.

[41] Prakash R, Parmley WW, Allen HN, Matloff JM. Effect of sotalol on clinical arrhythmias. Am J Cardiol 1972;29:379-400.

[42] Suttorp MJ, Kingma JH, Tjon Joe Gin RM, van Hemel NM, Koomen EM, Defauw JAM, Adan JM, Ernst JMPG. Efficacy and safety of low- and high-dose sotalol versus propranolol in the prevention of supraventricular tachyarrhythmias early after coronary artery bypass operations. J Thorac Cardiovasc Surg 1990;100:921-926.

[43] Suttorp MJ, Kingma JH, Peels JOJ, Koomen EM, Tijssen JGP, van Hemel NM, Defauw JAM, Ernst JMPG. Effectiviness of sotalol in preventing supraventricular tachyarrhythmias shortly after coronary artery bypass grafting. Am J Cardiol 1991;68:1163-1169.

[44] Charlier R, Deltour G, Baudine A, Chaillet F. Pharmacology of amiodarone, an antianginal drug with a new biological profile. Arzneim Forsch 1968;18:1408-1417.

[45] Rosenbaum MB, Chiale PA, Halpern MS, Nau GJ, Przybylski J, Levi RJ, Lazzari JO, Elizari MV. Clinical efficacy of amiodarone as an antiarrhythmic agent. Am J cardiol 1976;38:934-944.

[46] Salerno DM, Dias VC, Kleiger RE, Tschida VH, Sung RJ, Sami M, Giorgi LV, for the Diltiazem-Atrial Fibrillation/Flutter Study Group. Am J Cardiol 1989;63:1046-1051.

[47] Schamroth L, Krikler DM, Garrett C. Immediate effects of intravenous verapamil in cardiac arrhythmias. Br Med J 1972;1:660-662.

[48] Borgeat A, Goy JJ, Meandly R, Kaufmann U, Grbic M, Sigwart U. Flecal-nide versus quinidine for cardioversion of atrial fibrillation to sinus rhythm. Am J Cardiol 1986;58:496-498.

[49] Kayden HJ, Brodie BB, Steele JM. Procaine amide. Circulation 1957;15:118-126.

[50] Halpern SW, Ellrodt G, Singh BN, Mandel WJ. Efficacy of intravenous procainamide infusion in converting atrial fibrillation to sinus rhythm: relation to left atrial size. Br heart J 1980;44:589-595.

[51] Fenster PE, Comess KA, Marsh R, Katzenburg C, Hager WD. Conversion of atrial fibrillation to sinus rhythm by acute intravenous procainamide infusion. Am Heart J 1983;106:501-504.

[52] Deano DA, Wu D, Mautner RK, Sherman RH, Ehsani AE, Rosen KM. Antiarrhythmic efficacy of intravenous therapy with disopyramide phosphate. Chest 1977;71:597-606.

[53] Camm J, Ward D, Spurrell RAJ. The effect of intravenous disopyramide phosphate on recurrent paroxysmal tachycardias. Br J Clin Pharm 1979;8:441-449.

[54] Gavaghan TP, Feneley MP, Campbell TJ, Morgan JJ. Atrial tachyarrhythmias after cardiac surgery: results of disopyramide therapy. Aust NZ J Med 1985;15:27-32.

[55] Roden DM, Woosley RL. Drug therapy, flecainide. N Engl J Med 1986;315:36-41.

[56] Hellestrand KJ, Bexton RS, Nathan AW, Spurrell RAJ, Camm AJ. Acute electrophysiological effects of flecainide acetate on cardiac conduction and refractoriness in man. Br Heart J 1982;48:140-148.

[57] Nathan AW, Camm AJ, Bexton RS, Hellestrand KJ. Intravenous flecainide acetate acetate for the clinical management of paroxysmal tachycardias. Clin Cardiol 1987;10: 317-322.

[58] Suttorp MJ, Kingma JH, Jessurun ER, Lie-A-Huen L, van Hemel NM, Lie KI. The value of class IC antiarrhythmic drugs for acute conversion of paroxysmal atrial fibrillation or flutter to sinus rhythm. J Am Coll Cardiol 1990;16:1722-1727.

[59] Goy JJ, Grbic M, Hurni M, Finci L, Sigwart U. Cardioversion with flecainide in patients with atrial fibrillation of recent onset. Eur J Clin Pharmacol 1985;27:737-738.

[60] Crozier IG, Ikram H, Kenealy M, Levy L. Flecainide acetate for conversion of acute supraventricular tachycardia to sinus rhythm. Am J Cardiol 1987;59:607-609.

[61] Crijns HJGM, Wijk LM, Gilst WH, Kingma JH, Gelder IC, Lie KI. Acute conversion of atrial fibrillation to sinus rhythm: Clinical efficacy of flecainide acetate. Eur Heart J 1988;9:634-638.

[62] Harron DWG, Brogden RN. Propafenone: A review of its pharmacodynamic and pharmacokinetic properties, and therapeutic use in the treatment of arrhytmias. Drugs 1987;34:617-647.

[63] Dukes ID, Vaughan Williams EM, The multiple modes of action of propafenone. Eur Heart J 1984;5:115-125.

[64] Connolly SJ, Mulji AS, Hoffert DL, Davis C, Shragge BW. Randomized placebo-controlled trial of propafenone for treatment of atrial tachyarrhythmias after cardiac surgery. J Am Coll Cardiol 1987;10:1145-1148.

[65] Vita JA, Friedman PL, Cantillon C, Antman EM. Efficacy of intravenous propafenone for the acute management of atrial fibrillation. Am J Cardiol 1989;63:1275-1278.

[66] Bianconi L, Boccadamo R, Pappalardo A, Gentili C, Pistolese M. Effectiveness of intravenous propafenone for conversion of atrial fibrillation and flutter of recent onset. Am J Cardiol 1989;64:335-338.

[67] Benaim R, Uzan C. Les effects antiarythmiques de l'amiodarone injectable. Rev Med 1978;19:1959-1963.

[68] Faniel R, Schoenfeld Ph. Efficacy of i.v. amiodarone in converting rapid atrial fibrillation and flutter to sinus rhythm in intensive care patients. Eur Heart J 1983;4:180-185.

[69] Strasberg B, Arditti A, Sclarovsky S, Lewin R, Buimovici B, Agmon J. Efficacy of intravenous amiodarone in the management of paroxysmal or new atrial fibrillation with fast ventricular response. Int J Cardiol 1985;7:47-55.

[70] Gemmill JD, Howie CA, Meredith PA, Hillis WS, Rasmussen HS, Elliot HL. A dose-ranging study of UK-68-798, a novel class III antiarrhythmic agent in normal volunteers. Br J Clin Pharmacol 1991;32:429-432.

[71] Sedgewick M, Rasmussen HS, Walker DK, Cobbe SM. Pharmacokinetic and pharmocodynamic effects of UK-68-798, a new class III antiarrhythmic drug. Br J Clin Pharmacol 1991;31:515-519.

[72] Suttorp MJ, Polak PE, van 't Hof A, Rasmussen HS, Dunselman PH, Kingma JH. Efficacy and safety of a new selective class III antiarrhythmic agent dofetilide in paroxysmal atrial fibrillation or atrial flutter. Am J Cardiol 1992;69:417-419.

Chapter 7

DRUGS AFTER CARDIOVERSION TO PREVENT RELAPSES

OF CHRONIC ATRIAL FIBRILLATION OR FLUTTER

Harry J.G.M. Crijns

A.T. Marcel Gosselink

Isabelle C. van Gelder

Ans C.P. Wiesfeld

Maarten P. van den Berg

Ype S. Tuininga

Kong I. Lie

Department of Cardiology
Thoraxcenter
University Hospital Groningen
The Netherlands

J. H. Kingma et al. (eds.), Atrial fibrillation, a treatable disease?, 105–148.
© 1992 *Kluwer Academic Publishers.*

INTRODUCTION _____

Electrical cardioversion is the method of choice to restore sinus rhythm in patients with *chronic* atrial fibrillation or flutter. After this intervention, maintenance of sinus rhythm is a challenge to the clinician, since these arrhythmias have a high tendency to recur[1,2]. In addition, arrhythmic and hemodynamic complications associated with a recurrence, hazards of prophylactic drug therapy and risk of postcardioversion stroke are among the problems threatening these patients. This chapter deals with the pharmacologic treatment modalities in the prevention of recurrences of chronic atrial fibrillation and flutter. Prevention of thromboembolism is discussed elsewhere in this book.

WHY PROPHYLACTIC TREATMENT
AFTER CARDIOVERSION? _____

The most important reasons to convert atrial fibrillation and maintain sinus rhythm thereafter, are elimination of palpitations, fatigue, dyspnea or syncope, and prevention of left ventricular dysfunction. Atrial fibrillation or flutter have significant hemodynamic consequences. After onset of the arrhythmia loss of atrial systole, inadequate rate response with decreased filling time and reduction of stroke volume all contribute to the acute changes. Of even more importance are the long term hemodynamic effects of chronic arrhythmia, i.e. the development of an intrinsic *tachycardia related* cardiomyopathy. In this respect, reduction of the ventricular rate, especially during exercise, is a first prerequisite. However, rate control using digitalis, calcium-antagonists or ß-blockers, instituted to maintain an adequate rate response especially during exertion, does not readily improve exercise tolerance[3]. Several studies have shown long term improvement of exercise capacity after cardioversion[4-6], which was not reached with adequate rate control during atrial fibrillation (unpublished data).

It is well known that survival decreases after onset of chronic atrial fibrillation[7,8]. However, the impact of chronic prophylactic therapy on survival, after restoration of sinus rhythm, is less well known. Recently it appeared that patients on quinidine treatment[9] had an excess death rate compared to those on control treatment. In that metanalysis the duration of follow-up of the trials evaluated was 6 months at the most. For now it cannot be told if very long term (i.e. years, decades) maintenance of sinus rhythm, whether or not maintained with drugs, has a positive effect on survival. The same holds for the risk of thromboembolism after sinus rhythm has been reestablished. Most patients keeping sinus rhythm will stop oral anticoagulation. However, the risk for thromboembolism remains, since a recurrence may occur unexpectedly. Therefore it seems a rational approach, to maintain oral anticoagulation, not only in patients with an increased risk of thromboembolism for reasons other than atrial fibrillation, but also in the group with an expected high recurrence rate especially early after cardioversion.

PAROXYSMAL OR CHRONIC ATRIAL FIBRILLATION? _____

Determination of the value of antiarrhythmic drugs in atrial fibrillation from the literature, is hampered by the circumstance that in many trials both paroxysmal and chronic atrial fibrillation were studied at the same time[10-15]. One advantage of presenting mixed groups is the fact that 'large' numbers can be shown and conclusions toward general antiarrhythmic efficacy may be more valid. It also enables a direct comparison between episodic and persistent arrhythmia. However, paroxysmal is different from chronic not only by definition, but also the substrate, arrhythmogenic mechanisms and arrhythmogenicity differ profoundly and thus antiarrhythmic effects of drugs vary between these 2 *distinct* disease entities. If this distinction is not made, a rational approach towards the patient with atrial fibrillation is not possible. In the present chapter *only* chronic atrial fibrillation will be discussed.

DEFINITION OF CHRONIC ARRHYTHMIA _____

In clinical practice differentiation between chronic and paroxysmal atrial fibrillation is difficult. For practical purposes chronic atrial fibrillation or flutter may be defined as lasting *at least 24 hours*. In addition, sequential electrocardiograms should show the arrhythmia. This definition is based on clinical practice, since mostly Holter monitoring is the only readily available tool to document the continuous nature of the arrhythmia. It is especially valuable if adrenergic dependence (e.g. 'white coat' fibrillation) is suspected[16]. Obviously, this type of arrhythmia would lead to the diagnosis chronic atrial fibrillation and particularly these patients may appear intractable with frequent recurrences despite repeated electrical cardioversions.

RECURRENCE RATE WITH OR WITHOUT PROPHYLACTIC ANTIARRHYTHMIC TREATMENT

If left untreated atrial fibrillation relapses frequently after cardioversion [1,2], with a rate varying between 44 and 86% (Tables 1 and 2). However, with treatment recurrence rates are also high (Tables 1 and 2): 17 to 89%. Patients prone to recurrences have a long previous arrhythmia duration[1,2,12,14,17-19] or a long total arrhythmia history[20]. In addition, large left atrial size [14,21-26], high age[2,17,20] and specific cardiac diseases[20,27,28] may portend a negative arrhythmia prognosis. 'Lone' atrial fibrillation has also been associated with intractability[7,18,19,21,29] but occasionally with a favourable arrhythmia outcome[30]. In one study there was no difference in outcome between patients with or without underlying disease[31]. The discrepancies between these studies may reflect differences in characterization of 'lone' arrhythmia, possibly depending on the diagnostic effort put into identifying a specific underlying cause[31]. As positive clinical factors, atrial flutter, as opposed to atrial fibrillation[31], and a low NYHA class for exercise tolerance [14,17,32,31], have been demonstrated to predict preservation of sinus rhythm.

The relapse rate after cardioversion depends heavily on the degree of arrhythmia intractability. It must be noted that in most of the above mentioned studies intractability was determined on the basis of *pre-inclusion* data, obviously a retrospective method. This may have given a rather extensive and unknown selection bias. In a few recent studies intractability was determined during the course of the investigation[20,33,34]. In these studies a serial drug treatment approach was followed and thereby eventual determination of intractability of atrial fibrillation was possible on a prospective basis. It is conceivable that such a method may give an optimal insight into intractability which may not be gathered from a single cardioversion, single drug study.

POSTCARDIOVERSION ANTIARRHYTHMIC
DRUG STUDIES _____

Antiarrhythmic drug treatment is considered to improve arrhythmia outcome compared to control medication or no drug therapy (Tables 1 and 2). Unfortunately many studies on the value of prophylactic treatment have been inadequate: too few patients, uncontrolled therapy, or too short duration of follow-up. In addition, complications are not reported or only summarily presented.

Tables 1 and 2 show predominantly controlled trials, or trials in which 2 antiarrhythmics were compared. These studies have yielded varying results with respect to statistical and clinical significance of drug effects. Outcomes were different among studies depending on number of patients studied, dosage of the drug, underlying heart disease (easy-to-treat versus intractable) and the duration of follow-up. In addition, number of previous cardioversions and preventive drug trials (not shown) varied among investigations.

Trials showing a significant difference between quinidine and control treatment (Table 1) studied more patients than those not showing statistically significant results. With respect to previous duration of atrial fibrillation and the patient's age, there are no large differences, but the data are incompletely reported or presented differently from one study to the other. Concerning the underlying heart diseases, comparisons between studies are even more difficult. It appears as if the 'negative' trials studied more patients with valvular heart disease (studies 6,8,10), or, if only few valvular patients were included, the percentage of patients with hypertension was relatively high (studies 7,9).

An overall estimate of the patient's intractability in the different studies cannot be given from the data presented in the literature, since clinical characteristics considered to relate to intractability are not stated uniformly in each separate study. However, from a comparison of the earlier with the later studies (especially those on amiodarone), it may be inferred that the medically intractable patient is characterized by a high number of previous cardioversions and preventive drug trials.

Quinidine.   Quinidine has been studied most in the prophylaxis of recurrent atrial fibrillation. Of the 11 trials listed in Table 1, 5 showed a significant difference in favour of quinidine, whereas in the others quinidine was not

Table 1. Clinical controlled trials on *quinidine* prophylaxis of atrial fibrillation after electrical cardioversion. Only studies in which a control study group was incorporated were chosen. Studies presented in order of statistical significance and duration of follow-up. Atrial fibrillation duration represents the mean arrhythmia duration (if available) or the maximal arrhythmia duration allowed before inclusion. Concerning underlying heart disease only the large subgroups are given. (Modified after RWF Campbell [131])

Report (1st author)		Study	Year	Pts (n)	Duration AF (mnth)	Age (yr) (mean)	Underlying Heart Disease (%)			
							CAD	VHD	SH	lone
Hillestad	[132]	1	1971	100	< 24	54	10	69	–	8
Södermark	[133]	2	1975	176	< 36	58	35	27	9	8
Byrne-Q.	[134]	3	1970	92	<120	54	16#	56	#	20
Härtel	[135]	4	1970	175	NA	NA	24	38	0.5	14
Boissel	[136]	5	1981	212	NA	NA	1	64	3	18
Gunning	[137]	6	1970	85	< 24	NA	0	100	0	0
Rasmussen	[138]	7	1981	53	72%<24	NA	30	11	23	30
Hall	[28]	8	1968	84	79%<24	42-52	0	100	0	0
Edhag	[139]	9	1982	51	7.5	60	10	17	22	18
Lloyd	[43]	10	1984	53	< 36	44-48	11	70	5	6
Radford	[140]	11	1968	119	48%<12	NA	12#	54	#	15

= ischemic and/or hypertensive heart disease; AF = atrial fibrillation; CAD = coronary artery disease; NA = not available; Pts = patients; RhHD = rheumatic heart disease; SH = systemic hypertension; SR = sinus rhythm; VHD = valvular heart disease; Year = year of publication of the study.

Table 1. (continued)

Study	Double blind, Placebo	Follow-up (mnth)	Pts in SR Ctrl-----Drug		Stat Sign	Death on Ctrl------------drug (n/n)		Quinidine Related Death
1	No	12	15	31	Yes	0/ 52	1/ 48	0
2	Yes	12	28	51	Yes	2/ 75	5/ 91	0
3	Yes	12	16	54	Yes	0/ 43	1/ 45	1
4	No	3	34	59	Yes	0/ 87	1/ 88	1
5	No	3	56	75	Yes	1/105	2/105	0
6	No	24	25	11	No	1/ 42	0/ 43	–
7	No&	24	14&	29	No	0/ 36	2/ 45	0
8	No	12	56	54	No	0/ 40	0/ 54	–
9	No&	12	41&	46	No	0/ 22	1/ 29	0
10	Yes	6	39	48	No	0/ 25	2/ 26	1
11	No	3	42	59	No	1/ 85	2/ 34	2

& = comparison with verapamil; Stat Sign = statistically significant.

better than control treatment. In one study maintenance rates of sinus rhythm were even lower on quinidine. In their metanalysis Coplen et al.[9] showed that quinidine maintained sinus rhythm better than control treatment. This is not surprising since these investigators analyzed 6 of the 11 studies presented in Table 1, of which 5 were significant by themselves. Reports were excluded from their study if quinidine was *not given randomized*, if data were not available in a form permitting calculation of the percentage of patients in sinus rhythm at one or more predetermined times after cardioversion, or if *treatment regimens were not clearly described*. Also, *post-operative studies* were excluded, as well as those *comparing quinidine with another antiarrhythmic*. In view of the above mentioned, quinidine can be considered an effective agent in preventing relapse of atrial fibrillation after cardioversion.

Long acting preparations with more stable serum concentrations may be more effective in maintaining sinus rhythm than shorter acting ones[35]. It has also been suggested that higher serum levels may be more effective[36]. However, this has not been studied extensively and higher dosages presumably lead to more adverse events, among which heart failure.

Side effects. Frequently occurring side effects are gastrointestinal complaints, some of which can be prevented by simultaneous administration of an aluminium containing antacid or the addition of antidiarrheal agents. Gluconated or polygalacturonate formulations may be better tolerated. Less common side effects are cinchonism, allergic skin reactions and immunologically mediated blood disorders. A major concern with quinidine treatment is its proarrhythmic potential which has been known for a long time[37-41]. In the above mentioned metanalysis it was found that the total mortality for quinidine was significantly higher compared to control treatment[9] suggesting a negative effect of this drug on survival. Increased proarrhythmia on quinidine was also shown in another recent metanalysis in ventricular arrhythmias where quinidine appeared to be more arrhythmogenic than other class I anti-arrhythmics, including flecainide[42].

Disopyramide. Table 2 shows that disopyramide may be effective in preventing recurrent atrial fibrillation after cardioversion. In 1 direct comparison study[43] with quinidine neither drug was better than control. Numbers of patients in the treatment and control groups were rather small and the authors correctly point out that larger scale trials should be performed to decide on its efficacy. However, up to now no other controlled studies comparing quinidine and disopyramide and incorporating substantially large numbers of patients have been done.

Table 2. Clinical controlled trials on prophylaxis of atrial fibrillation after electrical cardioversion evaluating disopyramide, flecainide, propafenone, sotalol and amiodarone

Report (1st author)	Study	Year	Pts (n)	Duration AF (mnths)	Age (yr) (mean)	Underlying Heart Disease (%)			
						CAD	VHD	SH	Lone
Disopyramide 450-500 mg									
Härtel [141]	12	1974	48	81%<12	54-57	38	23	6	21
Karlson [142]	13	1988	90	< 12	60	16	13	13	40
Lloyd [43]	14	1984	54	< 36	44-45	9	76	6	7
Flecainide 150-300 mg									
Van Gelder [32]	15	1989	73	<120	57-60	27	37	10	18
Flecainide 200 mg versus quinidine 1100 mg									
Touboul [48]	16	1991	119	NA	NA	NA	NA	NA	NA
Flecainide 300 mg versus disopyramide 600 mg									
Rasmussen [47]	17	1988	60	NA	NA	NA	NA	NA	NA
Propafenone 450-1200 mg									
Porterfield [51]	18	1989	26	NA	70	35	27	19	12
Antman [11]	19	1988	60*)	30	62	−	25	28	15
Sotalol 160-320 mg versus quinidine sulphate 1200 mg									
Juul-Möller [52]	20	1990	183	5.1	59	16	6	26	≤52
Amiodarone 2000 mg/week versus quinidine 1200 mg									
Vitolo [60]	21	1981	54	79%<6*	53	56	44	0	0
Amiodarone, uncontrolled									
Horowitz [14]	22	1985	38*)	32$	60	34	29	0	24
Gold [12]	23	1986	68*)	NA	59	22	24	18	13
Blevins [59]	24	1987	25	75	62	44	12	−	4
Brodsky [22]	25	1987	28	45	61	18	46	0	0
Gosselink [61]	26	1991	89	30	63	37	55	20	10

Abbreviations as in *Table 1*; * = only available for the mitral disease group; *) = only 29% to 42% of patients with chronic atrial fibrillation; $ = for chronic atrial fibrillation only.

Table 2. (continued)

Study	Double blind, Placebo	Follow-up (mnth)	Pts in SR Ctrl-------Drug (%)		Stat Sign	Death on @-------------drug (n/n)		Drug Related Death
			Ctrl	Drug		@	drug	
12	Yes	3	30	72	Yes	0/20	0/18	–
13	Yes	12	30	54	Yes	0/46	2/44	0
14	Yes	6	35	50	No	0/23	0/18	–
15	No	12	36	49	No	0/37	0/36	–
16	Yes	6	40+	56	Yes	0/59+	1/60	1
17	No	6	44&	81	Yes	0/30&	1/30	1
18	No	15.6	–	46	–	–	0/26	–
19	No	6	–	40	–	–	0/60	–
20	No	6	42+	49	No	1/86+	1/97	0#
21	No	12	43+	83	Yes	0/26+	0/28	–
22	No	10$	–	46$	–	–	0/38	–
23	No	21	–	79++	–	–	0/68	–
24	No	≥ 3	–	40	–	–	0/25	–
25	No	22	–	36	–	–	0/28	–
26	No	36	–	53	–	–	1/89	0

@ = control drug; & = disopyramide; + = long-acting quinidine; # = 2 severe proarrhythmias, on each drug one; $ = for chronic atrial fibrillation only; ++ = by definition including also >75% reduction of paroxysms.

Side effects. Disopyramide, has rather potent negative inotropic effects[44]. Therefore the use of this drug in patients 'merely' treated for a supraventricular arrhythmia should be limited to those with normal left ventricular function. The clinical use of the drug is also limited by its potent dose related anticholinergic activity. In contrast to quinidine, disopyramide is less often associated with torsade de pointes.

Flecainide. Flecainide is one of the most extensively evaluated anti-arrhythmics for use in supraventricular tachycardia[45,46]. Its long-term efficacy in suppressing a variety of these arrhythmias has been reported between approximately 65 and 80%. Lower overall efficacy rates were found in atrial fibrillation and atrial flutter, varying between 52 and 63%[45,46].

To date 3 larger trials have been performed evaluating the efficacy of flecainide in preventing atrial fibrillation after cardioversion (Table 2)[32,47,48]. Van Gelder et al.[32] could not demonstrate a significant difference between flecainide and no treatment. However, looking at the time to recurrence, flecainide was significantly more effective in postponing this event. The study by Touboul et al.[48] was a comparison of flecainide 200 mg with 1100 mg long-acting quinidine daily. Flecainide was superior to quinidine in preventing recurrences after the cardioversion and was associated with significantly fewer side effects. However, 1 patient died suddenly 1 month after inclusion and the investigators conclude that flecainide may be the drug of choice for preventing recurrences of arrhythmia, but its use may be limited by proarrhythmia.

Rasmussen et al.[47] administered a fairly large dose of flecainide: 300 mg in a twice daily dosing scheme. They report a very high rate for maintenance of sinus rhythm (81%) at 6 months, which may have been due to the high dose used. Compared to disopyramide, flecainide was much more effective and had a significantly better profile of side effects. However, 1 patient died suddenly after 4 months treatment with flecainide. In this study death may have been dose-related. Van Gelder et al.[32] using only a mean of 199 mg daily did not find severe ventricular proarrhythmias or sudden death. However, the incidence of significant side effects in 58 patients still was 9%, consisting predominantly of complications due to negative dromotropism, with or without syncope. There were no tachyarrhythmic complications. This illustrates that significant adverse effects may occur at normal doses, and that the mechanism of syncope and sudden death is not necessarily related to a tachyarrhythmia, at least not in postcardioversion atrial fibrillation patients. In agreement with the above mentioned, Sihm et al.[49] found a 4% incidence of significant negative dromotropism with flecainide given for acute conversion or chronic prophylaxis in atrial flutter and fibrillation. Therefore, flecainide should be used with caution if intrinsic sinus node dysfunction or AV conduction disturbances exist. More data are needed in patients without extensive cardiac disease (particularly absent remote myocardial infarction), before the efficacy and safety of flecainide in preventing recurrent atrial fibrillation can be established.

Side effects. Flecainide shows dose related negative inotropic properties[50]. Especially patients with a previous history of heart failure and low left ventricular ejection fraction are susceptible to this complication. In turn, congestive heart failure predisposes to IC-related proarrhythmia. Therefore, like other class IC drugs, flecainide should be avoided in atrial fibrillation complicated by heart failure.

Propafenone. Propafenone is a class IC drug with mild ß-blocking activity. Although the effect is mild, the latter aspect of this drug may render it preferable to other IC drugs in socalled adrenergic dependent atrial fibrillation.

In an uncontrolled trial Porterfield and Porterfield[51] studied the effects of propafenone in preventing or suppressing attacks of chronic atrial fibrillation. In that report no other definition of chronic atrial fibrillation is given than that patients had developed 'sustained' arrhythmia. Of 26 patients 12 were successfully treated during a mean follow-up of 15.6 months. Recurrences were documented by telemetry monitoring or telephone transmission. Only 3 patients underwent electrical cardioversion. The fact that 77% of patients converted to sinus rhythm on the drug *alone* may be taken to indicate that the patient group was rather easy-to-treat. However, this is in contrast with the fact that all patients had failed several drugs previously, and that half of them had a history of congestive heart failure. Presumably, paroxysmal rather than chronic arrhythmia was present in most patients.

Antman et al.[11] studied a mixed group of 60 patients with episodic or chronic (25 patients) atrial fibrillation. The group was considered 'intractable' because of frequent recurrences before inclusion. The total dose tolerated by the patients was 795 mg/day on the average. All patients continued treatment chronically whether or not they had converted to sinus rhythm. Propafenone did not convert any of the 25 chronic patients, but in 21 sinus rhythm was restored by electrical cardioversion, whereas the other 4 had undergone chemical conversion with other antiarrhythmics before inclusion in the study. Unfortunately, no separate outcome data for the chronic patients are presented. For the whole group, 45% still had sinus rhythm after 6 months. Chronic, as opposed to paroxysmal atrial fibrillation, tended to be related to failure on propafenone, as were male sex, high number of previous unsuccessful drug trials, and large left atrial anteroposterior diameter.

No other larger scale trials evaluating the effects of propafenone have been reported. At present one Dutch multicenter trial is ongoing, comparing efficacy and safety of propafenone with disopyramide in postcardioversion atrial fibrillation.

Side effects. The most frequent side effects of propafenone are gastrointestinal and neurologic complaints. Since these are dose-dependent, dose reduction if possible, may abolish these side effects. Like other class IC drugs propafenone exerts a negative inotropic action and should be avoided in patients suffering from heart failure. Other adverse cardiac effects include conduction disturbances and ventricular proarrhythmia.

Sotalol. Recently much interest has arisen in class III antiarrhythmics. Sotalol has been available for many years in most European countries and gained wide clinical application. Due to its class III effect in combination with ß-blocking properties, it has proved effective in a variety of arrhythmias. In the specially postcardioversion prevention of atrial fibrillation only 1 controlled study[52] has been performed in a comparison with quinidine (Table 2). The dose of sotalol was relatively low, i.e. 160 to 320 mg daily. In that study data were elegantly presented by making a distinction between (a) recurrences (on intention-to-treat basis 37% with sotalol and 28% with quinidine, p=NS), (b) drug discontinuation for adverse effects (11 and 26% respectively, p<0.03) and (c) sinus rhythm while still treated with the drug (49 and 42% respectively, p=NS). Compared to baseline, the ventricular rate at relapse was significantly lower with sotalol if combined with digitalis (80 versus 68 bpm), but not with sotalol alone (81 versus 79 bpm). On the other hand, patients on quinidine had significantly higher ventricular rates at relapse whether (80 versus 109 bpm) or not (89 versus 109 bpm) treatment was combined with digitalis. This illustrates that facilitation of AV conduction as seen during quinidine does not seem to occur with sotalol. On the other hand, sotalol by itself seems less effective in controlling heart rate when no digitalis is given concomitantly. Sotalol was significantly better tolerated. Of note, 1 sotalol and 1 quinidine patient had a severe proarrhythmic response *early* after initiation of therapy, whereas no patient had a *late* proarrhythmic response. This underscores the notion that as long as patients are in a *stable* clinical condition, class IA and III related proarrhythmia is most likely to occur early after initiation of anti-arrhythmic therapy.

In an uncontrolled 3 stage serial approach we studied efficacy of sotalol in 39 patients after recardioversion for failure on flecainide. After a cumulative follow-up of 2 years sotalol had prevented relapse in 42% of these patients [20]. The mean dose was 269± 49 mg daily. Sotalol was moderately well tolerated, with 13% of patients developing side effects. Side effects related predominantly to the ß-blocking activity of sotalol. There was no ventricular proarrhythmia.

Side effects. Mostly these are related to sotalol's ß-blocking activity and have been reported in up to 50% of patients, leading to discontinuation in 20% of cases. Neurologic as well as gastrointestinal complaints are observed. Especially fatigue is a major problem leading to discontinuation of the drug. Due to its class III activity, sotalol may produce torsade de pointes. Despite its ß-blocking effect sotalol has only little influence on the inotropic state of the patient. This has been related to its class III effect, which produces a prolongation of the plateau phase of the action potential leading to an increased calcium influx[53].

Amiodarone. Amiodarone is a class III drug exhibiting also class I effects in addition to negative chronotropic (noncompetitive ß-blockade) and anti-ischemic actions. It is in widespread use for all types of arrhythmias in Europe. It seems particularly effective in acutely and safely terminating atrial fibrillation[54]. If conversion does not occur, the ventricular rate will be reduced significantly.

Intravenous but also oral amiodarone have not been studied extensively in controlled trials. Why? Amiodarone has significant side effects for which the drug is 'condemned' to last resort agent. Therefore it is used predominantly in intractable patients, in whom control treatment is deemed unethical. Another difficulty precluding proper evaluation in a controlled trial is the fact that most of its side effects take long to develop, since they occur predominantly after high *cumulative* doses[55]. Finally, the fact that a cross-over design is not possible because of its complicated pharmacokinetics further limits feasibility of controlled trials with amiodarone.

Amiodarone has been reported to be effective in the treatment of atrial fibrillation, with success rates ranging from 53% to 97%[12-14,56-59]. These studies evaluated predominantly patients with paroxysmal atrial fibrillation or included only relatively small numbers of patients with chronic atrial fibrillation. In addition, the daily maintenance dose was relatively high in most of them. In subgroups with chronic atrial fibrillation, maintenance rates of sinus rhythm were somewhat lower than the above mentioned figures (range 44% to 75%), indicating that chronic atrial fibrillation is more difficult to treat than recurrent episodic atrial fibrillation.

The only controlled trial on the efficacy of amiodarone in postcardioversion prevention of atrial fibrillation has been performed by Vitolo and coworkers[60], who compared amiodarone with quinidine (Table 2). After the electrical cardioversion, but before randomization, patients were stratified according to age, duration of atrial fibrillation, mitral valve disease and cardiac surgery. After 6 months treatment amiodarone was more effective than quinidine. With amiodarone 83% of patients remained in sinus rhythm versus 43% on quinidine. In addition, amiodarone was associated with fewer side effects, but this should be viewed against the above mentioned background, that most side effects occur only in the very long term. In this respect, it must be noted that a relatively high dose of 2000 mg/week was used, potentially leading to a high rate of *late* side effects. In contrast, in a nonrandomized study from our department[61], only an average of 211 mg daily was administered. In that study, the actuarial results were 61% and 53% of 89 patients were still in sinus rhythm after 1 and 3 years respectively. Effective plasma concentrations averaged 1.7 mg/L for amiodarone and 1.3 mg/L for desethylamiodarone. Severe side effects occurred in only 1 patient. On one hand the low dose may have precluded side effects, but on the other it may also have caused the lower success rate in maintaining sinus rhythm as compared to the study by Vitolo et al. However, the lower success rate of amiodarone in our population may also have been due to the more chronic and refractory nature of the arrhythmia with a high number of previous cardioversions and a long previous arrhythmia duration (Table 2). Therefore, high dosages need not necessarily be given to these patients to obtain clinically significant efficacy. Also other studies have shown that low dose amiodarone may be effective[62-64].

Gold et al.[12] studied 68 atrial fibrillation patients of whom at least 28 had chronic arrhythmia according to the above mentioned definition. Only these 28 patients underwent electrical cardioversion during the study after at least one month amiodarone pretreatment. In 79% of cases amiodarone prevented recurrent atrial fibrillation at a mean follow-up of 21 months. Maintenance of sinus rhythm was less in patients with atrial fibrillation lasting more than 1 year: 57%. As many as 35% of patients had side effects, and amiodarone was stopped in 10% for that reason. Again, the relatively high incidence of severe side effects, as well as the high success rates in this study may have been due to the high dose used (up to 400 mg). It is important to note that in this study incidence of side effects was high despite the fact that drug therapy was guided by amiodarone plasma concentrations. The target concentration was between 1.0 and 2.5 mg/l.

Brodsky et al.[22] studied the efficacy of amiodarone in 28 chronic atrial fibrillation patients with an enlarged left atrium. Patients were treated for at least one month with amiodarone and if chemical cardioversion had not occurred by that time electrical cardioversion was performed. Only 16 patients underwent direct current cardioversion (i.e. primary success of amiodarone 57%). During long-term follow-up patients with a left atrial dimension in excess of 46 mm (arbitrary cutoff point) appeared relatively resistant to amiodarone.

Horowitz et al.[14] studied 38 patients of whom only 11 had chronic atrial fibrillation. Overall efficacy was 67% in the 27 patients with paroxysmal and 45% in 11 patients with chronic atrial fibrillation. Especially patients with increased left atrial dimension, low left ventricular ejection fraction and patients with chronic atrial fibrillation with a long previous arrhythmia duration appeared refractory to amiodarone.

Blevins et al.[59] studied 38 patients of whom 25 had chronic atrial fibrillation. They concluded that amiodarone is safe and effective. Only four patients (11%) developed intolerable side effects. The average dose was 232 ± 80 mg/d. During long term treatment with a mean follow-up of 16 months 53% of the patients remained in sinus rhythm, i.e. 11 of 25 patients with chronic atrial fibrillation and 9 of 13 patients with paroxysmal atrial fibrillation.

The latter 4 reports illustrate the diversity of clinical characteristics of the patients in trials studying prevention of atrial fibrillation. The patients included in these studies appear to have only one common denominator, i.e. intractability. Strength of these studies is flawed predominantly by the fact that no distinction is made between chronic and periodic atrial fibrillation. This confounds the efficacy issue and in addition, makes these studies less suitable for identificati-on of factors associated with arrhythmia intractability.

Side effects. The clinical use of amiodarone is limited by its side effects. Virtually all patients develop skin photosensitivity and some a dermatitis or blue-gray skin discoloration. All of these effects are reversible. Apart from this, gastrointestinal and neurologic complaints including peripheral neuropathy and proximal muscle weakness, may occur. Slight elevations of T_4 and TSH levels are frequently found in association with low T_3 and the incidence of clinical hyperthyroidism may amount to 5-10% of patients. Pulmonary toxicity is most troublesome, presenting either as an acute onset hypersensitivity early after initiation of therapy or (more commonly) as a slowly progressing diffuse bilateral pulmonary fibrosis or infiltration. The patients at risk for this serious complication cannot be predicted. Chest X-ray is the best way to produce the diagnosis in combination with the clinical picture. Heart failure due to amiodarone may occur but is uncommon, and the relation with amiodarone therapy mostly is difficult to establish.

AMIODARONE IN ATRIAL FIBRILLATION COMPLICATED BY HEART FAILURE

Development of congestive heart failure, especially with disopyramide, the IC drugs and sotalol may be a major concern. Heart failure was not reported in the earlier studies evaluating quinidine. However, quinidine as a class IA drug may also have profound effects on cardiac function[44,65]. The same holds for the IB drugs[66].

Interestingly, in the above mentioned study by Gosselink et al.[61] logistic regression analysis suggested that amiodarone was especially effective in patients with a compromised left ventricular function. This is in contrast with the study of Horowitz and coworkers[14], who found that the lower the left ventricular ejection fraction the worse the response to amiodarone. Hamer et al. showed that amiodarone compared to placebo improved left ventricular function in heart failure patients after a 6 months observation period[67]. Whether this also played a role in our postcardioversion atrial fibrillation patients remains obscure. After the cardioversion many hemodynamic changes take place, posing a difficulty in separating out the effects of amiodarone. The role of amiodarone in this condition still needs further elucidation. Whether in the future the newly developed potassium channel blockers (a.o. dofetilide, sematilide, almokalant) with exclusive class III actions will be of special benefit in this condition, remains to be established. Especially the safety aspect in these patients, intrinsically prone to ventricular proarrhythmia, might be of major concern.

SERIAL TREATMENT

Figure 1 depicts schematically a 'serial treatment' approach   toward the postcardioversion atrial fibrillation patient. There are several possibilities:

- **serial electrical cardioversion**: serial electrical cardioversions only, *without* institution of prophylactic drugs;

- **serial drug treatment**: serial electrical cardioversions with change to a different class of antiarrhythmic drug after each repeat cardioversion.

Figure 1. Scheme of Serial Electrical Cardioversion or Serial Drug Treatment in patients with chronic atrial fibrillation or flutter.

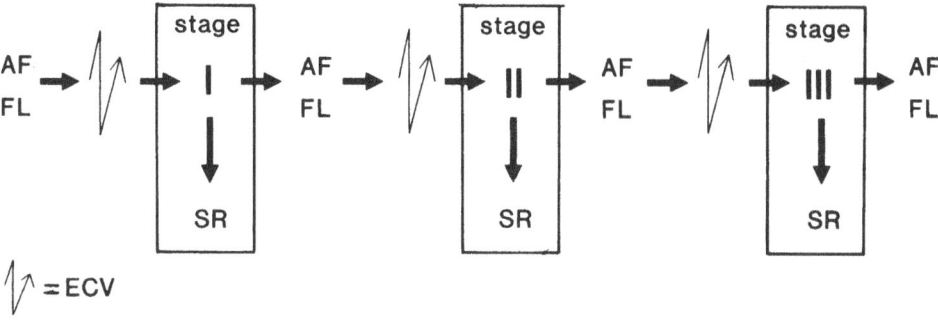

AF = atrial fibrillation; FL = atrial flutter; SR = sinus rhythm; ECV = electrical cardioversion.

The *serial electrical* approach is attractive since it avoids the use of potentially harmful antiarrhythmics. The rationale to perform serial electrical cardioversion lies in the fact that after the cardioversion several beneficial effects enhancing the preservation of sinus rhythm may take place. Among these are a decrease of atrial dimensions[68] and improvement of left ventricular function[4,5,31]. These changes develop within one week to one month. Therefore, it seems reasonable to state that patients are eligible for this approach only if the interval in sinus rhythm after the shock is at least 1 month. The above mentioned beneficial changes are less likely to occur in patients with severe mitral valve disease, especially stenosis[20] and these patients should not be considered candidates for serial electrical cardioversion.

The rationale for *serial drug* treatment is that the underlying arrhythmogenic mechanism at the atrial level may differ between patients. Since in most cases the arrhythmogenic mechanism cannot be determined beforehand, it is impossible to tell which drug is best for which patient. The patient failing a conduction slowing drug may respond to a drug exhibiting predominantly action potential prolongation or vice versa. Sometimes the combined effects of atrial premature beat suppression, conduction slowing (at fast rates) and action potential prolongation (at the onset of arrhythmia) may be beneficial. The sequence of drug types to be instituted, is arbitrary. In the serial treatment study from this institution[20], we used sequentially flecainide, followed by sotalol or quinidine, and as a last resort treatment amiodarone. Amiodarone was used as the last agent for its potentially severe side effects. In view of recent studies[9,42,52] we would advise to use first sotalol, then flecainide or propafenone (if no CAST-like[69] clinical characteristics are present) and lastly amiodarone. In the future, new pure class III drugs will become available. However, their efficacy and safety remain to be established. Serial drug treatment may also include serial shocks and reinstitution of the *same* anti-arrhythmic drug, especially if there was a long period in sinus rhythm while using the drug, whereas the patient had early recurrence(s) without anti-arrhythmics.

For both approaches applies that patients should be carefully selected. In the above mentioned serial drug treatment study[20] we found that apart from the presence of mitral valve disease, also a high age (e.g. >70 years), a long previous arrhythmia duration (e.g. >5 years) and a history of multiple episodes of chronic arrhythmia (e.g. ≥3) all predicted intractability despite serial treatment.

The serial *electrical* approach is especially feasible in patients with a very low recurrence rate, e.g. once per year. Instead of posing these patients chronically to the threat of drug-related proarrhythmia, exclusively repeated electrical cardioversion may be performed. However, if atrial fibrillation relapses early after the shock, or if multiple recurrences have dominated the clinical picture, it seems reasonably to carry out serial *drug* treatment. This should be considered only in severely symptomatic patients. In others institution of negative chronotropic drugs may be sufficient to control symptoms. In patients

who remain severely symptomatic despite adequate inhibition of AV conduction, but who are considered prone to develop proarrhythmic effects, ablation of
AV conduction may be an alternative. When deciding which strategy to follow,
the risks of catheter ablation of the AV junction also have to be taken into
consideration[70].

DIFFERENTIAL EFFECTS OF CLASS I AND CLASS III ANTIARRHYTHMICS ON VENTRICULAR RATE DURING ATRIAL FIBRILLATION: IMPLICATION FOR CLINICAL PRACTICE

It has been known for long that quinidine[71] and disopyramide[72]
may cause rapid AV conduction during atrial fibrillation or flutter. This may be
caused by a decrease of intrinsic atrial rate leading to diminished concealed
conduction in the AV node, and by facilitation of AV conduction due to an
anticholinergic action. It is an important side effect, limiting the applicability of
these agents in the prophylaxis of atrial fibrillation, since *unexpected* relapses
may be more troublesome **with** these drugs than without them. The same has
been described for lidocaine[73,74], ajmaline[75], flecainide (Figure 2)[10,76-
81], encainide[81], propafenone[75,82] and cibenzoline[75]. To prevent this
complication the concomitant use of digitalis or verapamil has been advocated.
At this point it cannot be stressed enough that, **after** a patient has developed
permanent atrial fibrillation or flutter, *all class I drugs become contraindicated.*
This holds not only for class IA or IB, but also for class IC drugs. Despite the
fact that it has been reported that flecainide (only in combination with digoxin)
may reduce the maximum heart rate during exercise while in atrial fibrillation,
this effect was only modest and was obtained at the cost of significant ventricular proarrhythmia in 2 of 12 patients, of whom 1 required ventricular defibrillation[83,84]. Apart from this, *there also is no electrophysiologic rationale for
the use of these drugs in established chronic atrial fibrillation.* Instead, effective negative chronotropic medication should be instituted and its effect evaluated by exercise testing and 24 hour ambulatory monitoring. In this respect it is
also important to note that the above mentioned deleterious effects of class I
drugs may not always be evident at rest, i.e. in the absence of a significant
neurohumoral drive. In some instances 1:1 AV conduction of atrial flutter or
rapid AV nodal transmission of impulses during atrial fibrillation (Figure 2) may

be evident only with exercise[83,84]. Therefore, when using class I drugs in the *prevention* of relapses of these supraventricular arrhythmias, the patient should be instructed to temporarily avoid vigorous exercise if symptoms of arrhythmia recurrence have presented.

Table 3. Comparison negative chronotropic actions of digoxin, combination digoxin and verapamil, and amiodarone in 10 patients undergoing sequential maximal exercise tests while in atrial fibrillation

		Drug Regimens		
		Digoxin	Digoxin & Verapamil	Amiodarone
Heart Rate Rest	(mean, bpm)	106	93	93
Peak Exercise	(mean, bpm)	184	154*	146*
Exercise Level	(mean, Watts)	115	117	100

* Statistically significant compared to digoxin

The above mentioned disadvantage of class I drugs does not seem to apply for class III agents. Patients in atrial fibrillation treated with sotalol or amiodarone may even benefit from a negative chronotropic action on the AV node[15,52,85]. Slowing of AV conduction by sotalol may become enhanced by digitalis[52]. On the other hand, it has been shown that some of the electrophysiologic effects of amiodarone are acutely reversible by an increase in neurohumoral drive[86]. Presumably the same holds for sotalol. This means that despite the fact that at a recurrence acceptable heart rates are found, the heart rate may still become high during exercise. This is also illustrated by Table 3. Others have demonstrated that both resting and peak exercise heart rate decrease with amiodarone[87]. Thus, in patients treated chronically with amiodarone or sotalol while having established atrial fibrillation, exercise heart rate should be evaluated before deciding on continued therapy with these drugs. If maximum rate is high, class III drug treatment may not be feasible and the usual negative chronotropic drugs or catheter ablation should be considered.

Figure 2.

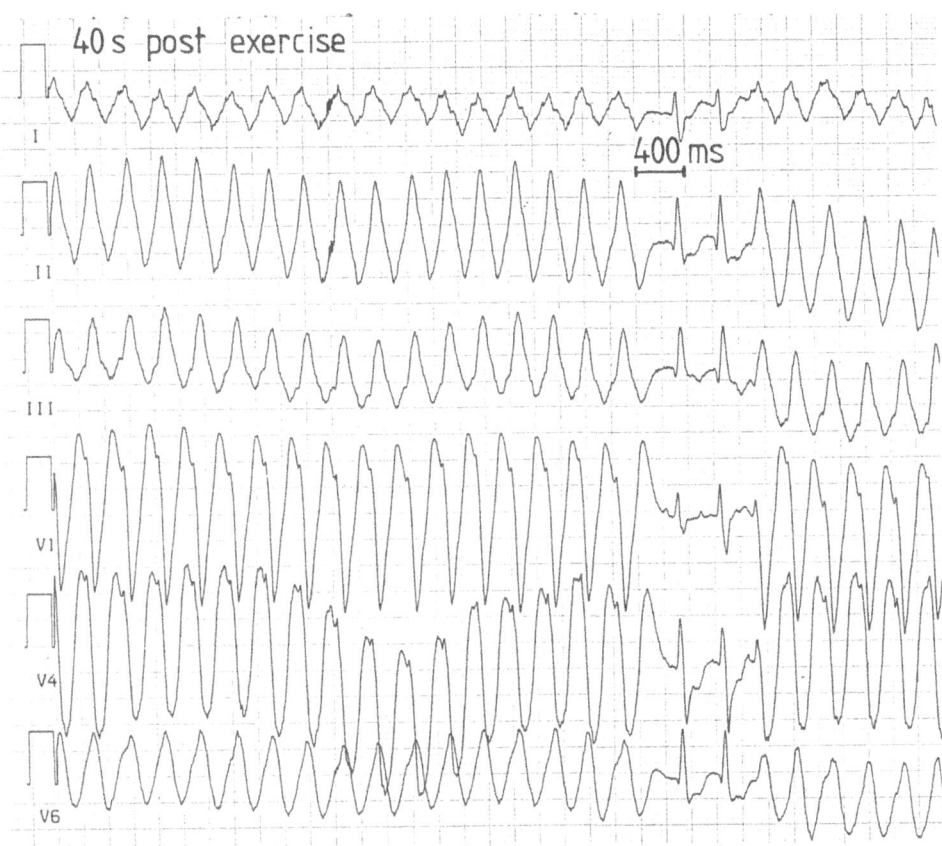

Aberrant conduction due to 1:1 AV conduction in a patient with an atrial tachycardia/flutter with a cycle length of approximately 280 ms 40 seconds after stopping exercise. Note match between atrial rate (right hand side of the figure) and rate of the wide QRS tachycardia.

ANTIARRHYTHMICS IN THE PREVENTION OF ATRIAL FIBRILLATION IN THE WPW-SYNDROME _____

In the WPW-syndrome complicated by atrial fibrillation, it is well known that drugs slowing atrioventricular nodal conduction (digitalis, non-dihydropyridine calciumantagonists and ß-blockers) are contraindicated. This holds for both acute termination of a paroxysm and chronic prophylactic therapy. AV nodal conduction may be slowed more than that over the accessory pathway. This may result in an increased ventricular rate due to rate-related facilitation of pathway conduction and diminished retrograde concealed conduction into it. Deleterious acceleration of the ventricular rate in this syndrome has also been described for lidocaine[89] and amiodarone[90].

Flecainide has been used in patients with the WPW-syndrome to convert *acute* attacks of atrial fibrillation with rapid conduction over the accessory pathway[77]. Before conversion a significant reduction of the ventricular rate from 280 to a mean of 130 beats per minute, with relief of symptoms was noted. In the electrophysiology laboratory the influence of this drug on the properties of the abnormal pathway in patients with atrial fibrillation has been studied extensively[91-94]. It was demonstrated that flecainide prolonged both the refractory period of the accessory pathway as well as the shortest RR interval during atrial fibrillation. These studies indicated that class IC drugs may be effective and safe for chronic prophylaxis of atrial fibrillation in the setting of the Wolff-Parkinson-White syndrome, which was subsequently demonstrated by several studies[94,95]. However, it must be recognized that at an attack of atrial fibrillation exercise-related reversal of antiarrhythmic activity may occur and render the patient at risk for rapid ventricular rate due to facilitated conduction over the AV node as well as over the accessory pathway.

Most of the above mentioned also holds for amiodarone[86,96] and disopyramide[97]. Amiodarone prolongs refractoriness in the atrium as well as in the accessory pathway and slows the ventricular response to atrial fibrillation by an average of 50%[96]. This drug seems safe in this condition, although deleterious acceleration of ventricular rate has been reported in a single case of a WPW patient with an old inferior myocardial infarction and atrial fibrillation [90]. The long term effects of sotalol in this syndrome have not been studied extensively. It is conceivable that sotalol through its ß-blocking effects may be harmful in some patients.

PROARRHYTHMIA DURING TREATMENT OF ATRIAL FIBRILLATION OR FLUTTER

The most important proarrhythmic effect occurring during therapy for atrial fibrillation is new onset ventricular tachycardia, fibrillation or torsade de pointes. However, several other types of proarrhythmia, among which those occurring at the supraventricular level, should be considered. Table 4 presents the most common types.

Ventricular proarrhythmia. This complication, occurring in patients not having had sustained ventricular tachycardia, fibrillation or torsade de pointes before, is of major concern and limits the clinical applicability of all anti-arrhythmic drugs. It expresses either as a polymorphic ventricular tachycardia of the torsade de pointes type, or as a monomorphic tachycardia. The former is predominantly caused by class IA[9,40,98-100], or class III drugs[101] and may also occur with the calciumchannel blocker bepridil. Monomorphic ventricular tachycardias in atrial fibrillation patients are mostly caused by IC drugs[49,69,84,102,103].

Table 4. **Proarrhythmia during treatment of chronic atrial fibrillation or flutter**

Ventricular proarrhythmia
    Torsade de pointes (ref @)
    Sustained monomorphic ventricular tachycardia (ref $)
    Sustained polymorphic ventricular tachycardia without long QT
Atrial proarrhythmia
    Provocation recurrence ?
    Conversion of atrial fibrillation to flutter
Abnormalities of conduction or impulse formation
    Acceleration of ventricular rate
    – enhancement of AV nodal conduction
    – preferential accessory pathway conduction
    AV block
    Abnormal sinus mechanisms after conversion to sinus rhythm

@ references (40, 98, 99, 100, 109, 9)
$ references (102, 122, 123, 69, 95, 103, 84, 49, 20)

Torsade de pointes. Quinidine. The proarrhythmic potential of quinidine has been known for a long time[37-40]. In fact as early as 1923 quinidine was implicated in the precipitation of sudden death[104]. Roden et al. estimated the annual risk at at least 1.5%[100]. The incidence of torsade de pointes with quinidine administered for atrial fibrillation may amount 8.5% of consecutive patients[41].

In the metanalysis by Coplen et al.[9] it was found that the total mortality for quinidine was 2.9 % compared to only 0.8 % in the control group.

There were 12 deaths in a total of 413 quinidine treated patients. However, in only 7 cases the mode of death was clear and in 3 out of these 7 patients death was sudden, suggesting proarrhythmia of quinidine in these few cases only. Whether negative inotropic effects of the drug played a role in the others, is unclear. In the control group there were only 4 deaths in 387 patients. The cause of death was known in 3, of which non was sudden.

The pooled data presented in Table 1 corroborate the findings of Coplen et al.[9]. In 11 studies there were 17 deaths (2.8%) during quinidine treatment in a total of 608 patients versus 5 deaths (0.8%) in 612 control patients. While 5 of 17 deaths in the active treatment group were ascribed to quinidine, there were no sudden deaths in the untreated cohort.

Comparing the death rates on quinidine (Table 1) to other drugs (Table 2) this suggests that quinidine may be more toxic, presumably due to a higher proarrhythmic potential. Whereas quinidine was considered to have caused 5 deaths in 608 (0.8%) treated patients, there were only 2 deaths in 665 (0.3%) patients on active treatment in the pooled data of studies on disopyramide (n=80), flecainide (n=120), propafenone (n=86), sotalol (n=97) or amiodarone (n=276). This difference is even more outspoken when looking at total mortality (2.8% with quinidine versus 0.9% on the other drugs). When comparing these figures it must be noted that quinidine trials were done in an earlier era in a different type of patients. On the other hand, it still suggests that quinidine has a more toxic effect including a higher proarrhythmic potential. This was also demonstrated by a recently published metanalysis on quinidine versus other class I antiarrhythmics, evaluating mortality in short-to-median term trials in patients with benign or potentially lethal ventricular arrhythmias[42]. In 502 quinidine treated patients there were 12 deaths and 20 early proarrhythmic events (not fatal), versus 4 deaths and 11 early proarrhythmias in 504 patients treated with flecainide (n=141), mexiletine (n=246), tocainide (n=67) or propafenone (n=53). The risk difference for quinidine versus the other drugs was 0.16 and the odds ratio was 3.08 for death on quinidine compared with the other drugs. The authors state that the exact mechanism of enhanced mortality with quinidine is not known. However, looking at the cause of death, 10 of 12 deaths on quinidine were due to an arrhythmia mechanism (unspecified, sudden cardiac death or ventricular fibrillation). In addition, considering the relative potential of quinidine to cause early proarrhythmia in this metanalysis, an arrhythmia mechanism as cause of the terminal event becomes very likely.

Factors predisposing to torsade de pointes. Predisposing factors for drug-induced torsade de pointes with special reference to quinidine are listed in Table 5. Preexisting prolonged QT interval has for long been associated with an intrinsic propensity to develop torsade de pointes on class IA anti-arrhythmics[98-100,105-109]. However, the QT interval during therapy has no predictive value. Hypokalemia and hypomagnesemia may produce by themselves electrocardiographic changes indistinguishable from those of quinidine and other class IA or III antiarrhythmics. It is therefore not surprising that low serum concentrations of these electrolytes predispose for quinidine toxicity since effects most likely are additive.

For the clinician it is extremely important to recognize the role of (relative) bradycardia preceding the onset of quinidine induced torsade de pointes. In the atrial fibrillation patient relatively slow heart rates may occur due to (paroxysmal) AV block or at the very moment of conversion of atrial fibrillation to sinus rhythm. Sinus node dysfunction may play an additional role. As early as 1922, the relation between slow heart rate and 'quinidine syncope' was recognized[110]. Also others have pointed to the fact that bradycardia predisposes to arrhythmias induced by quinidine[100,101,105,106,108,109]. The same was seen with disopyramide in the example in this chapter (Figure 3).

Table 5. **Factors predisposing to drug-induced torsade de pointes**

Preexisting QT prolongation, 'concealed' long QT syndrome
Low potassium, low magnesium
Bradycardia or relative bradycardia
    – after development of AV block
    – after conversion of atrial fibrillation to sinus rhythm
    – associated with ectopy producing short-long RR sequences
Structural heart disease ?
Rapid dose increase ?

A classic description of the effects of bradycardia and the relation with conversion to sinus rhythm can be found in the paper by Selzer and Wray

[40]. In their case seven, high dose quinidine was administered uneventfully until conversion. After resumption of sinus rhythm however, torsade de pointes developed. Clearly, before this attack a relatively high dosage had been used. However, on a separate occasion this patient had a second attack of torsades after a low cumulative dose, this time not long after electrical restoration of sinus rhythm. Of note, the authors remark that postshock sinus rhythm was accompanied by frequent premature beats in this patient (which may have introduced significant pauses with short-long RR cycles, setting the stage for pause dependent torsade de pointes, see below). The same sequence of events occurred in their case number eight: 990 mg was administered over 18 hours, whereafter a successful electrocardioversion took place. After two days of maintenance therapy with 1200 mg quinidine per day, torsade de pointes occurred during an episode of sinus rhythm with frequent ventricular prematu-re beats. Roden et al.[100] and later on also Jackman et al.[101] have reemphasized the role of conversion from 'rapid' atrial fibrillation to 'slow' sinus rhythm.

Apart from bradycardia also short-long RR cycles preceding drug-induced torsade de pointes play a pivotal role[99,100,108,111]. In fact, this cycle length perturbation, incorporating at least 1 long cycle, represents an acute bradycar-dia. This pattern of RR interval changes was found to be remarkably consis-tent[100] and can also be seen in Figure 3.

Recently other electrocardiographic characteristics have been associated with the development of torsade de pointes. These include the emergence of a 'slow diastolic wave'[41], postpause U wave accentuation[101] and new postpause ventricular premature beats in a bigeninal pattern[41,101]. Also the induction of a Q-peak T duration of ≥ 400 ms by quinidine has been related to proarrhythmia with this agent[100]. Finally, in patients prone to IA related proarrhythmia, Kadish et al.[112] found that the QT interval may fail to shorten normally (or may even lengthen paradoxically) during exercise[112], but this was not confirmed by others[113].

Ejvinsson and Orinius[41] described U wave like 'slow diastolic waves' during quinidine therapy for attempted chemical conversion for atrial fibrillation. It was present in 5 of the 6 patients developing torsade pointes and in none of the other 65 patients, and preceded arrhythmia onset with a time interval between 13 and 185 minutes. Before torsades occurred ventricular premature beats had emerged from these 'slow waves' in a bigeminal pattern. Jackman et al. found postpause U wave accentuation (see also Figure 3) in 42 of 46 cases of drug-induced torsade de pointes a median of 24 hours before its onset (range 2 minutes to 15 days). They also found new postpause ventricular premature beats in a bigeminal pattern in 43 of the 46 cases, beginning 2 minutes to 60 days (median 7 hours) before onset of torsade. Although both latter 'warning signs' were highly sensitive, they lacked significant specificity since e.g. postpause U wave accentuation was not invariably associated with the arrhythmia. Whether arrhythmias may present more often in these patients in the presence of other provoking factors like hypokalemia is not known [101]. It is also unknown if post pause U wave alterations in the *drug free* state predispose a patient to torsade on drugs. Obviously this might be a valuable 'warning sign' facilitating the identification of high risk patients[101].

It is uncertain whether specific underlying heart diseases predispose to torsades de pointes with quinidine. Although it is frequently assumed that the severity of structural heart disease by itself is a risk factor, it must always be kept in mind that quinidine proarrhythmia may occur in the normal heart [101,105,114]. Congestive heart failure may enhance this type of proarrhythmia[111] because of the fact that it is associated with an increased arrhythmogenicity by itself and through the use of diuretics. However, the relative risk for developing proarrhythmia in this condition has not been established. Webb et al.[109] suggested that children after corrective surgery for transposition of the great arteries might be at particular risk because of an age-related increase in bradyarrhythmias typically associated with intermittent tachyarrhythmias.

Patients developing torsade de pointes on one quinidine-like drug are likely to show the same on another member of this subclass[115], but may be safely treated with IB drugs[116,117].

The role of digitalis in development of quinidine induced torsades is vague. In many reports digitalis therapy (no intoxication) has been incriminated as a cofactor, but others could not support this. Nevertheless it is advocated by many to diminish the dose if quinidine therapy is initiated. Interestingly, Morganroth and Goin[42] revive the discussion on the potential negative effects of the quinidine-digitalis combination. In one trial 5 of 7, and in another 2 of 3 deaths on quinidine occurred while the patients used a 'therapeutic' dose of digitalis. In the patients treated with the other drugs, this relation was

Figure 3.

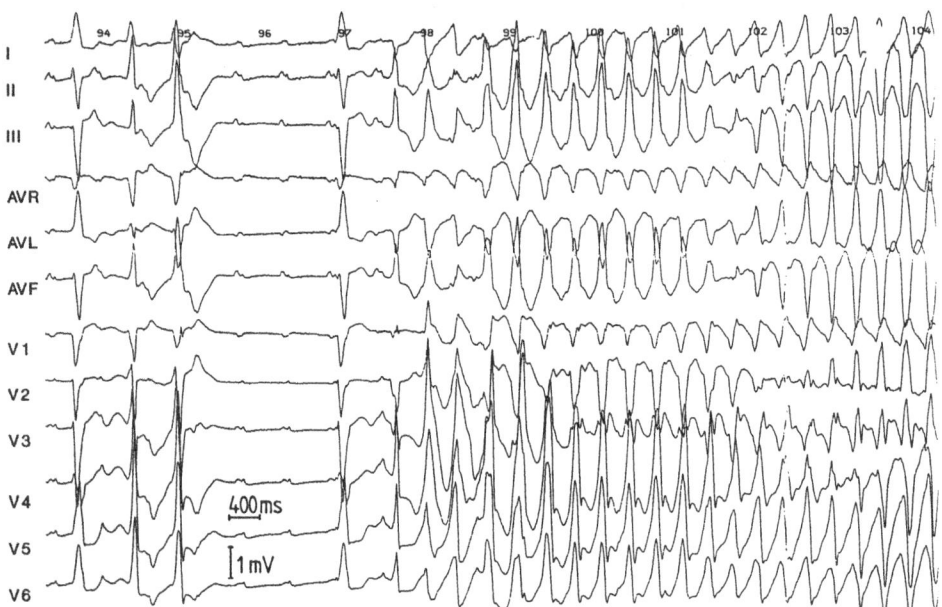

Due to disopyramide intoxication (high levels) this patient had paroxysmal AV block with slow escape rhythm. Only **after** the development of the slow rate torsade de pointes emerged. Therefore bradycardia seemed a prerequisite for the development of the tachyarrhythmia. Note the post pause U wave accentuation associated with slight decrease of the T wave in the 4th beat from the left, particularly visible in leads V4 and V5 (compare with TU complex of 1st beat).

less evident (despite comparable use of digitalis), obviously due to the low incidence of death.

Factors associated with late proarrhythmia on quinidine. Of major concern is 'late' proarrhythmia occurring during chronic quinidine therapy (Table 6).

Table 6. **Factors predisposing to late proarrhythmia with quinidine**

- change of dose/preparation
- addition of drugs:
  diuretics
  other antiarrhythmics
  tricyclic, tetracyclic antidepressants
  ketanserin
  ß-blocker ?
- reinitiation after short discontinuation
- intercurrent hypokalemia/hypomagnesemia
- intercurrent 'bradycardia'
  conversion from tachycardia to sinus rhythm
  sick sinus syndrome
  AV block

As many as half of all torsades may develop only after 4 days treatment. In their series of 38 patients developing torsade on quinidine, procainamide or disopyramide, Jackman et al. noted that 18 had their proarrhythmia after 4 days treatment, of whom 7 developed it after 1 month. Late onset torsade de pointes has been associated with a change in dose or preparation, addition of drugs (e.g. diuretics, other antiarrhythmic, ketanserin, tricyclic and tetracyclic antidepressants, ß-blocker?) and reinitiation of therapy after a brief discontinuation[100,101]. Furthermore, intercurrent hypokalemia, hypomagnesemia and bradyarrhythmias may play a role[100,101,109]. Late onset (relative) bradycardia is especially important in the atrial fibrillation patient. As mentioned above, the mere conversion to sinus rhythm, may expose torsade de pointes in susceptible individuals. It follows that if a patient is *sent home* on quinidine while still in atrial fibrillation, he or she may develop out of hospital torsade de pointes the very moment conversion to sinus rhythm occurs. The most prudent way to follow is to actually see how the patient responds to the drug not only while in atrial fibrillation but especially after conversion to sinus rhythm. Obviously, this implies electrical cardioversion if necessary. Only then one may be sure that quinidine or other IA drugs do not provoke torsade during 'bradycardia' per se. If the patient has no adverse response while in sinus rhythm, chronic therapy may be safe provided other provoking factors are prevented.

Torsade de pointes. Other class IA and III drugs. Most of the above mentioned not only holds for quinidine but also for other class IA or III drugs. Whereas torsade with quinidine occurs predominantly at low or normal serum levels, its incidence with sotalol clearly increases with dose[118-120]. It occurs only infrequently at low dosages[52]. As a general guideline it is advocated that the dose should not exceed 480 mg daily[120]. Also amiodarone has been implicated in torsade de pointes, but its proarrhythmic potential seems less than with other antiarrhythmics. In the compiled data from Table 2, no torsade de pointes occurred with this drug. In contrast, classic pause-dependent torsades de pointes were found in 4% of 180 patients in a series of Jackman et al.[101].

Monomorphic or polymorphic ventricular tachycardia unassociated with long QT. This is an unusual proarrhythmic response in patients treated for atrial fibrillation or flutter, since it presupposes an established substrate in the ventricular myocardium. This substrate is either due to an old myocardial infarction or a cardiomyopathy with or without overt heart failure. Among the mechanisms causing monomorphic ventricular tachycardia reentry is the most important and especially IC drugs, producing significant frequency dependent conduction slowing are likely to provoke this unexpected proarrhythmia in atrial fibrillation patients. Particularly during the sinus tachycardia of exercise, rate-dependent slowing of intraventricular conduction may become outspoken [103]. Thus, exercise can set the stage for reentry and might be a useful tool to uncover unexpected IC-related ventricular proarrhythmia[84,103,121,122]. The number of cases with monomorphic or polymorphic ventricular tachycardias unassociated with long QT reported in the literature occurring during IC drugs given for supraventricular arrhythmias, is however small[20,49,84,95, 103,122,123]. Most cases did show hemodynamic deterioration during the proarrhythmia, depending on rate and degree of ventricular dysfunction. In our experience among 127 patients receiving flecainide for prevention of recurrent atrial fibrillation after cardioversion 1 patient, not known with ventricular tachycardia before, developed a severe proarrhythmia. She had a hypertensive cardiomyopathy with LVEF 18%. A hemodynamically significant monomorphic ventricular tachycardia with sinusoidal QRS complexes with a left bundle branch block, left axis morphology at a ventricular rate of 198 beats per minute was seen 23 hours after initiation of 100 mg flecainide b.i.d. (Figure 4). Repeated electrical cardioversions were necessary. Between cardioversions she had atrial fibrillation with a mean ventricular rate of 120 beats per minute. After cessation of flecainide recovery was uneventful. She did not have coronary artery disease. Before onset of the proarrhythmia there were no overt signs of heart failure. Sihm et al.[49] retrospectively found severe pro-arrhythmia in 9 of 100 atrial fibrillation or flutter patients receiving flecainide for acute conversion or chronic prophylaxis after cardioversion. Most occurred within the first 5 days of therapy including all severe tachyarrhythmias: ventri-cular tachycardia and fibrillation in 2 patients each and there was 1 patient with sudden death. The other 4 patients had negative dromotropic effects: sinus arrest in 2 and asystole and bradycardia in another 2 patients.

Risk factors for IC proarrhythmia. Factors predisposing to ventricular proarrhythmia with IC drugs are (a) previous sustained ventricular tachycardia, (b) rapid dose increase and high dosage and (c) structural heart disease [124]. Previous myocardial infarction[69] is an example of the latter factor. Although these factors mainly have been identified in the ventricular arrhythmia population, it is reasonable to assume that these also apply for patients with atrial arrhythmias. On the other hand, it is important to note that in contrast to the quinidine-like drugs, ventricular proarrhythmia or sudden death is virtually absent in patients without overt heart disease.

CAST[69] has shown that proarrhythmia with IC drugs does not exclusively occur early after initiation of therapy but appeared ongoing throughout follow-up. Which factors relate to late (out-of-hospital) pro-arrhythmia or sudden death during IC drug therapy are not completely clear. In CAST[69] several have been suggested: late development of ischemia which may be more arrhythmogenic in the presence of IC drugs; congestive heart failure whether or not elicited by the drug; and cumulation of the drug to toxic levels. It is reasonable to assume that for supraventricular tachycardia patients with CAST-like clinical characteristics (particularly ischemic myocardial disease) similar risk factors for late proarrhythmia apply.

Aberrant conduction. One diagnostic pitfall potentially leading to over-diagnosis of ventricular proarrhythmia with class IC drugs, deserves attention. Aberrant conduction in the presence of IC drugs may be very difficult to differentiate from ventricular tachycardia[77,75,80,81] (Figures 2 and 5). In our own experience with wide QRS tachycardias during IC drugs, classic rules [125,126], but also recently developed ones[127], always favoured ventricular tachycardia. In all cases however, we were able to diagnose aberrancy on the basis of observations on prolonged rhythm recordings. These may reveal (a) rate-dependent offset of aberrancy, (b) a match between supraventricular and ventricular rate in the cases with regular tachycardias, or (c) irregularity of the ventricular rhythm strongly suggesting atrial fibrillation as the dominant rhythm.

Aberrant ventricular conduction may occur in virtually every patient with atrial fibrillation. Different types may be present: rate-related or interval-dependent (Ashman phenomenon or phase IV aberrancy)[128]. In some patients its onset is not compatible with one of these mechanisms and may be due to 'fatigue' or overdrive suppression[129]. This phenomenon has been observed during flecainide treatment in atrial fibrillation patients[130] and may be typical for IC drugs. Its clinical importance lies in the fact that aberrancy with IC drugs does not always conform to the normal rules for aberrant conduction, thereby enhancing the above mentioned confusion when differentiating between aberrancy and ventricular tachycardia.

Atrial proarrhythmia. An increase in the propensity to develop chronic atrial fibrillation during prophylactic therapy is extremely difficult to establish. In fact, a recurrence of chronic arrhythmia may indicate inefficacy of the drug or a proarrhythmic response. In a serial electrical approach, followed by serial drug treatment some patients might be identified who have proarrhythmia in that they have recurrences earlier after cardioversion **with** drugs than without them. In our own experience with pirmenol, a class I antiarrhythmic, a young female with ventricular arrhythmias in the setting of mitral valve prolapse syndrome, developed chronic atrial fibrillation on this antiarrhythmic which was never recorded before and which reverted to sinus rhythm after withdrawal of

Figure 4.

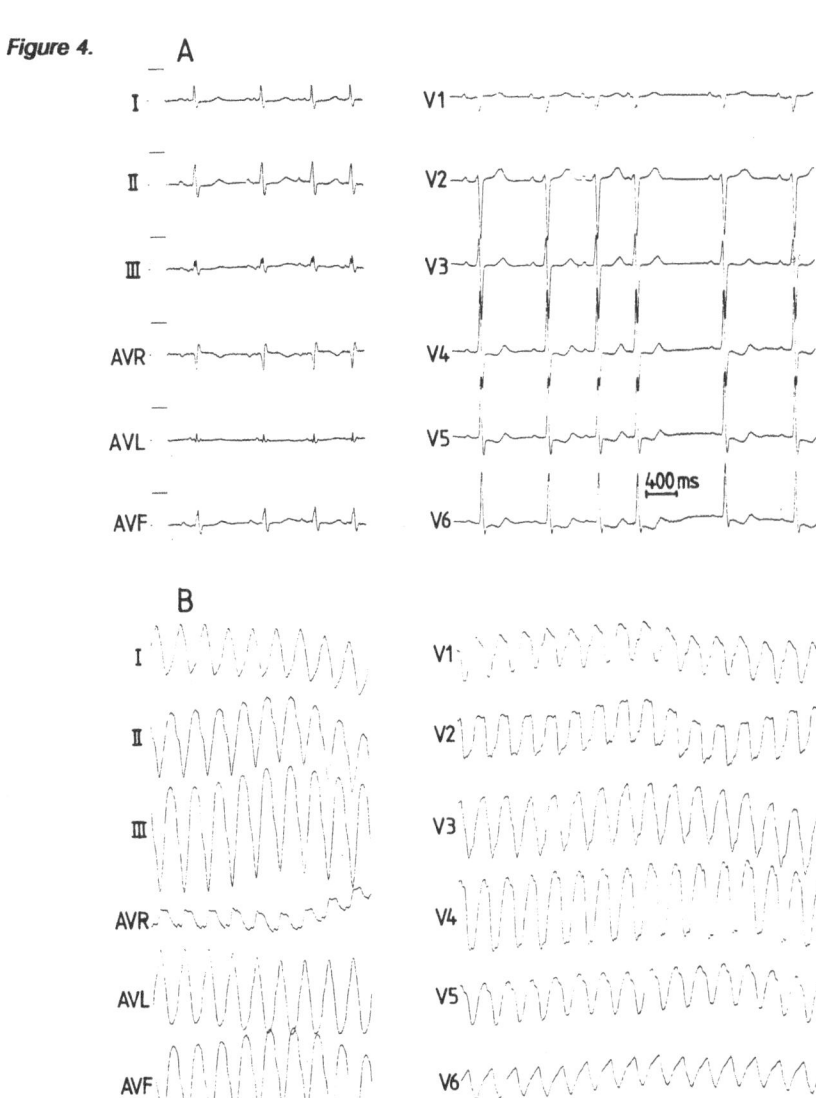

Proarrhythmic event in a 61 year old female, during stage I. Panel A shows the 12 lead ECG after DC electrical cardioversion for chronic atrial fibrillation: sinus rhythm with frequent premature atrial complexes; minimal intraventricular conduction delay with QRS duration 0.09 s, presumably due to the combination of initial conduction delay (absent 'septal' q-wave in leads I and V6) and a terminal delay (r-wave lead aVR). Aspecific ST-T wave abnormalities, unchanged compared to previous ECGs. Panel B: ventricular tachycardia with a left bundle branch block, left axis morphology, 23 hours after initiation of 100 mg flecainide b.i.d.. Most leads show a sinusoidal QRS morphology. Lead V1 shows a 2:1 relationship between QRS-complexes and P-waves, presumably due to 2:1 VA conduction (see text for details).

Figure 5.

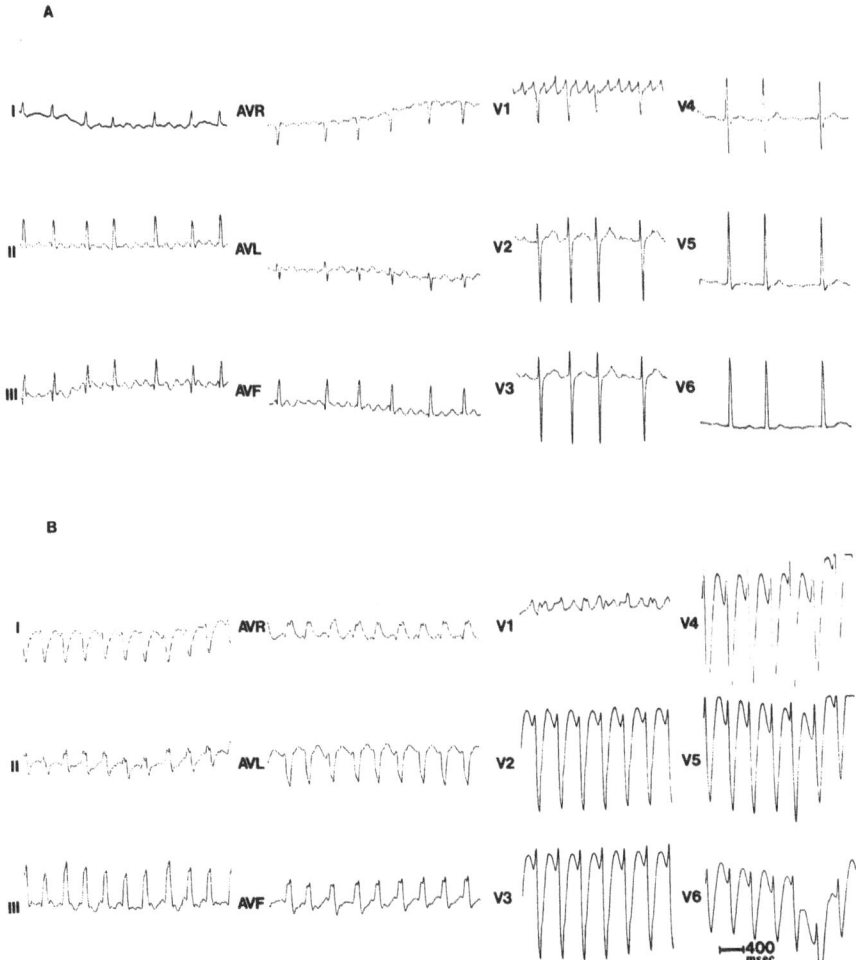

Panel A: control ECG showing atrial flutter. Panel B: Wide QRS tachycardia 1 minute after 150 mg flecainide intravenously for termination of atrial flutter. Flutter slowed but was not converted. 1:1 AV conduction was diagnosed during carotid sinus massage during continuous rhythm recording, showing match between tachycardia rate and flutter rate as well as interval-dependent normalization of intraventricular conduction. Calibration: 10 mm/mV.

the drug. This sequence of events could be observed several times in this patient. In general however, this may be considered a rare complication and therefore presumably has only minor clinical significance.

Acceleration of ventricular rate. Antiarrhythmics may facilitate AV conduction by slowing the intrinsic atrial rate in atrial fibrillation or causing a more organised atrial rhythm (flutter) thereby diminishing concealed antegrade AV nodal conduction. In addition, anticholinergic effects of some drugs may lead to increased conduction velocity and shortened refractoriness in the AV node. In case of atrial fibrillation in the Wolff-Parkinson-White syndrome accessory pathway conduction may become enhanced after shortening of its refractoriness (digitalis, lidocaine, adrenergic influences) or after decreased retrograde concealed conduction into the abnormal pathway due to reduced transmission of impulses over the AV node (all drugs hampering AV nodal conduction). Clinical implications, particularly with respect to the differential effects of class I and class III antiarrhythmics, have been mentioned above.

Bradycardia. A substantial number of atrial fibrillation patients may suffer from underlying sick sinus syndrome. All antiarrhythmics may aggravate sinus arrests in this condition. Sometimes concomitant AV nodal conduction disturbances exist further decreasing safety of drug therapy. In some cases precardioversion AV node conduction problems may be evident, and in these electrical cardioversion may be abandoned in the first place. If drug treatment is considered unavoidable, implantation of a permanent pacemaker will be necessary in a few cases.

GENERAL GUIDELINES FOR DRUG TREATMENT AFTER CARDIOVERSION

Before instituting an antiarrhythmic drug after cardioversion the benefit-to-risk ratio of drug therapy should be determined, taking the above mentioned efficacy rates and risk factors into account. Obviously, provoking factors like heart failure, hypertension and ischemia should be corrected first. If antiarrhythmic therapy is deemed unavoidable, early and late proarrhythmia should be prevented.

Since all antiarrhythmics, may provoke significant proarhythmia electrical cardioversion without postshock institution of class I or III antiarrhythmics is advocated (especially if low recurrence risk). If a fast ventricular rate during atrial fibrillation caused symptoms, simple and safe negative chronotropic drugs (digitalis, calcium antagonist, ß-blocker) may be given after the shock.

However, if frequent recurrences are expected during a serial *electrical* approach, institute *serial drug treatment*. This should be considered only in severely symptomatic patients. In others, accepting atrial fibrillation as the dominant rhythm and institution of negative chronotropic drugs may be sufficient to control symptoms and prevent a tachycardiomyopathy. In patients with established chronic arrhythmia: *never* use class I drugs to control the ventricular rate. If risk for drug related proarrhythmia is deemed too high, and patients cannot be controlled with negative chronotropic drugs, consider AV ablation.

During a serial drug treatment approach, we propose sotalol as first line agent; in patients without significant myocardial disease the IC drugs flecainide or propafenone may be an alternative; and as a last resort amiodarone. IC drugs should be avoided if the patient has CAST-like clinical characteristics. Occasionally quinidine(-like) drugs may be useful.

Serial electrical treatment should be avoided in significant mitral valve disease especially stenosis (no beneficial effects on left ventricular and left atrial function). Serial drug treatment should not be carried out in old patients and those who had more than 3 previous episodes of chronic arrhythmia (primary inefficacy of drugs).

If after restoration of sinus rhythm significant and persisting signs of sick sinus syndrome are found, long term prophylactic therapy using whatever antiarrhythmic may be hazardous and should be avoided. Pacemaker implantation may be warranted in some cases after which drug treatment sometimes is attempted.

Atrial fibrillation and heart failure. All antiarrhythmics should be avoided in atrial fibrillation associated with congestive heart failure. In these patients optimal heart failure therapy and adequate rate control is indicated. Especially these patients may benefit from a serial electrical approach keeping the intercardioversion intervals as short as possible in order to maintain beneficial hemodynamic effects gained during the previous period of sinus rhythm. Finally, if necessary, amiodarone may be used as prophylactic agent in resistant cases. Especially if a *serial electrical* approach is chosen and the interval to relapse is too short (<1 month), this agent may be helpful in prolonging the period in sinus rhythm and provoke a hemodynamic improvement which in turn may enhance maintenance of sinus rhythm.

Prevention of late proarrhythmia is of extreme importance. In this respect, special attention should be paid to intercurrent ischemia and congestive heart failure, and intercurrent hypokalemia or hypomagnesemia. With quinidine-like drugs intercurrent bradycardia or its equivalents (sudden pauses) are of special importance and their effects on the rhythm should be known before discharging the patient. For prevention of late proarrhythmia with IC drugs it seems especially important to avoid rapid ventricular rates which may occur during a recurrence. Patients likely to develop rapid AV conduction should receive negative chronotropics and the advise to temporarily avoid vigorous exercise at an arrhythmia relapse. Finally, addition of other drugs should be avoided or if necessary, carefully evaluated. Also, too low (quinidine) and too high dosages (sotalol, IC drugs) should be avoided.

References

[1]   Morris Jr JJ, Peter RH, McIntosh HD. Electrical cardioversion of atrial fibrillation. Immediate and long term results and selection of patients. Ann Int Med 1966;65:216-231.
[2]   Waris E, Kreus KE, Salokannel J. Factors influencing persistence of sinus rhythm after DC shock treatment of atrial fibrillation. Acta Med Scand 1971;189:161-166.
[3]   Lewis RV, Laing E, Moreland TA, Service E, McDevitt DG. A comparison of digoxin, diltiazem and their combination in the treatment of atrial fibrillation. Eur Heart J 1988;9-:384-390.
[4]   Lipkin DP, Frenneaux M, Stewart R, Joshi J, Lowe T, McKenna WJ. Delayed improvement in exercise capacity after cardioversion of atrial fibrillation to sinus rhythm. Br Heart J 1988; 59:572-77.
[5]   Atwood JE, Myers J, Sandhu S, Lachterman B, Friis R, Oshita A, Forbes S, Walsh D, Froelicher V. Optimal sampling interval to estimate heart rate at rest and during exercise in atrial fibrillation. Am J Cardiol 1989;63:45-48.
[6]   Van Gelder IC, Landsman MJ, Crijns HJ. Delayed improvement in exercise capacity after electrical cardioversion of atrial fibrillation to sinus rhythm. Circulation 1989;80:II-609.
[7]   Kannel WB, Abbott RD, Savage DD, McNamara PM. Epidemiologic features of chronic atrial fibrillation. N Engl J Med 1982;306:1018-1022.
[8]   Petersen P, Godtfredsen. Atrial fibrillation-a review of course and prognosis. Acta Med Scand 1984;216:3-9.
[9]   Coplen SE, Antman EM, Berlin JA, Hewitt P, Chalmers TC. Efficacy and safety of quinidine therapy for maintenance of sinus rhythm after cardioversion. A meta-analysis of randomized controlled trials Circulation 1990;82:1106-1116.
[10] Berns E, Rinkenberger RL, Jeang MK, Dougherty AH, Jenkins M, Naccarelli GV. Efficacy and safety of flecainide acetate for atrial tachycardia or fibrillation. Am J Cardiol 1987;59:1337-1341

[11]   Antman EM, Beamer AD, Cantillon C, McGowan N, Goldman L, Friedman PL. Long-
        term oral propafenone therapy for suppression of refractory symptomatic atrial
        fibrillation and atrial flutter. J Am Coll Cardiol 1988;12:1005-1011.
[12]   Gold RL, Haffajee CI, Charos G, Sloan K, Baker S, Alpert JS. Amiodarone for refractory
        atrial fibrillation. Am J Cardiol 1986;57:124-127.
[13]   Graboys TB, Podrid PJ, Lown B. Efficacy of amiodarone for refractory supraventricular
        tachyarrhythmias. Am Heart J 1983;106:870-876.
[14]   Horowitz LN, Spielman SR, Greenspan AM et al. Use of amiodarone in the treatment of
        persistent and paroxysmal atrial fibrillation resistant to quinidine therapy. J Am Coll
        Cardiol 1985; 6:1402-1407.
[15]   Blomström P, Edvardsson N, Olsson B. Amiodarone in atrial fibrillation. Acta Med
        Scand 1984;216:517-524.
[16]   Coumel P. Role of the autonomic nervous system in paroxysmal atrial fibrillation. In:
        Touboul P, Waldo AL, eds. Atrial Arrhythmias. Current concepts and management.
        Mosby-Year Book Inc. 1990: 248-61.
[17]   Flugelman MY, Hasin Y, Gotsman MS. Restoration and maintenance of sinus rhythm
        after mitral valve surgery for mitral stenosis. Am J Cardiol 1984; 54:617-619.
[18]   Resnekov L, McDonald L. Appraisal of electroconversion in treatment of cardiac
        dysrhythmias. Br Heart J 1968;30:786-811.
[19]   Bjerkelund C, Orning OM. An evaluation of DC shock treatment of atrial arrhythmias.
        Acta Med Scand 1968;184:481-491.
[20]   Crijns HJ, Van Gelder IC, Van Gilst WH, Hillege H, Gosselink ATM, Lie KI. Serial
        antiarrhythmic drug treatment to maintain sinus rhythm after electrical cardioversion for
        chronic atrial fibrillation or atrial flutter. Am J Cardiol 1991;68:335-341.
[21]   DeSilva RA, Lown B. Cardioversion and defibrillation. Am Heart J 1980;100:881-895.
[22]   Brodsky MA, Allen BJ, Walker CJ, Casey TP, Luckett CR, Henry WL. Amiodarone for
        maintenance of sinus rhythm after conversion of atrial fibrillation in the setting of a
        dilated left atrium. Am J Cardiol 1987;60:572-575.
[23]   Brodsky MA, Allen BJ, Capparelli EV, Luckett CR, Morton R, Henry WL. Factors
        determining maintenance of sinus rhythm after chronic atrial fibrillation with left atrial
        dilatation. Am J Cardiol 1989;63:1065-1068.
[24]   Henry WL, Morganroth J, Pearlman AS, Clark CE, Redwood DR, Itscoitz SB, Epstein
        SE. Relation between echocardiographically determined left atrial size and atrial
        fibrillation. Circulation 1976;53:273-279.
[25]   Höglund C, Rosenhamer G. Echocardiographic left atrial dimension as a predictor of
        maintaining sinus rhythm after conversion of atrial fibrillation. Acta Med Scand 1985;
        217:411-415.
[26]   Resnekov L, McDonald L. Electroversion of lone atrial fibrillation and flutter including
        hemodynamic studies at rest and on exercise. Br Heart J 1971;33:339-350.
[27]   Dittrich HC, Erickson JS, Schneiderman T, Blacky R, Savides T, Nicod PH. Echocardi-
        ographic and clinical predictors for outcome of elective cardioversion of atrial fibril-
        lation. Am J Cardiol 1989;63:193-197.
[28]   Hall JI, Wood DR. Factors affecting cardioversion of atrial arrhythmias with special
        reference to quinidine. Br Heart J 1968;30:84-90.
[29]   Gajewski J, Singer RB. Mortality in an insured population with atrial fibrillation. JAMA
        1981; 245:1540-44.
[30]   Ewy GA, Ulfers L, Hager D, Rosenfeld AR, Roeske WR, Goldman S. Response of atrial
        fibrillation to therapy: role of etiology and left atrial diameter. J Electrocardiol 1980;13:
        119-124.
[31]   Van Gelder IC. Management of chronic atrial fibrillation in the nineties. Thesis. Universi-
        ty of Groningen, The Netherlands, 1991.

[32] Van Gelder IC, Crijns HJ, Van Gilst WH, Van Wijk LM, Hamer JPM, Lie KI. Efficacy and Safety of Flecainide Acetate in the Maintenance of Sinus Rhythm After Electrical Cardioversion of Chronic Atrial Fibrillation or Atrial Flutter. Am J Cardiol 1989;64:1317-1321.

[33] Lundström T, Ryden L. Chronic atrial fibrillation. Long term results of direct current cardioversion. Acta Med Scand 1988;223:53-59.

[34] Antman EM, Beamer AD, Cantillon C, McGowan N, Friedman PL. Therapy of refractory atrial fibrillation and atrial flutter: A staged care approach with new antiarrhythmic drugs. J Am Coll Cardiol 1990;15:698-707.

[35] Normand JP, Legendre M, Kahn JC, Bourdarias JP, Mathivat A. Comparative efficacy of short-acting and long-term quinidine for maintenance of sinus rhythm after electrical conversion of atrial fibrillation. B Heart J 1976;38:381-387.

[36] Sokolow M, Ball RE. Factors influencing conversion of chronic atrial fibrillation with special reference to serum quinidine concentration. Circulation 1956;14:568-583.

[37] Binder MJ, Rosove L. Paroxysmal ventricular tachycardia due to quinidine. Am J Med 1952;12:491.

[38] Baker CG, Robinson BHB, Trounce JR. Ventricular tachycardia and fibrillation following quinidine. Guy's Hosp. Rep. 1956;105:433.

[39] Thompson GW. Quinidine as a cause of sudden death. Circulation 1956;14:757-65.

[40] Selzer A, Wray HW. Quinidine syncope: Paroxysmal ventricular fibrillation occurring during treatment of chronic atrial arrhythmias. Circulation 1964;30:17-26.

[41] Ejvinsson G, Orinius E. Prodromal ventricular premature beats preceded by a diastolic wave. Acta Med Scand 1980;208:445-450.

[42] Morganroth JL, Goin JE. Quinidine-related mortality in the short-term treatment of ventricular arrhythmias. A meta-analysis. Circulation 1991;84:1977-1983.

[43] Lloyd EA, Gersh BJ, Forman R. The efficacy of quinidine and disopyramide in the maintenance of sinus rhythm after electrocaonversion from atrial fibrillaion. A double-blind study comparing quinidine, disopyramide and placebo. S Afr Med J 1984;65:367-369.

[44] Podrid PJ, Schoenberger A, Lown B. Congestive heart failure caused by oral disopyramide. N Eng J Med 1980;302:614-617.

[45] Anderson JL, Jolivette DM, Fredell PA. Summary of efficacy and safety of flecainide for supraventricular arrhythmias. Am J Cardiol 1988;62:62D-66D.

[46] Benditt DG, Dunnigan A, Buetikofer J, Milstein S. Flecainide acetate for long-term prevention of paroxysmal supraventricular tachyarrhythmias. Circulation 1991;83:345-349.

[47] Rasmussen K. Andersen A, Abrahamsen AM, Overskeid K, Bathen J. Flecainide versus disopyramide in maintaining sinus rhythm following conversion of chronic atrial fibrillation (abstract). Eur Heart J 1988;9(suppl 1):52.

[48] Touboul P, Aliot E, Brembilla-Perrot B. Flecainide in the prevention of atrial fibrillation after cardioversion: Comparison with quinidine. Circulation 1991;84:II-127.

[49] Sihm I, Hansen FA, Rasmussen J, Pedersen AK, Thygesen K. Flecainide acetate in atrial flutter and fibrillation. The arrhythmogenic effects. Eur Heart J 1990;11:145-148.

[50] Josephson MA, Ikeda N, Singh BN. Effects of flecainide on ventricular function: Clinical and experimental correlations. Am J Cardiol 1984;53:95B-100B.

[51] Porterfield JG, Porterfield LM. Therapeutic efficacy and safety of oral propafenone for atrial fibrillation. Am J Cardiol 1989;63:114-116.

[52] Juul-Möller S, Edvardsson N, Rehnqvist-Ahlberg N. Sotalol versus quinidine for the maintenance of sinus rhythm after direct current cardioversion of atrial fibrillation. Circulation 1990;82:1932-1939.

[53]   Hutton I, Lorimer AR, Hillis WR, McCall D, Reid JM, Lawrie TDV. Haemodynamics and myocardial function after sotalol. Br Heart J 1972;34:787-790.

[54]   Cowan JC, Gardiner P, Reid DS, Newell DJ, Campbell RWF. A comparison of amiodarone and digoxin in the treatment of atrial fibrillation complicating suspected acute myocardial infarction. J Cardiovasc Pharmacol 1986;8:252-256.

[55]   Kopelman HA and Horowitz LN. Efficacy and toxicity of amiodarone for the treatment of supraventricular tachyarrhythmias. Prog Card Vasc Dis 1989;31:355-366.

[56]   Ward DE, Camm AJ, Spurrell RAJ. Clinical antiarrhythmic effects of amiodarone in patients with resistant paroxysmal tachycardias. Br Heart J 1980;44:91-95.

[57]   Haffajee CI, Love JC, Canada AT, Lesko LJ, Asdourian G, Alpert JS. Clinical pharma-cokinetics and efficacy of amiodarone for refractory tachyarrhythmias. Circulation 1983;67;6:1347-1355.

[58]   Rosenbaum MB, Chiale PA, Halpern MS, et al. Clinical efficacy of amiodarone as an antiarrhythmic agent. Am J Cardiol 1976;38:934-944.

[59]   Blevins RD, Kerin NZ, Benaderet D, et al. Amiodarone in the management of refractory atrial fibrillation. Arch Intern Med 1987;147:1401-1404.

[60]   Vitolo E, Tronci M, Larovere MT, Rumolo R, Morabito A. Amiodarone versus quinidine in the prophylaxis of atrial fibrillation. Acta Cardiologica 1981;36:431-444.

[61]   Gosselink ATM, Crijns HJ, Van Gelder IC, Hillige H, Lie KI. Long term safety of low dose amiodarone after cardioversion of atrial fibrillation. Circulation 1991;84:II-411.

[62]   Kerin NL, Blevins RD, Kerner N, et al. A low incidence of proarrhythmia using low-dose amiodarone. J Electrophysiol 1988;2:289-295.

[63]   Kowey PR, Friehling TD, Marinchak RA, Sulpizi AM, Stohler JL. Safety and efficacy of amiodarone. The low-dose perspective. Chest 1988;93:54-59.

[64]   Kerin NZ, Aragon E, Faitel K, Frumin H, Rubenfire M. Long term efficacy and toxicity of high- and low-dose amiodarone regimens. J Clin Pharmacol 1989;29:418-423.

[65]   Gottlieb SS, Kukin ML, Medina n, et al. Comparative hemodynamic effects of procaina-mide, tocainide and encainide in severe chronic heart failure. Circulation 1990;81:860-864.

[66]   Gottlieb SS, Weinberg M. Cardiodepressant effects of mexitil in patients with severe left ventricular dysfunction.: Relation to plasma concentrations. Circulation 1989;80:II-429.

[67]   Hamer AW, Arkles LB, Johns JA. Beneficial effects of low dose amiodarone in patients with congestive heart failure: A placebo-controlled trial. J Am Coll Cardiol 1989;14:1-768-74.

[68]   Van Gelder IC, Crijns HJ, Van Gilst WG, Hamer JPM, KI Lie. Decrease of Atrial Sizes after DC Electrical Cardioversion in Patients with Chronic Atrial Fibrillation. Am J Cardiol 1991;67:93-95.

[69]   The Cardiac Arrhythmia Suppresion Trial (CAST) investigators. Preliminary report: effect of encainide and flecainide on mortality in a randomized trial of arrhythmia suppression after myocardial infarction. N Engl J Med 1989;321:406-412.

[70]   Evans GT, Scheinman MM, Bardy G, et al. Predictors of in-hospital mortality after DC catheter ablation of atriaoventricular junction: Results of a prospective, international, multicenter study. Circulations 1991;84:1924-1937.

[71]   London F, Howell M. Atrial flutter: 1 to 1 conduction during treatment with quinidine and digitalis. Am Heart J 1954;48:152-155.

[72]   Robertson CE, Miller HC. Extreme tachycardia complicating the use of disopyramide in atrial flutter. Br Heart J 1980;44:602-603.

[73]   Adamson AR, Spracklen FH. Atrial flutter with block: contraindication to use of lignocai-ne. Br Med J 1968;2:223

[74]   Marriott HJL, Bieza CF. Alarming ventricular acceleration after lidecaine administration. Chest 1972;61:682-687.

[75]   Fauchier JP, Cosnay P, Babuty RD. Drug-induced atrial arrhythmias. In: Touboul P, Waldo AL, eds. Atrial Arrhythmias. Current concepts and management. St. Louis: Mosby Year Book, 1990:288-310.

[76]   Nathan AW, Hellestrand KJ, Bexton RS, Banim SO, Spurrel RAJ, Camm AJ. Proarrhythmic effects of the new antiarrhythmic agent flecainide acetate. Am Heart J 1984;107: 222-228.

[77]   Crijns HJ, Den Heijer P, Van Wijk LM, Lie KI. Successful use of flecainide in atrial fibrillation with rapid ventricular rate in the Wolff-Parkinson-White syndrome. Am Heart J 1988;115:1317-1319.

[78]   Priestley KA et al. Experience with flecainide for the treatment of cardiac arrhythmias in children. Eur Heart J 1988;9:1284.

[79]   Ziegler V, Gillette PC, Ross BA, Ewing L. Flecainide for supraventricular and ventricular arrhythmias in children and young adults. Am J Cardiol 1988;62:818-820.

[80]   Naccarelli GV, Rinkenberger RL, Dougherty AH, Fitzgerald DM, Jenkins M. Occurrence of atrial flutter with 1:1 atrioventricular nodal conduction during encainide and flecainide therapy (abstract). Circulation 1989;80:II-634(A).

[81]   Feld GK, Chen PS, Nicod P, Meyer DB, Fleck RP. Possible atrial proarrhythmic effecs of Class 1C antiarrhythmic drugs. Am J Card 1990;66:378-383.

[82]   Murdock CJ, Kyles AE, Yeung-Lai-Wah JA, Qi A, Vorderbrugge S, Kerr CR. Atrial flutter in patients treated for atrial fibrillation with propafenone. Am J Cardiol 1990;15:755-757.

[83]   Timm CT, Knowlton AA, Battinelli NJ, Falk RH. Flecainide for heart rate control in atrial fibrillation. J Am Coll Cardiol 1989;13:164A.

[84]   Falk RH. Flecainide-induced ventricular tachycardia and fibrillation in patients treated for atrial fibrillation. Ann Intern Med 1989;111:107-111.

[85]   Rowland E, Krikler D. Electrophysiologic assessment of amiodarone in treatment of resistant supraventricular arrhythmias. Br Heart J 1980;44: 82-90.

[86]   Wellens HJJ, Brugada P, Abdollah H. Effect of amiodarone in paroxysmal supraventricular tachycardia with or without Wolff-Parkinson-White syndrome. Am Heart J 1983;106:876-880.

[87]   Perelman MS, McKenna WJ, Rowland E, Krikler Dm. A comparison of bepridil with amiodarone in the treatment of established atrial fibrillation. Br Heart J 1987;58:339-344.

[89]   Akhtar M, Gilbert CJ, Shenasha M. Effect of lodocaine on atrioventricular response via the accessory pathway in patients with Wolff-Parkinson-White syndrome. Circulation 1981;63:435-441.

[90]   Sheinman BD, Evans T. Acceleration of ventricular rate by amiodarone in atrial fibrillation associated with the Wolff-Parkinson-White syndrome. Br Med J 1982;285:999-1000.

[91]   Neuss H, Buss J, Schlepper M, Berthold R, Mitrovic V, Kramer A, Musial WJ. Effects of flecainide on electrophysiological properties of accessory pathways in the Wolff-Parkinson-White Syndrome. Eur Heart J 1983;4:347.

[92]   Kappenberger LJ, Fromer MA, Shenasa M, Gloor HO. Evaluation of flecainide acetate in rapid atrial fibrillation complicating Wolff-Parkinson-White Syndrome. Clin Cardiol 1985;8:321.

[93]   Hellestrand KJ, Nathan AW, Bexton RS, Camm AJ. Electrophysiological effects of flecainide acetate on sinus node function, anomalous atrioventricular connections, and pacemaker thresholds. Am J Cardiol 1984;53:   30B.

[94]   Kim SS, Smith P, Ruffy R. Treatment of atrial tachyarrhythmia and preexcitation syndrome with flecainide acetate. Am J Cardiol 1988;62:29D-34D.

[95] Van Wijk LM, Crijns HJ, Van Gilst WH, Wesseling H, Lie KI. Flecainide acetate in the treatment of supraventricular tachycardias; value of programmed electrical stimulation for long term prognosis. Am Heart J 1989;117:365-369.

[96] Feld GK, Nademanee K, Stevenson W, Weiss J, Klizner T, Singh BN. Clinical and electrophysiological effects of amiodarone in patients with atrial fibrillation complicating the Wolff-Parkinson-White syndrome. Am Heart J 1988;115:102-107.

[97] Fujimura O, Klein GJ, Sharma AD, Yee R, Szabo T. Acute effects of disopyramide on atrial fibrillation in the Wolff-Parkinson-White syndrome. J Am Coll Cardiol 1989;13:113-117.

[98] Koster RW, Wellens HJJ. Quidinine-induced ventricular flutter and fibrillation without digitalis therapy. Am J Cardiol 1976;38:519-23.

[99] Bauman JL, Bauernfeind RA, Hoff JV, Strassberg B, Swiryn S, Rosen KM. Torsade de Pointes due to quinidine: Observations in 31 patients. Am Heart J 1984;107:425-430.

[100] Roden DM, Woosley RL, Primm RK. Incidence and clinical features of the quinidine-associated long QT syndrome: implications for patient care. Am Heart J 1986;111:1088-1093

[101] Jackman WM, Friday KJ, Anderson JL, Aliot EM, Clark M, Lazzara R. The long QT syndromes: a critical review, new clinical observations and a unifying hypothesis. Prog Cardiovasc Dis 1988;31:115-172.

[102] Crijns HJ, Van Wijk LM, Van Gelder IC, Lie KI. Observations on flecainide-induced ventricular tachycardias. PACE 1987; 10: 596.

[103] Ranger S, Talajic M, Lemery R, Roy D, Nattel S. Amplification of flecainide-induced ventricular conduction slowing by exercise. Circulation 1989;79:1000-1006.

[104] Viko LE, Marvin HM, White PD. Clinical report of the use of quinidine sulfate. Arch Intern Med 1923;345-363.

[105] Smith WM, Gallagher JJ. "Les torsade de pointes": An unusual ventricular arhhythmia. Ann Intern Med 1980;93:578.

[106] Keren A, Tzivoni D, Gavish D, et al. Etiology, warning signs and therapy of Torsade de Pointes. A study of 10 patients. Circulation 1981;64:1167-74.

[107] Moss AJ, Schwartz PJ. Delayed repolarization (QT or QTU prolongation) and malignant ventricular arrhythmias. Mod Concepts Cardiovasc Dis 1982;51:85-90.

[108] Kay GN, Plumb VJ, Arciniegas et al. Torsades de pointes: The long-short initiating sequence and other clincial features. Observations in 32 patients. J Am Coll Cardiol 1983;2:806-817.

[109] Webb CL, Dick M, Rocchini AP, Snider AR, Crowly DC, Beekman RH, Spicer RL, Rosenthal A. Quinidine syncope in children. J Am Cardiol 1987;9:1031-1037.

[110] Kerr WJ, Bender WL. Paroxysmal ventricular fibrillation with cardiac recovery in a case of auriculari fibrillation and complete heart block while under quinidine sulphate therapy. Heart 1922;9:269-81.

[111] Denes P, Gabster A, Huang SK. Clinical electrocardiographic and follow-up observations in patients having ventricular fibrillation during Holtermonitoring. Role of quinidine therapy. Am J Cardiol 1981;48:9-16.

[112] Kadish AH, Weisman HF, Veltri EP, Epstein AE, Slepian MJ, Levine JH. Paradoxical effects of exercise on the QT interval in patients with polymorphic ventricular tachycardia receiving type Ia antiarrhythmic agents. Circulation 1990;81:14-19.

[113] Hii JTY, Gillis AM, Wyse DG, Ramadan D, Mitchell BL. Torsade de pointes by class Ia drugs: Incidence and predictive value of exercise testing in 175 consecutive patients (abstract). Circulation 1990;III-55.

[114] Nguyen PT, Scheinman MM, Seger J. Polymorphous vnentricular tachycardia: clinical characterization, therapy and the QT interval. Circulation 1986;74:17-26.

[115]   Clark M. Friday K, Anderson N, Jackman W, Aliot E, Lazarra R. Drug induced torsade de pointes: high concordance rate among type IA antiarrhythmic drugs and amiodarone (abstract). J Am Coll Cardiol 1985;5:450.
[116]   Maloney JD, Nissen RG, McGolgan BS. Open clinical studies at a referral center: Chronic maintenance therapy in patients with recurrent sustained ventricular tachycardia refractory to conventional antiarrhythmic agents. Am Heart J 1980;100:1023-1030.
[117]   Shah A, Schwartz H. Mexiletine for treatment of torsade de pointes. Am Heart J 1984;107:589-591.
[118]   Neuvonen PJ, Elonen E, Vuorenmaa T, et al. Prolonged QT interval and severe tachyarrhythmias, common features of sotalol intoxication. Eur J Clin Pharmacol 1981;20:85-89.
[119]   Kuck KH, Kunze KP, Roewer N, et al. Sotalol-induced torsade de pointes. Am Heart J 1984;107:179-180.
[120]   Falk RH. Proarrhythmic responses to atrial antiarrhythmic therapy. In: Falk RH, Podrid PJ, eds. Atrial fibrillation. Mechanisms and Management. Raven Press, Ltd. 1992:287.
[121]   Anastasiou-Nana MI, Anderson JL, Stewart JR, Crevey BJ, Yanowitz FG, Lutz JR, Johnson TA. Occurrence of exercise-induced and spontaneous wide complex tachycardia during therapy with flecainide for complex ventricular arrhythmias: A probable proarrhythmic effect. Am Heart J 1987; 113:1071-1077.
[122]   Hoffmann A, Wenk M, Follath F. Exercise-induced ventricular tachycardia as a manifestation of flecainide toxicity. Int J Card 1986;11:353-355.
[123]   Rinkenberger RL, Naccarelli GV, Miles WM, Markel ML, Dougherty AH, Prystowsky EN, Heger JJ, Zipes D. Encainide for atrial fibrillation associated with Wolff-Parkinson-White syndrome. Am J Cardiol 1988;62:26L-30L.
[124]   Morganroth JL. Risk factors for the development of proarrhythmic events. Am J Cardiol 1987;59:32E-37E.
[125]   Wellens HJJ, Bär FW, Vanagt EJ, Brugada P, Farré J. The differentiation between ventricular tachycardia and supraventricular tachycardia with aberrant conduction: The value of the 12-lead electrocardiogram, in Wellens HJJ, Kulbertus HE(eds): What's New in Electrocardiography? The Hague, Martinus Nijhoff Publishing, 1981; pp 184-199.
[126]   Kindwall KE, Brown J, Josephson ME. Electrocardiographic criteria for ventricular tachycardia in wide complex left bundle branch block morphology tachycardias. Am J Card 1988;61:1279-1283.
[127]   Brugada P, Brugada J, Mont L, Smeets J, Andries EW. A new approach to the differential diagnosis of a regular tachycardia with a wide QRS complex. Circulation 1991;83:1649-1659.
[128]   Fisch C. Aberration: seventy five years after Sir Thomas Lewis. Br Heart J 1983;50:297-302.
[129]   Fisch C. Bundle branch block after ventricular tachycardia: a manifestation of "fatigue" or "overdrive suppression". J Am Coll Cardiol1984;6:1562-1564.
[130]   Crijns HJ, Van Gelder IC, De Langen C, Lie KI. Use-dependent aberrant conduction during flecainide treatment: A manifestation of "fatigue" (abstract). PACE 1989;12:643.
[131]   Campbell RWF. Drug prophylaxis of atrial fibrillation. In Kulbertus HE, Ollson SB, and Schlepper M, editors: Atrial fibrillation, Mölndal, 1982, AB Hässle.
[132]   Hillestad L, Bjerkelund C, Dale J, Maltau J, Storstein O. Quinidine in maintenance of sinus rhythm after electroconversion of chronic atrial fibrillation. A controlled clinical study. Br Heart J 1971;33:518-521.
[133]   Södermark T, Edhag O, Sjögren A, Jonsson B, Olsson A, Orö L, Danielsson M, Rosenhamer G, Wallin H. Effect of quinidine on maintaining sinus rhythm after conversion of atrial fibrillation or flutter. A multicenter study from Stockholm. Br Heart J 1975;37:486-492.

[134] Byrne-Quinn E, Wing AJ. Maintenance of sinus rhythm after DC reversion of atrial fibrillation. Br Heart J 1970;32:370-376.

[135] Härtel G, Louhija A, Konttinen A, Halonen PI. Value of quinidine in maintainance of sinus rhythm after electric cardioversion of atrial fibrillation. Br Heart J 1970;32:57-60.

[136] Boissel JP, Wolf E, Gillet J, Soubrane A, Cavallaro A, Mazoyer G, Delahaye JP. Controlled trial of a long-acting quinidine for maintenance of sinus rhythm after conversion of sustained atrial fibrillation. Eur Heart J 1981;2:49-55.

[137] Gunning JF, Kristinsson A, Miller G, Saunders K. Long-term follow-up of direct current cardioversion after cardiac surgery with special reference to quinidine. Br Heart J 1970;32:462-466.

[138] Rasmussen K, Wang H, Fausa D. Comparative efficiency of quinidine and verapamil in the maintenance of sinus rhythm after DC conversion of atrial fibrillation. A controlled clinical trial. Acta Med Scand 1981;Suppl 645:23-28.

[139] Edhag O, Erhardt LR, Lundman T, Södermark T, Sjögren A. Verapamil and quinidine in maintaining sinus rhythm after electroconversion of atrial fibrillation. Opuscula Medica 1982;27:22-24.

[140] Radford MD, Evans DW. Long term results of DC reversion of atrial fibrillation. Br Heart J 1968;30:91-96.

[141] Härtel G, Louhija A, Konttinen A. Disopyramide in the prevention of atrial fibrillation after electroconversion. Clin Pharm Ther 1974;15:551-555.

[142] Karlson BW, Torstensson I, Åbjörn C, Jansson SO, Peterson LE. Disopyramide in the maintenance of sinus rhythm after electrocardioversion of atrial fibrillation. A placebo controlled one-year follow-up study. Eur Heart J 1988;9:284-290.

Chapter 8

EPISODIC TREATMENT OF

PAROXYSMAL ATRIAL FIBRILLATION

Loraine Lie-A-Huen

J. Herre Kingma

Departments of Clinical Cardiology
and
Research & Development Cardiology
St Antonius Hospital
Nieuwegein
The Netherlands

J. H. Kingma et al. (eds.), Atrial fibrillation, a treatable disease?, 149–157.
© 1992 *Kluwer Academic Publishers*.

INTRODUCTION _____

Most symptoms of diseases are exhibited by an irregular course of attacks. For example there is asthma, epilepsy, cluster headache, migraine and different types of tachycardia. All of these examples have a chronic and episodic form. It is the irregular pattern of the attacks which affects the patients quality of life. How to cope with the sudden onset of an attack is not only uncomfortable for the patient but a source of anxiety and concern over the ability to continue to function as usual. However, there is the old cliché: "You will have to live with it".

Hitherto, treatment of these diseases had a prophylactic and routine character. Patients were instructed to take the drug of choice, several times a day, in order to prevent the next attack. However, it is the very irrigular incidence of the attacks which makes routine and chronic treatment less attractive. Patients motivation to take their medication on a regular basis for a long period of time, without even experiencing an attack of a disease, is low. This reason for patients noncompliance is well understood[1].

In order to improve patients compliance to therapy, pharmaceutical industries now develop different formulations of drugs with a retarded delivery of the active drug component in the required pharmaceutical dosage. Modern dosage regimens are based on an once a day schedule. Another feasible possibility is the development of drug delivery systems which deliver a bolus dose controlled by a trigger manually initiated by the patient, such as the management of pain by a morphine pump or automatically triggered by a measured physiologic parameter such as the delivery of insulin by a pump, depending on the blood sugar concentration in a diabetes patient. When maintenance therapy is required because of too frequent attacks, episodic intermittent drug therapy may still be of value in the treatment of breakthrough episodes.

DEVELOPMENT OF EPISODIC
TREATMENT UNTIL NOW _____

Treatment of an acute attack rather than prophylactic treatment on a regular basis can also be accomplished by selfadministration by the patient of a dose of the drug at the onset of the very first symptoms of an attack. For the comfort of the patient it is important that the patient can selfadminister the drug in an outpatient situation.

In 1980 [2] episodic drug treatment in the management of paroxysmal arrhythmias was reported by using a cocktail with a combination of different antiarrhythmic agents. Failure of episodic high-dose oral verapamil therapy to convert supraventricular tachycardia was also reported[3]. In noncomparative clinical trials, adenosine terminated 85% to 100% of induced or spontaneous episodes of paroxysmal supraventricular tachycardias involving the AV node in the reentrant circuit[4]. Adenosine is an ideal drug for episodic treatment due to its short half-life of 0.6 to 10 seconds, however, the possibility of only intravenous administration limits its episodic use to the clinical setting. Further- more the intermittent use of sublingual nitrates in angina is well known. Apart from cardiology, the management of other diseases by episodic treatment is investigated. Treatment of acute, episodic asthma in preschool children using intermittent high dose inhaled steroids at home is described[5]. Finally, the management of migraine is described by acute rectal administration of 600 mg pirprofen capsules in a double-blind within patient randomized study[6]. Pirprofen significantly reduced the duration of headache attack and associated symptoms, but not the peak of pain intensity. Recently a new drug, sumatrip- tan, has entered the drug market for the acute management of migraine attacks. The claimed innovative success of this drug has been established by patients knowing the discomfort of migraine attacks on their quality of life.

(DIS)ADVANTAGES _____

Apart from the patients compliance, other disadvantages are related to chronic, prophylactic drug treatment. The adverse effects of the drug, developed during chronic treatment, may tempt the patient to change the dosage or even to discontinue the medication in the course of treatment. In case of paroxysmal supraventricular tachycardia, the alternative of frequent cardioversions requiring repeated hospitalizations is both costly and inconvenient for patients. A similar comparison, in terms of cost, can be made for the chronic regular maintenance treatment of other diseases. As demonstrated above, the development of episodic drug treatment in the management of specific diseases has started. Before applying this episodic treatment, both the pharmaceutical dosage formulation and the disease have to meet several criteria. Episodic treatment is defined as enteral selfadministration of the drug on the basis of the appearance of an attack when anticipated by the patient or shortly after onset of such an attack. This implies irregular drug intake but at the same time the absolute requirement of rapid and reproducible absorption in order to ensure a rapid build up of therapeutic serum concentrations. The clinician and the patient should be provided with a dosage form, that guarantees an adequate effect under many different circumstances. Irrespective of whether the patient has just taken food or has an empty stomach, the extent and rate of absorption should be reproducible.

When considering to which diseases episodic drug treatment may be applied, it is obvious that patients must be able to indicate the sudden onset of the attack in advance. Furthermore the severity of the attack must not be a great risk to patients health. In other words the management of the attack may last for a certain time period, during which effective therapeutic drug concentrations are attained.

PAROXYSMAL ATRIAL FIBRILLATION _____

Paroxysmal atrial fibrillation seems to meet these criteria for episodic treatment. A study of the feasibility of episodic rather than chronic treatment of atrial fibrillation seemed worthwhile. Although not severe initially, treatment of paroxysmal atrial fibrillation may become necessary either if an attack is longstanding and very symptomatic or if it occurs in the setting of heart failure, which even may constitute a life threatening event. It is said that all of us could experience at least one attack of atrial fibrillation in our life, for instance after a heavy meal or drinking. However, some patients with atrial fibrillation experience attacks of atrial fibrillation several times a year or even several times a day.

Currently, patients with frequent attacks of atrial fibrillation have to be frequently hosptalized to obtain acute conversion to sinus rhythm either by DC cardioversion, intravenous administration of an antiarrhythmic drug or a combination of both. For the prevention of recurrences, the clinician traditionally relies on prescribing an oral maintenance dosage regimen of antiarrhythmic drugs to be taken two to four times daily.

Figure 1.   **Flecainide**

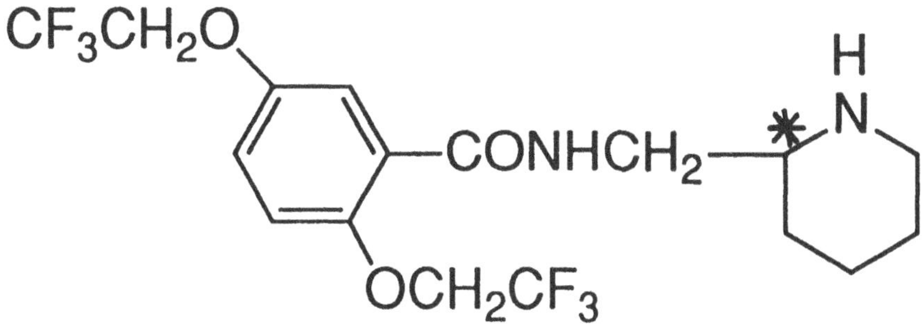

Flecainide (Fig.1) has shown promising results in the conversion of attacks of atrial fibrillation to normal i.e. sinus rhythm. Flecainide was compared with other antiarrhythmic drugs such as verapamil and propafenone. Apart from the lower efficacy of these antiarrhythmic drugs in terminating paroxysmal atrial fibrillation, the absorption kinetics of verapamil and propafenone are less suitable for episodic treatment, since both drugs exhibit an extensive first-pass effect. Based upon these arguments flecainide was chosen as a model drug to study the feasibility of episodic treatment in patients with atrial fibrillation[7]. Flecainide is marketed in the European Community for oral and intravenous administration and is available in ampoules containing 150 mg flecainide acetate and tablets containing 100 mg flecainide acetate.

Considering the requirements for episodic treatment, an optimal dosage form for antiarrhythmic medication to be used at the onset of the arrhythmia had to be initially developed. Various enteral dosage forms are in principle possible. Rectal administration of the drug in a solution seems appropriate in this respect, since this administration route lacks some of the potential problems of oral administration in which the rate of absorption may vary greatly with feeding conditions and or the dissolution rate of tablets. In order to decide which enteral dosage form of flecainide could be easily used by the patient in his own surrounding, the absorption profiles after oral and rectal administration were studied in seven healthy volunteers (Fig.2)[8]. The mean absolute bioavailability was 98%, 78% and 81% for the rectally administered solution, the oral solution and the tablet containing 100 mg flecainide. The lagtime found after administration of an oral solution was 0.33 h, after the tablet 0.86 h and only 0.18 h after administration of the rectal solution.

Figure 2.

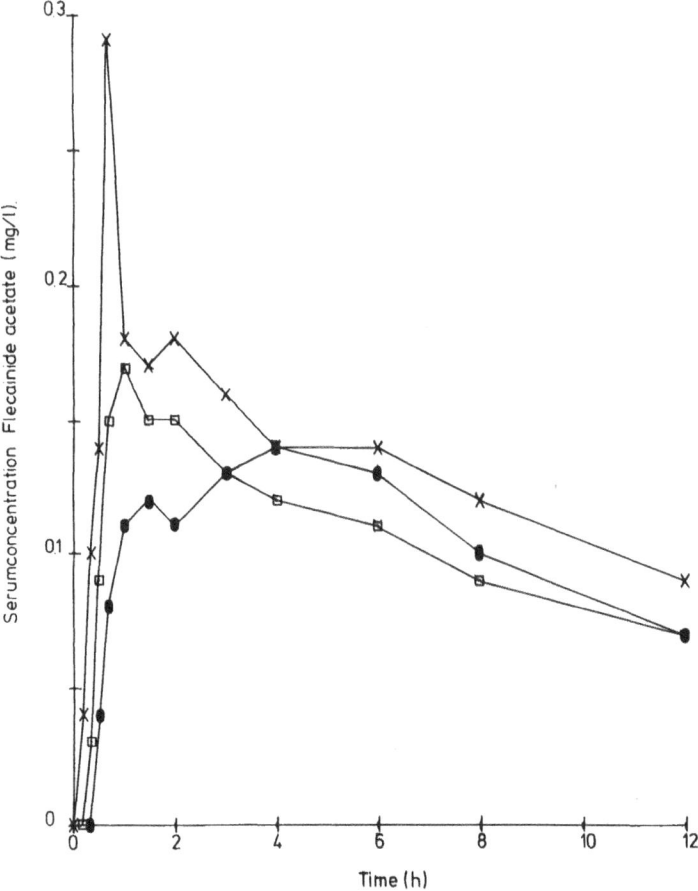

Mean serumconcentration(mg/l) versus time(h) profiles after administration of oral solution(□), rectal solution (X) and tablet (●) containing 100 mg flecainide acetate each.

The mean time to reach a maximum serum concentration (tmax) after administration of the rectal solution (0.67 h) was shorter compared to tmax after either a tablet (4 h) or the oral solution (1 h). The maximum serum concentration, Cmax, found were 0.29 mg/l after administration of the rectal solution, 0.14 mg/l after administration of the tablet and 0.17 mg/l after administration of the oral solution. Based upon reliable and complete bioavailability and a significant higher rate of absorption, rectal solution of flecainide seemed a suitable form for episodic treatment of paroxysmal atrial fibrillation so far.

THE 'IDEAL' FORMULATION

Since the relative lack of ease in administering the rectal solution in the outclinic situation is a major disadvantage, the search for a suitable oral dosage form of flecainide continued. In trying to avoid major variability in presentation rate as much as possible, the influence on the absorption kinetics of the addition of a gastric emptying promoter, the prokinetic drug cisapride, to the oral solution of flecainide was studied[9]. Cisapride is known to promote gastric motility in man by stimulating the release of acetylcholine on the myenteric plexus. By virtue of this property it accelerates the absorption of other drugs such as benzodiazepine, morphine, digoxin and H2-receptorblocking agents. To the same seven volunteers that already participated in the absorption study mentioned above an oral solution of 100 mg flecainide in combination with 20 mg cisapride was administered and the absorption profiles with and without the addition of a gastric emptying promotor were compared (Figure 3). The bioavailability of the oral solution without cisapride was 75% compared to 84% for the oral solution with cisapride. The addition of cisapride raised the maximun serum concentration Cmax from 0.17 to 0.27 mg/l, an increase of approximately 60%. The absorption rate constant after administration of the oral solution with cisapride was two times ($p < 0.05$) higher (1.74 1/h) compared to the absorption rate constant after oral solution without cisapride (0.83 1/h). A clearly stimulating effect of cisapride on the absorption rate of flecainide was demonstrated. On the basis of these results it can be concluded that the addition of cisapride to an oral solution of flecainide is a favourable enteral formulation in the episodic treatment of paroxysmal atrial fibrillation. Considering the practical convenience for the outclinic patient confronted with a sudden attack of atrial fibrillation in the daily situation, administration of the oral solution rather than the rectal solution should probably be preferred.

Figure 3.

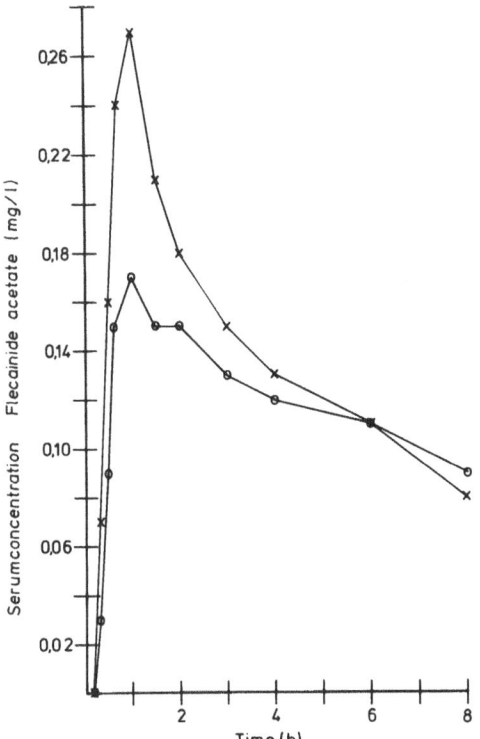

Mean serum concentration of Flecainide acetate (mg/l) versus time (h) after administration of an oral solution with (x) and without (o) 20mg cisapride containing 100 mg flecainide

Finally, the oral solution of flecainide containing cisapride was adminis- tered to patients in the hospital with paroxysmal atrial fibrillation[10]. In an open study the feasibility of episodic treatment of paroxysmal atrial fibrillation was tested in six patients with a single dose of 400 mg flecainide. Treatment was considered successful if sinus rhythm was obtained within 2 hours after dosing. Conversion to sinus rhythm was achieved in 4 of 6 (66%) patients. The average time to conversion was 0.9 h. Therapeutic effective serum concen- trations were measured in all patients 40 minutes after dosing. The mean maximum serum concentration Cmax was 0.80 mg/l, 80 minutes following the administration of the flecainide solution. Combined with cisapride, flecainide can be used in an oral solution for episodic treatment of paroxysmal atrial fibrillation. A dose-finding study in a larger group of patients is necessary to define the feasibility and the adequate dose.

CONCLUSION

Although the number of patients that participated in this part of the study was not large enough to be conclusive, the preliminary results seem promising. If these results would be confirmed, patients with paroxysmal atrial fibrillation could be discharged from the hospital with a solution of oral flecainide at hand and instructed to take this medication only at the first symptoms of an attack of atrial fibrillation. If this flecainide solution proves to be successful in the treatment of paroxysmal atrial fibrillation, such patients could be relieved of lifelong, daily, intake of antiarrhythmic agents.

References

[1]   Squire A, Goldman ME, Kupersmith J, Stern EH, Fuster V et al. (1984) Long-term antiarrhythmic therapy: problem of low drug levels and patients noncompliance. Am J Med 77: 1035-1038.

[2]   Margolis B, DeSilva RA, Lown B (1980) Episodic drug treatment in the management of paroxysmal arrhythmias. Am J Cardiol 45:621-626.

[3]   Hamer AW, Tanasescu DE, Marks JW, Peter T, Waxman AD, Mandel WJ (1987) Failure of episodic high-dose oral verapamil therapy to convert supraventricular tachycardia: a study of plasma verapamil levels and gastric motility. Am Heart J 114: 334-42.

[4]   Parker RB, McCollam PL (1990) Adenosine in the episodic treatment of paroxysmal supraventricular tachycardia. Clin Pharm 9:261-271.

[5]   Wilson NM, Silverman M (1990) Treatment of acute, episodic asthma in preschool children using intermittent high dose inhaled steroids at home. Arch Dis Child 65:407-410.

[6]   Guidotti M, Zanasi S, Garagiola U (1989) Pirprofen in the treatment of migraine and episodic headache attacks: a placebo-controlled crossover clinical trial. J Int Med Res 17:48-54.

[7]   Suttorp MJ, Kingma JH, Jessurum ER, Lie-A-Huen L, van Hemel NM, Lie KI (1990) The value of class IC antiarrhythmic drugs for acute conversion of paroxysmal atrial fibrillation or flutter to sinus rhythm. J Am Coll Cardiol 16:1722-1727.

[8]   Lie-A-Huen L, Proost JH, Kingma JH, Meijer DKF (1990) Absorption kinetics of oral and rectal flecainide in healthy subjects. Eur J Clin Pharmacol 38:595-598.

[9]   Lie-A-Huen L, Proost JH, Kingma JH, Meijer DKF The gastric emptying promoter cisapride improves the absorption rate of oral flecainide: a useful interaction for anti-arrhythmic treatment of the outclinic patient. submitted for publication.

[10]   Lie-A-Huen L, Suttorp MJ, van 't Hof AWJ, Hulst RM, Meijer DKF, Kingma JH Is episodic treatment of paroxysmal atrial fibrillation feasible with an oral solution of flecainide? submitted for publication.

Chapter 9

AN AICD FOR ATRIAL FIBRILLATION?

Andrew M. Tonkin

Jonathan M. Kalman

* Norma Gilli

Department of Cardiology
Austin Hospital, Melbourne
and
* Telectronics Pty. Ltd., Sydney
Australia

J. H. Kingma et al. (eds.), Atrial fibrillation, a treatable disease?, 159–165.

INTRODUCTION

Some 20 years ago, Mirowski, Mower and coworkers showed the feasibility of achieving low energy transcatheter reversion of atrial fibrillation in canines[1]. They found that the delivery of 0.05-0.5 joules was usually effective and 1-3 joules always effective in terminating atrial fibrillation in animals in whom the arrhythmia was initiated by topical application of acetyl choline and gentle traction of the atrial appendage. In the same model, 40-100 joules were needed for cardioversion with transthoracic shock. These findings relating to the success of low energy defibrillation have been corroborated by a number of other investigators[2,3].

The possible extension of this technique to clinical practice is again being investigated because of the general acceptance of the implantable defibrillator as a treatment modality for patients with ventricular tachyarrhythmi-as, and the suboptimal nature of pharmacological approaches. In addition, implantation of a defibrillator for the treatment of ventricular arrhythmias is followed by the development of new-onset atrial fibrillation in up to 20% of patients[4]. This occurs because shock delivery may occur within the atrial vulnerable period. Also, the benefits of maintenance of sinus rhythm in decreasing thromboembolic events and in optimising cardiac performance in patients with heart failure are well known.

Various aspects of the technique of transcatheter atrial defibrillation will be discussed in this article, and data relating to testing of a newer lead system in canines and a patient are presented.

ANIMAL EXPERIMENTATION

A number of aspects which might influence the efficacy and extension to clinical practice of transcatheter defibrillation have been studied in grey-hounds.

a. Shock delivery. Work by a number of investigators has shown that in general, energy requirements for ventricular fibrillation are less with delivery of a single capacitor biphasic waveform than double capacitor biphasic or monophasic waveforms[5,6].

Comparative studies for atrial defibrillation are unavailable and in the succeeding experiments investigating purpose-built leads in different configurations, a biphasic truncated exponential pulse with width 12msec and interpulse delay of 0.5 msec was delivered from a single capacitor (150 microfarad).

b. Electrode systems and configurations: Energy requirements and lead impedance. Investigation of low-energy cardioversion for ventricular tachycardia has often utilised a purpose - built Medtronics 6880 lead with a larger electrode surface area than conventional[7]. Recent studies of atrial defibrillation in patients[8,9] have generally used a standard USCI electrode catheter. This has a surface area of 8-10 mm^2. Our studies of impedance with this lead have shown much higher values than with the lead which we have studied.

Use of the electrode system we have employed has previously been described for ventricular defibrillation. The electrode is of titanium and constructed as an endocardial tube which provides a surface area of 600 mm^2. A 90 cm "J" lead is employed for positioning against the wall of the right atrial appendage and a 100 cm straight lead sited at the right ventricular apex. The electrodes are 8F and were introduced via the internal jugular vein.

We tested these leads in a number of configurations in anaesthetised greyhounds. In addition to the right atrial appendage and right ventricular leads, in other experiments either a straight braided endocardial lead was tunnelled subcutaneously between the left fourth and sixth ribs or fifth and seventh ribs, or an R_2 patch electrode sited over the left hemithorax.

After bilateral vagotomy, atrial fibrillation was initiated by AOO pacing, at a rate 20bpm above intrinsic sinus rate during vagal stimulation of the right vagosympathetic trunk. Atrial defibrillation was attempted if the arrhythmia had persisted for >60 sec, using a purpose-built support device (Telectronics 4510).

It has been shown that the efficacy of defibrillation is unrelated to its timing relative to atrial activity[2] and energy was delivered synchronously with ventricular electrograms to avoid possible initiation of ventricular fibrillation[2,10]. Atrial defibrillation was first attempted at a level of 0.1 joules. If this was unsuccessful, other configurations were tested at this energy level and if these were also unsuccessful, progressively higher energy levels were then tested. The order of lead configurations tested was not randomized and not all configurations were tested in each animal. Therefore, although a total of 653 shocks were given in 8 greyhounds, the number with each configuration varied considerably. The dose-ranging nature of the studies and these other aspects make comparisons of relative success rates and required energy levels difficult. However, there was considerable intra-animal and interanimal variation in the minimal successful energy level and the most successful configuration. All episodes of atrial fibrillation were terminated by energy <0.83 joules. The data suggested that individual episodes of atrial fibrillation might equally be terminated by delivery of energy between two intracardiac electrodes (right atrium and right ventricle) or one intracardiac electrode and an R2 patch electrode.

Although others have reported possible pathological changes with focal subendocardial necrosis[2], in a series of 3 animals, no gross or microscopic changes were found on pathological examination of the heart. In 2 animals, no significant ventricular arrhythmias could be induced by programmed ventricular stimulation undertaken seven days after the atrial defibrillation experiment.

APPLICATION TO HUMANS

Recently, Levy et al.[8] and other investigators[9] have observed that atrial fibrillation may be terminated during transcatheter AV node ablation. Their technique of selective atrial defibrillation entails shock delivery via the proximal electrode after withdrawal of a standard USCI catheter across the tricuspid valve until the His bundle electrogram can no longer be recorded. They used a backplate as the anode. Their method deliberately avoids contact with the atrial wall, and they described reversion of atrial fibrillation with energy levels of 200-300 joules when transthoracic DC shock has been unsuccessful. However, these levels of energy are suboptimal for any implantable device and instead we have elected to investigate the use of lower energy levels.

Figure 1 shows a series of ECG rhythm strips obtained from the first patient in whom we have attempted low energy catheter reversion. The patient developed atrial fibrillation 36 hours following coronary bypass surgery. He had no previous history of atrial arrhythmia. He remained in atrial fibrillation after digitalisation until he reverted to atrial flutter approximately one week later.

He remained in this rhythm until attempted catheter reversion on the eleventh post -operative day. Under general anaesthesia, 8F braided endocardial leads were introduced by the internal jugular vein to the right atrium and right ventricular apex. Initial delivery of 0.5 joules between the right ventricular and right atrial leads had no effect other than a transient increase in the degree of AV block. However the next delivery of 1.0 joules initially resulted in change in the cycle length and morphology of regular atrial activity. Approximately one minute later, the atrial rhythm reverted to a pattern similar to that seen original- ly and this was followed by restoration of sinus rhythm.

Figure 1.

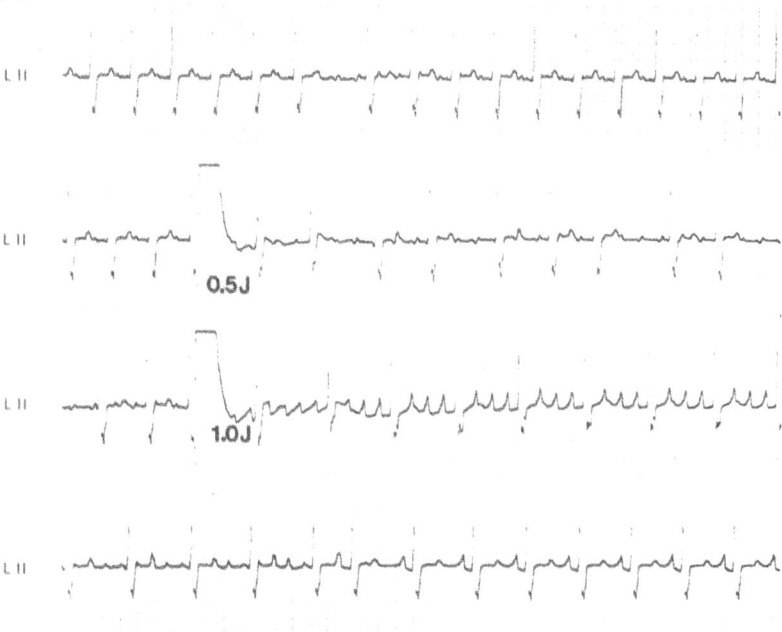

Series of ECG rhythm strips in the patient in whom low energy cardioversion was attempted for atrial fibrillation and flutter following coronary bypass surgery.

Late reversion was first noted by Mower and Mirowski[10] and has also been commented upon by others. The change in atrial cycle length and P wave morphology in our patient was consistent with initial alteration in functio- nal properties of the atrium.

Nathan et al.[11] described similar termination of atrial flutter in one patient amongst their series of patients with atrial fibrillation or flutter. They delivered energy via a Medtronics 6880 lead. However shocks were ineffective in the other patients and also ineffective in the successfully treated patient after atrial flutter was reinitiated, even using higher energy levels. They also noted that patients may experience considerable discomfort with defibrillation, contrary to the initial report of Mirowski and Mower[1]. This may be greater than with similar energies used to treat ventricular arrhythmias[11].

SENSING ALGORITHMS _____

Implantable devices used for the treatment of life-threatening ventricular arrhythmias must if necessary sacrifice specificity to allow very high sensitivity. For the treatment of atrial arrhythmias, because of their varied and frequently non-sustained nature and usual absence of gross haemodynamic compromise, specificity will also be very important.

Atrial rate, power spectral analysis and amplitude probability density functions may all allow recognition of atrial fibrillation from electrograms and its differentiation from sinus tachycardia for example[12]. Algorithms based on these might be incorporated in an implantable device. It is quite probable that analysis in the frequency domain will better describe functional properties of the atrium, and may even allow recognition of atrial fibrillation from which spontaneous reversion is likely[13] perhaps obviating any requirement for energy discharge.

CONCLUSIONS _____

In summary, low energy defibrillation should be feasible in patients and the availability of a dual chamber defibrillator is a realistic prospect in the near future. Cost-effectiveness considerations make it much less likely that a single chamber system for atrial defibrillation will be freely available, despite the clinical benefits of maintenance of sinus rhythm. It is unlikely that the additional algorithms for sensing of atrial fibrillation and capacity for delivery of low energy shock for atrial defibrillation will add substantial cost to the current implantable defibrillator.

The technique of low energy atrial defibrillation may also have significant applications in the electrophysiology laboratory for termination of unwanted atrial fibrillation and possibly also for management of the arrhythmia in other situations, such as in patients following cardiac surgery.

References

[1] Mirowski M, Mower MM, Langer AL. Low-energy catheter cardioversion of atrial tachycardias. Clin Res 1974;22:290A.

[2] Dunbar DN, Tobler G, Fetter J, et al. Intracavitary electrode catheter cardioversion of atrial tachyarrhythmias in the dog. J Am Coll Cardiol 1986;7:1015-1027.

[3] Kumagai K, Yamanouchi N, Hiroki T, Arakawa K. Low energy syndronous transcatheter cardioversion of atrial flutter/fibrillation in the dog.
J Am Coll Cardiol 1990;16:497-501.

[4] Gartman DM, Bardy GH, Allen MD, et al. Short-term morbidity and mortality of implantation of automatic implantable cardioverter-defibrillator. J Thorac Cardiovasc Surg 1990;100:353-359.

[5] Kavanagh KM, Tang ASL, Rollins DL, et al. Comparison of the internal defibrillation thresholds for monophasic and double and single capacitor biphasic waveforms. J Am Coll Cardiol 1989;14:1343-1349.

[6] Saksena S, Scott SE, Accorti PR, et al. Efficacy and safety of monophasic and biphasic waveform shocks using a braided endocardial defibrillation systems. Am Heart J 1990;120:1342-1347.

[7] Jackman WM, Zipes DP. Low energy synchronous cardioversion of ventricular tachycardia using a catheter electrode in a canine model of subacute myocardial infarction. Circulation 1982;66:187-195.

[8] Levy S, Lacombe P, Conte R, Bru P. High energy transcatheter cardioversion of chronic atrial fibrillation. J Am Coll Cardiol 1988;12:514-518.

[9] Kumagai KM, Yamanouchi Y, Hiroki T, Arakawa K. Effects of transcatheter cardioversion on chronic lone atrial fibrillation. PACE 1991;14:1571-1575.

[10] Mower MM, Mirowski M. Phenomenon of delayed reversion following atrial cardioversion. Circulation 1974;50:III-194.

[11] Nathan AW, Bexton RS, Spurrell RAJ, Camm AJ. Internal transvenous low energy cardioversion for the treatment of cardiac arrhythmias. Br Heart J 1984;52:377-384.

[12] Slocum S, Sahakian H, Swiryn S. Computer discrimination of atrial fibrillation and regular atrial rhythms from intra-atrial electrograms. PACE 1988;11:610-21.

[13] David D, Lang RM, Neumann A, et al. Parasympathetically modulated antiarrhythmic action of lidocaine in atrial fibrillation. Am Heart J 1990; 119:1061-68.

Chapter 10

THE 'CORRIDOR' OPERATION AS AN ALTERNATIVE IN THE

TREATMENT OF ATRIAL FIBRILLATION

Jo A.M. Defauw

Norbert M. van Hemel

J. Herre Kingma

Wybren Jaarsma

Freddy E.E. Vermeulen

Jacques M.T. de Bakker

Gérard M. Guiraudon

Departments of Cardiology and Cardiothoracic Surgery
St Antonius Hospital
Nieuwegein
The Netherlands

Department of Experimental Cardiology
University Medical Center Amsterdam
and
Interuniversity Cardiology Institute
The Netherlands

Department of Surgery
University of Western Ontario
London Ontario
Canada

J. H. Kingma et al. (eds.), Atrial fibrillation, a treatable disease?, 167–181.
© 1992 Kluwer Academic Publishers.

INTRODUCTION _____

Atrial fibrillation without structural heart disease[1] or pre-excitation syndrome[2] is an arrhythmia which does not markedly affect life expectancy but may strongly alter exercise capacity and quality of life. This arrhythmia is highly prevalent among cardiac arrhythmias, particularly in older people, and becomes frequently manifest without demonstrable cause ('lone atrial fibrillation'). In circumstances of drug refractoriness of disabling atrial fibrillation today two alternative electrophysiologic interventions are available: His-bundle ablation followed by chronic cardiac pacing[3,4], or the surgical exclusion of the anatomical substrate of atrial fibrillation[5,6,7].6

This study addresses the result of cardiac surgery using the 'corridor' procedure[5,8,9,10], which aims to preserve physiologic activation of the ventricles. The left atrium is electrically isolated from an anatomical conduit containing the sinus node - atrioventricular node axis (the 'corridor') and can fibrillate without any influence on the sinus node activity. To prevent atrial fibrillation to occur in the 'corridor' the dimension of the 'corridor' is surgically reduced by isolation of a part of the right atrial free wall. This approach does not permit atrial fibrillation to emerge into the 'corridor' because its surface cannot harbour a sufficient number of wavelets of atrial fibrillation to occur, and hence the arrhythmogenic conditions for atrial fibrillation as formulated by Moe[11] and Allessie[12] cannot be fulfilled.

Short-term results of the 'corridor' procedure have already shown the feasibility of the surgical concept[5,8], but refinement of the technique, and in particular the approach of the coronary sinus[8], is needed while patient selection has to be further defined. In this review long-term efficacy of the 'corridor' procedure is evaluated, taking into consideration the absence of atrial fibrillation, sinus node function, the hemodynamic behaviour of the 'corridor' and quality of life.

METHODS _____

Between 1987 and 1991, 24 patients with *paroxysmal* lone atrial fibrillation underwent the 'corridor' operation at the St Antonius Hospital. Patients with sick-sinus syndrome or other supraventricular or ventricular arrhythmias than paroxysmal atrial fibrillation were excluded from this surgery. In addition, only patients with no documented severe structural heart disease and normal atrial size as documented by echocardiography, were accepted. Paroxysmal atrial fibrillation was observed in all patients for at least 1 year prior to surgery (Table 1) and caused disabling symptoms such as dizziness, loss of exercise capacity and extreme fatigue during the attacks. These symptoms frequently forced patients to stop working. Between the attacks of arrhythmia, all patients experienced a normal life style and physical capacity. In all patients consent for surgery was obtained following extensive information about the investigational character of this surgical intervention.

This study reports the long-term results of 20 of 24 (83%) successively operated patients with successful electrical isolation of the 'corridor' from the residual right and left atrium. The baseline characteristics are depicted in Table 1. In the remaining 4 patients a permanent electrical isolation between the 'corridor' and the left atrium could not be achieved despite reoperation and consequently the His bundle was ablated, followed by pacemaker implantation-[8].

Table 1. **Baseline characteristics of 20 'corridor' patients**

male/female	12/8
age at surgery	mean 55±11 years
years of paroxysmal atrial fibrillation	mean 7±5 years
organic heart disease	0
extracorporeal circulation	mean 136±24 min
aortic cross clamp time	mean 82±8 min
supplementary surgery, all without	
extracorporeal circulation	5/12
follow-up time	mean 32±15 months
loss of follow-up or death	0

Standard electrocardiography (ECG), 24 hrs 2-channel Holter recordings and bicycle stress testing were used to document paroxysmal atrial fibrillation and to exclude sinus node disease, abnormal atrioventricular (AV) conduction and accessory AV nodal pathways. Sinus node function was considered normal when its rate varied from 60 to 120 bpm during Holter monitoring without medication and when the corrected sinus node recovery time was <550 ms, determined with the conventional method[13]. In 10 of 20 patients electrocardioversion was needed during programmed electrical stimulation to permit the investigation of sinus node function. Normal AV conduction was defined 1:1 AV conduction to at least 140 bpm at spontaneous sinus rhythm or driven atrial rhythm at programmed electrical stimulation. Accessory AV nodal pathways, atrial flutter and tachycardia were excluded with programmed electrical stimulation using standard methods[13]. The invasive studies were carried out after withdrawal of antiarrhythmic drugs of at least 2.5 times half lifetime. The therapy with amiodarone was terminated at least 4 months before electrical programmed stimulation and surgery.

Routine 2-Dimensional echocardiography and Doppler echocardiographic studies were performed to define the size of both atria[14] and to exclude presence of mitral and tricuspid incompetence and other structural heart diseases. This examination was repeated in all patients at the end of follow-up (October 1991). For examination of transvalvular flow velocity spectra, postoperatively 2-Dimensional and pulsed wave Doppler echocardiographic examination was done in all patients with a 2.5 mHz transducer and a Hewlett Packard cardiac ultrasound (77020 A) imaging system. For Doppler assessment of the transvalvular flow spectrum in the apical 4 chamber view the sample volume was placed between the mitral and tricuspid leaflet tips and adjusted until flow velocities were maximal. Doppler recordings were made together with electrogram tracings and recorded at 25 or 50 mm/sec. Attention was paid to the presence of the second peak of the velocity curve which represents an increase in velocity following atrial contraction. In sinus rhythm the second peak is usually present whereas in atrial fibrillation it is absent[15]. In all cases left and right heart catheterization and coronary angiography was performed to rule out cardiac abnormalities.

SURGICAL PROCEDURE AND IN-HOSPITAL ELECTROPHYSIOLOGIC STUDIES

Patients undergoing the 'corridor' procedure are prepared as for routine open cardiac surgery. After median sternotomy, institution of cardiopulmonary bypass and cold cardioplegic cardiac arrest, the 'corridor' procedure is carried out in two steps. The right atrium is incised next to the atrial appendage down to the interatrial groove. This incision is extended to the anterior and to the posterior side of the atrioventricular junction. Hence the sinus node area lies superior to the incision in the right atrium. The incision lies just lateral to the fossa ovalis and reaches the posterior atrioventricular junction just lateral of the orifice of the coronary sinus. On the anterior side the incision reaches the tricuspid ring as medial as possible, preserving the sinus node artery (Fig. 1).

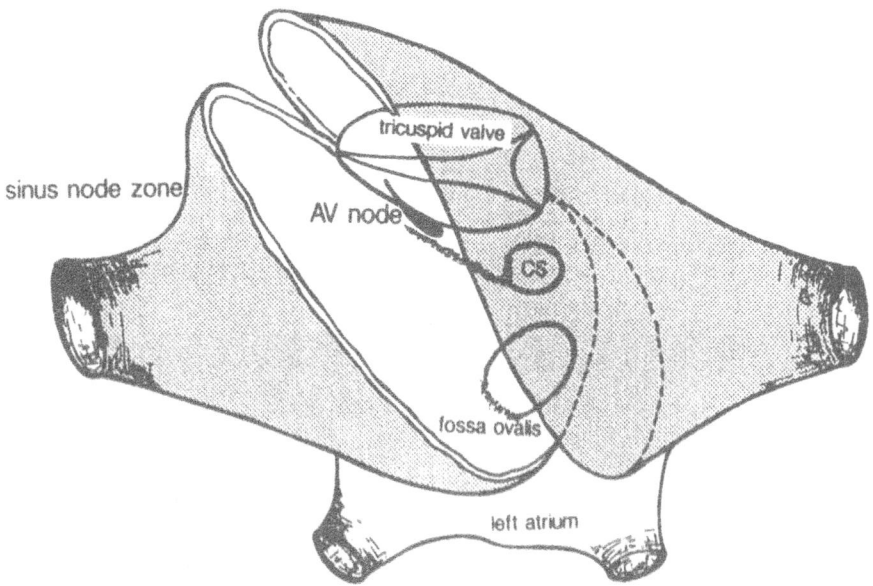

Figure 1. Schematic display of the right atrial incision. The right atrium is incised next to the atrial appendage down to the interatrial groove. The fossa ovalis is kept at the medial side of the incision as well as the orifice of the coronary sinus (CS). The incision is extended to reach the tricuspid ring at the atrioventricular junction, at which site an additional cryoablation is performed. The atrial part that becomes the 'corridor' comprises the sinus node zone, the atrioventricular nodal (AV node) region, and the orifice of the coronary sinus[8]. (With permission)

In the second step the left atrial incision is started in the interatrial groove, and carried out further to the roof of the left atrium under the superior caval vein. It is prolonged behind the aorta, cutting the atrial wall from the inside, until it reaches the mitral valve ring which lies in front of the left atrial appendage. On

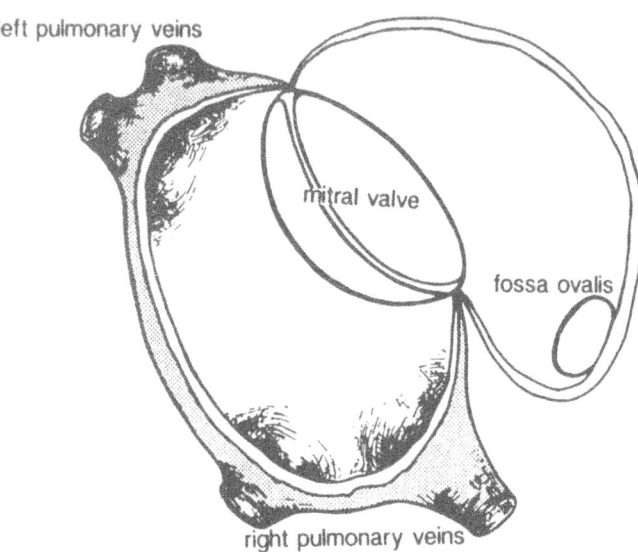

Figure 2. Schematic display of the left atrial incision. The left atrium is incised anterior to the right pulmonary veins in the interatrial groove. The incision is extended upward, under the superior caval vein to the roof of the left atrium, and extended to reach the mitral valve ring, anterior to the orifice of the left atrial appendage. The incision is extended posteriorly to reach the mitral valve ring next to the interatrial septum. An additional cryoablation is performed at the site where the incision reaches the mitral ring[8] (with permission).

Figure 3. Detail of the posterior side of the left atrial incision. The incision of the atrial wall is carried out from the inside and the coronary sinus is visualized. Care is taken to sever this structure. An additional freezing of the coronary sinus at this point is performed[8] (with permission).

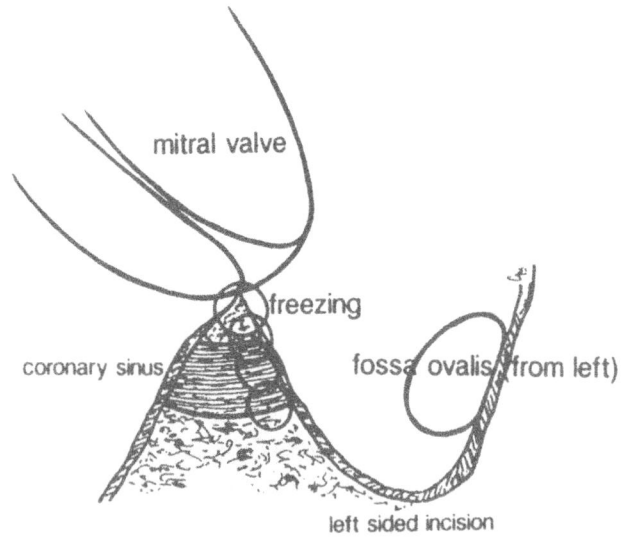

the inferior side the incision is extended downwards to reach the mitral valve ring next to the interatrial septum, near the posteromedial commissure (Fig. 2). This is also performed from within the left atrium. The coronary sinus is identified (Fig. 3), and great care is taken to strip the coronary sinus from all muscular fibers. Before resuturing the atrial incisions to restore the atrial anatomy, cryocoagulation is carried out at the 4 sites where the incisions reach the AV sulcus to ensure complete electrical isolation. Additionally, the coronary sinus is thoroughly cryoablated at the site where it is devoid of muscular fibers to ensure complete electrical isolation. The suturing of the left atrium is performed in a single layer with Prolene (R) 3-0 and the right atrium is sutured with Prolene (R) 4-0. Before unclamping the aorta, the left and right ventricle are thoroughly debubbled to avoid air emboli.

The methods of per- and postoperative electrophysiological studies have been reported[8]. To summarize, using temporary epicardial atrial leads the isolation of the 3 atrial compartments is tested per and postoperatively by stimulation of each compartment. When incomplete surgical isolation became apparent in the immediate postoperative phase, reoperation was always performed (Table 1). The residual electrical connection was uniformly found adjacent to the coronary sinus in all reoperated patients[8]. The connection could be interrupted by additional dissection and cryoablation of that area, which was always done without extracorporeal circulation (Table 1). Postoperative induction of atrial fibrillation was attempted in any atrial compartment. The postoperative behaviour of the sinus node and AV node was evaluated before discharge. In addition to standard postoperative care, all patients received anticoagulant therapy with coumadine, starting on the first postoperative day and continued up to 3 months after discharge, at which time aspirine therapy was initiated.

All patients have been followed at 3 to 6 months intervals. Patients were asked in particular for palpitations and symptoms of cerebrovascular accidents. In addition, Holter recordings and bicycle stress testing were regularly used to detect arrhythmias, particularly atrial fibrillation, and for the evaluation of the activity of the sinus and AV node. Postoperative incompetent chronotropy of the sinus node was defined as symptomatic sinus bradycardia at rest <60 bpm requiring pacemaker therapy or as an insufficient increase in sinus rate at stress testing arbitrarily chosen at <80% of predicted value according to gender and age criteria[16] without any antiarrhythmic drug.

RESULTS _____

After a mean follow-up of 32 ± 15 months after surgery 17 of 20 (85%) patients remained free of any supraventricular arrhythmia without drug therapy (Table 2).

Table 2. **Rhythm results of 'corridor' surgery of 20 patients**

		Number of patients	%
Free of arrhythmias and drugs		17	85
New arrhythmias and drugs*		3	15
paroxysmal atrial flutter	2		
paroxysmal atrial tachycardia	1		
Normal sinus node at rest (>60 pbm)		16	80
stress testing:			
>80% predicted sinus rate		13	65
<80% predicted sinus rate		3	15
Abnormal sinus node at rest (<60 bpm)			
pacemaker rhythm		4	20
stress testing:			
>80% predicted sinus rate		4	20
<80% predicted sinus rate			0
Normal AV conduction		20	100

* In 1 patient paroxysmal atrial fibrillation reoccurred temporarily (see text)

Paroxysmal atrial fibrillation in the 'corridor' occurred in only 1 patient 4 months after discharge. After a period of 2 months these attacks disappeared spontaneously during 19 months of follow-up. Other tachycardia in the 'corridor' after discharge were paroxysmal flutter with a rate of 360 bpm (2 patients), and paroxysmal atrial tachycardia with a rate of 180 and 190 bpm respectively (1 patient), which could be easily suppressed with a single antiarrhythmic drug. The actuarial freedom of supraventricular arrhythmias was 79 ± 9% at 1 year after surgery and remained unchanged during the next years of follow-up. Follow-up shows that new arrhythmias emerged more frequently within the first half year after surgery.

A normal sinus node activity at rest was observed in 16 of 20 (80%) patients, whereas 13 of these 16 patients showed a sufficient increase in sinus rate at exercise (Table 2). In 3 of these 16 patients an incompetent chronotropic response at exercise became manifest. However, in all 4 cases of required artificial cardiac pacing due to symptomatic insufficient sinus node activity at rest (<60 bpm) a sufficient rise of heart rate at exercise was observed. The actuarial proportion of patients with sufficient chronotropic competence of the sinus node was 90 ± 6% at 1 year after surgery and 78 ± 9% during the following 2 years. Follow-up shows that deterioration of sinus node activity occurred gradually after surgery. An impairment of the AV conduction was never observed.

Pulsed-wave Doppler examination of the mitral valve showed absence of left atrial contraction (i.e., A wave) in all 20 patients (Table 3). Frequently the left atrium showed mechanical standstill or very slow activity. However, an

Table 3. Long-term echocardiographic results of 'corridor' surgery

(N = 20)

			N
left atrioventricular synchrony			0
right atrioventricular synchrony			15
dissociation due to bradycardia			5
left atrial size increased			14
right atrial size increased			13
mitral incompetence	grade	0	16
	grade	1/4	2
	grade	2/4	2
tricuspid incompetence	grade	0	16
	grade	1/4	2
	grade	2/4	2

obvious right atrial contraction (i.e., presence of A wave) was observed in 15 patients (Table 3). A slow rhythm in the 'corridor' with temporary nodal rhythm or a ventricular pacemaker rhythm at rest caused mechanical asynchrony between the right atrium and right ventricle (4 cases). At the end of this study the left atrium dimension was slightly increased in a majority of the patients (Table 3). This was also observed in the right atrium. In only a limited number of patients new mild mitral (4 patients) and tricuspid valve incompe-tence (4 patients) was observed with colour Doppler flow mapping.

Two patients experienced a transient ischemic attack, 1 patient after reoperation and 1 patient 4 months after discharge. In the first patient anti-coagulant therapy was diminished prior to the attack, and started again on the day of reoperation. Presumably the degree of anticoagulant therapy was insufficient when the transient ischemic attack occurred. In the second patient coumadin therapy was terminated 1 month before this event. Echocardio-graphy performed immediately after this complication showed a normal left atrial size in the first, and a slight enlargement in the second patient. A full neurological recovery was noted at the end of this study.

Finally, although no specific questionnaires were used, clinical judgement disclosed a clear improvement of lifestyle in all patients. Seven of the 12 male patients returned to their original profession while the remaining 5 patients were already retired or rejected for duties due to other medical problems. Two years after surgery one of the younger patients was able to accomplish a complete marathon run, which he was used to perform before the surgical intervention.

DISCUSSION

The surgical approach of drug-refractory atrial fibrillation was reported for the first time in 1981 by Seally and coworkers, who used cryo-ablation to interrupt the His bundle[4]. Since 1982 closed chest ablation of the His bundle with catheter electroshocks became a widely used treatment for drug refrac-tory atrial fibrillation[3]. However, these procedures implicate the exclusion of the physiologic cardiac pacemaker to drive the ventricles, the interruption of hemodynamic AV synchrony and life-long artificial pacemaker dependency.

Surgery for atrial fibrillation

Left atrial surgical isolation done in canine hearts and reported in 1980 by Williams and coworkers, circumvents the interruption of sinus node activity[17]. After the isolation of the body of the left atrial mass from the remainder of the heart, sinus node firing and AV synchrony remain undisturbed and hemodynamics unimpaired. A draw back of this method is that the fibrillating left atrium might constitute the origin of thromboembolism. As far as we know, this method has never been applied to human atrial fibrillation.

Because it cannot be ignored that atrial fibrillation can also emerge in the right atrium, in 1985 Guiraudon and coworkers introduced 'corridor' surgery in humans, in which a conduit of atrial tissue connecting the sino-atrial node area and the AV node was isolated from the right and left atrium[5]. By reduction of the right atrial mass to construct the 'corridor', its size may not contain a sufficient number of atrial wavelets to allow atrial fibrillation to occur or perpetuate[11,12]. This surgical method preserves physiological driving of the ventricles, but left atrial contribution to left ventricular filling ('atrial kick') is lost. Because the left atrium is independent and shows standstill or atrial fibrillation a vulnerability for thromboembolism remains. Hence, anti-coagulant therapy using coumadines or aspirin is recommended after 'corridor' surgery.

Finally, in 1991, the electrical 'maze' procedure was introduced by Cox and coworkers[6,7]. Multiple atrial incisions associated with subtotal exclusion of the left atrium prevent the emergence of fibrillation, permit normal sinus node action in the included atrial tissue as well as in the ventricles resulting in left and right sided atrial transport. This surgical procedure claims to preserve normal hemodynamics and to show no risk of thromboembolism because both atria contract actively as suggested by the preliminary results of a small series of patients[7].

'Corridor' results

Because paroxysmal atrial fibrillation reoccurred for a short interval in only 1 of the 20 successfully operated patients, the concept of 'corridor' surgery to eliminate atrial fibrillation appears to be valid. When new supraventricular arrhythmias arose after surgery, they were limited to paroxysmal atrial flutter and tachycardia in the 'corridor', which had not been documented prior to the intervention. Long-term follow-up could demonstrate that 'corridor' surgery does not impair the AV node function. An important concern of 'corridor' surgery is the long-term postoperative behaviour of the sinus node. In our series normal sinus node activity at rest was present in 80%, and at exercise in 85% of the patients at the end of follow-up. It is emphasized that the 4 patients with ventricular pacing at rest, displayed sufficient rise of heart rate at stress testing. This observation reveals a characteristic behaviour of the sinus node function in sick-sinus syndrome[18]. Furthermore, this study shows that the hazard of deterioration of the sinus node function is not particularly associated to the early postoperative phase, but that the failure appears to be a gradual process.

The early results of the Guiraudon group showed a higher incidence of sinus node disease: in 4 of 9 patients a very long sinus node recovery time or sporadic sinus node activity had been observed in the early phase after surgery[5,9]. This finding was not specifically related to the preoperative pattern of chronic or paroxysmal atrial fibrillation[9]. However, these results cannot precisely be compared with ours due to a difference in the time window of follow-up. Long-term sinus node activity of the 7 patients with the 'maze' procedure remained normal in 5 patients: the 2 patients with preoperative documented sick-sinus syndrome required demand artificial cardiac stimulation[7]. Considering the initial data, it is today still unclear whether the maintenance of the sinus node function after cardiac surgery for atrial fibrillation is determined by the direction and extension of atrial incisions[19], or an unfavourable selection of patients who had silent sinus node disease at the time of surgery. It can be assumed that much care is spent to spare the circulatory supply of the sinus node during atrial surgery[7,8]. It is clinically recognized that chronic or paroxysmal atrial fibrillation is sometimes one limb of an ongoing sick-sinus syndrome, which initially manifests exclusively with tachycardia. Therefore, the selection of surgical candidates with regard to long-term preservation of normal sinus node function is very critical. Because many surgical candidates are on drugs, which hampers appropriate investigation of the sinus node function, or without drugs, which necessitates electrical cardioversion to restore sinus rhythm providing false or very limited information, frequently sinus node function can only be tested superficially.

Hemodynamic consequences of 'corridor' surgery

Doppler pulsed-wave examination during follow-up clearly demonstrated right atrial transport in the majority of 'corridor' patients (Table 3), suggesting that the 'corridor' indeed contracts actively. Absence of an active filling of the right ventricle was only observed in cases of pacemaker rhythm (4 patients) and in 1 patient with asymptomatic episodic sinus bradycardia with AV nodal escape rhythm. As was expected, left atrial contraction was absent in all cases and therefore the left atrium does not contribute to maintenance of cardiac output. However, experimental hemodynamic studies have shown that absence of left atrial contribution to left ventricular filling does not adversely affect cardiac output[17]. In addition, in the presence of normal left ventricular function, the ability to increase heart rate appears to be more important than atrial contraction per se for an increase in cardiac output[20]. Therefore, it is not surprising that in these series of 20 'corridor' patients the exercise capacity remained unimpaired during follow-up. Finally, long-term hemodynamic studies are needed to define the clinical significance of slight postoperative mitral and tricuspid valve incompetence as shown by colour Doppler flow velocity studies. So far these findings did not ask for medical or surgical therapy (Table 3).

Thromboembolism

The risk of thromboembolism is unaltered after 'corridor' surgery because the left atrium can continue to fibrillate. In this respect it is worthwhile to note that echocardiography showed a slight increase in diameter and size of both atria in the majority of patients. A gradual enlargement of the left atrium after surgery can be easily explained as a result of paroxysmal or chronic fibrillation in that compartment[21], while the increase in size of the right atrium can be attributed to asystole of the excluded right atrial free wall as was frequently observed in the early postoperative phase using epicardial electrocardio-graphic recordings, or due to the atrial incisions. Considering these findings, long-term anticoagulant therapy after 'corridor' surgery is presently recommended.

CONCLUSIONS

Of the various surgical methods to treat drug refractory atrial fibrillation, the 'corridor' procedure offers a valid alternative, at least in patients with paroxysmal atrial fibrillation with preoperative normal sinus node function. Long-term follow-up did not disclose adverse sequelae of 'corridor' surgery in terms of deterioration of the cardiac function. Contrarily, the majority of patients experienced an improvement of life style because of elimination of paroxysmal atrial fibrillation without antiarrhythmic drugs. Presence of right sided atrial flutter, atrial tachycardia or atrial fibrillation in the setting of sick-sinus syndrome do not qualify to the concept of 'corridor' surgery and need an alternative non-pharmacological solution in case of drug refractoriness.

References

[1] Gajewski J, Singer RB. Mortality in an insured population with atrial fibrillation. JAMA 1981;245:1540-1544.
[2] Torner Montoya P, Brugada P, Smeets J, Talajic M, Della Bella P, Lezaun R, v.d. Dool A, Wellens HJJ, Bayés de Luna A, Oter R, Breithardt G, Borggrefe M, Klein H, Kuck KH, Kunze K, Coumel P, Leclercq JF, Chouty F, Frank R, Fontaine G. Ventricular fibrillation in the Wolff-Parkinson-White syndrome. Eur Heart J 1991;12:144-150.
[3] Gallagher JJ, Svenson RH, Kasell JH, et al. Catheter technique for closed chest ablation of the atrioventricular conduction system. N Engl J Med 1982;306:194-200.
[4] Sealy WC, Gallagher JJ, Kasell JH. His bundle interruption for control of inappropiate ventricular responses to atrial arrhythmias. Ann Thorac Surg 1981;32:429-438.
[5] Guiraudon GM, Campbell CS, Jones DL, McLellan DG, MacDonald JL. Combined sino-atrial node atrio-ventricular isolation: a surgical alternative to His bundle ablation in patients with atrial fibrillation. Circulation 1985;72:III-220.
[6] Cox JL. The surgical treatment of atrial fibrillation. IV. Surgical technique. J Thorac Cardiovasc Surg 1991;101:584-592.
[7] Cox JL, Schuessler RB, D'Agostino HJ, Stone CM, Byung-Chul Ch, Cain ME, Corr PB, Boineau JP. The surgical treatment of atrial fibrillation. III. Development of a definitive surgical procedure. J Thorac Cardiovasc Surg 1991;101:569-583.
[8] Defauw JJAMT, Guiraudon GM, van Hemel NM, Vermeulen FEE, Kingma JH, de Bakker JMT. Surgical therapy of paroxysmal atrial fibrillation with the 'corridor' operation. Ann Thorac Surg 1992;53:564-571.
[9] Leitch JW, Klein G, Yee R, Guiraudon GM. Sinus node-atrioventricular node isolation: Long-term results with the 'corridor' operation for atrial fibrillation. JACC 1991;17:970-5.
[10] van Hemel NM, Defauw JAM, Kingma JH, Jessurun ER, de Bakker J, Guiraudon G. Longterm efficacy of surgical treatment for drug refractory paroxysmal atrial fibrillation using the 'corridor' procedure. Circulation 1991;84:II-194 (abstract).
[11] Moe GK. On the multiple wavelet hypothesis of atrial fibrillation. Arch Int Pharmacodyn Ther 1962;140:183-188.

[12] Allessie MA, Lammers WJEP, Bonke FIM, Hollen J. Experimental evaluation of Moe's multiple wavelets hypothesis of atrial fibrillation. In: Cardiac electrophysiology and arrhythmias. Zipes DP and Jalife J, eds., New York: Grune and Stratton, 1985, 265-275.

[13] Josephson ME, Seides SF. Clinical cardiac electrophysiology, Techniques and interpretations. Lea & Febiger, Philadelphia 1979, pp 64-70.

[14] Weyman AE, Gillam LD. Normal adult cross-sectional echocardiographic values: linear dimensions and chamber areas. Echocardiography 1984;1:403-426.

[15] Hatle L, Angelsen B. (1985) Dopller ultrasound in cardiology, 2nd edn, Lea and Febiger, Philadelphia, pp 74-96.

[16] Recommandations and standard guidelines for exercise testing. Eur Heart J 1988;9: Supp K, 3-37.

[17] Williams JM, Ungerleider RM, Lofland GK, Cox JL. Left atrial isolation: new technique for the treatment of supraventricular arrhythmias. J Thorac Cardiovasc Surg 1980;80:373-380.

[18] Kallryd A, Kruse I, Rydén L. Atrial inhibited pacing in the sick-sinus node syndrome: clinical value and the demand for rate responsiveness. PACE 1989;12:954-961.

[19] Boineau JP, Canavan TE, Schuessler RB, Cain ME, Corr PB, Cox JL. Demonstration of a widely distributed atrial pacemaker complex in the human heart. Circulation 1988;77: 1221-1237.

[20] Rydén L, Karlson O. Kristensson BE. The importance of different atrioventricular intervals for exercise capacity. PACE 1988;11:1051-1061.

[21] Sanfilippo AJ, Abascal VM, Sheehan M, Oertel LB, Harrigan P, Hughes RA, Weyman AE. Atrial enlargement as a consequence of atrial fibrillation, a prospective echocardiographic study. Circulation 1990;82:792-797.

Chapter 11

TACHYCARDIOMYOPATHY IN PATIENTS

WITH SUPRAVENTRICULAR TACHYCARDIA

Hein J.J. Wellens

Luz-Maria Rodriquez

Joep L.R.M. Smeets

Emile C. Cheriex

Frans Pieters

Karel den Dulk

Department of Cardiology
Academic Hospital Maastricht
University of Limburg
Maastricht
The Netherlands

J. H. Kingma et al. (eds.), Atrial fibrillation, a treatable disease?, 183–193.

INTRODUCTION _____

Chronic supraventricular tachycardias may lead to cardiac enlargement and depressed cardiac function[1-9]. That observation has resulted in the introduction of the term tachycardiomyopathy, indicating that deterioration in cardiac function can be caused by the arrhythmia per se and that normal heart function may be restored by cure of the arrhythmia.

In this chapter we will concentrate on the three types of supraventricular tachycardia who are now known as possible causes of a tachycardiomyopathy. It is essential for the cardiologist to be aware of this possibility because cure of the arrhythmia will usually lead to spectacular improvement in cardiac function.

PATHOPHYSIOLOGIC BACKGROUND _____

Recently, Spinale et al.[10,11] showed that in the pig heart 3 weeks of rapid atrial pacing leads to right and left sided chamber dilatation and a decrease in wall thickness. They quantified changes in myocyte morphology by studying myocyte composition, size and shape. Myocytes became longer and thinner and were found to have a higher water content than control cells. The percent volume of myocytes decreased, especially in the subendocardial layer.

OBSERVATIONS IN THE HUMAN HEART _____

Incessant atrial tachycardia, incessant circus movement tachycardia using a slowly conducting accessory atrio-ventricular pathway and long lasting paroxysmal or chronic primary (idiopathic) atrial fibrillation may cause a tachycardiomyopathy. Our experience with each of these arrhythmias over a 15 year period will be discussed below in more detail.

A. *Incessant atrial tachycardia.* From 1977-1992 53 patients with atrial tachycardia were studied in the clinical electrophysiology laboratory of the Academic Hospital Maastricht. In 19 patients an incessant or permanent atrial tachycardia was present. The diagnosis of incessant tachycardia was made when the arrhythmia was present more than 12 per 24 hours. As discussed elsewhere in the incessant or permanent form of atrial tachycardia the arrhythmia cannot reproducibly be initiated and terminated by programmed electrical stimulation of the heart and is most likely based upon abnormal automaticity [12]. Table 1 shows that in 5 of the 19 patients with incessant atrial tachycardia a dilated cardiomyopathy with diminished cardiac function was present. A comparison between patients with and without a tachycardiomyopathy revealed no differences in sex, age at presentation in our clinic, duration of the arrhythmia and tachycardia rate. Duration of the arrhythmia, however, was significantly longer in patients with the cardiomyopathy.

Table 1. **Characteristics of patients with incessant atrial tachycardia with (+) or without (-) congestive cardiomyopathy**

	CMP +	CMP -	P
Nb	5	14	
Age (yrs)	11- 43 (28±12)	2-66 (22±14)	
Sex (M/F)	3/2	9/5	
Duration Arrh (yrs)	5- 40 (18±13)	1-13 (4 ± 3)	<0,001
Tachy rate/min	140-200 (162±25)	150-220 (175±20)	NS

Arrh = Arrhythmia; CMP = congestive cardiomyopathy; F = female;
M = male. Mean values within brackets.

Figures 1 and 2 illustrate 2 features present in patients with incessant atrial tachycardia developing a dilated cardiomyopathy: 1) inability to prevent 1 to 1 AV conduction by pharmacological means during atrial tachycardia and 2) an increase in atrial rate (accompanied by 1 to 1 AV conduction) during exercise.

Table 2 indicates the improvement in left heart dimensions and function after surgical cure of the arrhythmia. All 5 patients had surgical removal or cryoablation of their tachycardia focus after atrial mapping. It is unclear at this point in time whether similar results can be obtained by radiofrequency catheter ablation of the area of abnormal impulse formation.

Table 2. Incessant atrial tachycardia in 5 patients with congestive cardiomyopathy

		Effect of surgical treatment		
		before	after	P
LVEF	(%)	25-48 (38±9)	45-76 (55±12)	<0,05
LA size	(mm)	37-48 (41±4)	34-45 (34± 4)	<0,05
LVESD	(mm)	25-41 (35±6)	29-40 (31± 4)	NS
LVEDD	(mm)	35-56 (49±8)	35-58 (48± 5)	NS

LA = left atrium; LVEF = left ventricular ejection fraction; LVEDD = left ventricular end diastolic diameter; LVESD = left ventricular systolic diameter. Mean values within brackets.

Table 3. Characteristics of patients with incessant circus movement tachycardia using a slowly conducting accessory pathway with (+) and without (-) congestive cardiomyopathy (CMP)

		CMP +	CMP -	P
Nb		11	13	
Age	(yrs)	11- 55 (27±15)	14 - 58 (33±14)	NS
Sex	(M/F)	4/7	10/3	NS
Duration Arrh	(yrs)	2- 30 (13 ± 8)	1 - 18 (9 ± 6)	
Tachy rate/min		125-165 (143±11)	100-150 (134±17)	NS

Arrh = Arrhythmia; CMP = congestive cardiomyopathy; F = female; M = male. Mean values within brackets.

B. *Incessant circus movement tachycardia using a slowly conducting accessory atrio-ventricular pathway.* Of 463 patients (seen in Maastricht from 1977 to 1992) with accessory atrio-ventricular pathways, 24 patients were found to have a circus movement tachycardia using a slowly conducting accessory atrio-ventricular pathway for ventriculo-atrial conduction. Clinically, these patients suffered from incessant or permanent tachycardia with approximately half of them showing a dilated cardiomyopathy. In 1990, our institution

Figure 1.

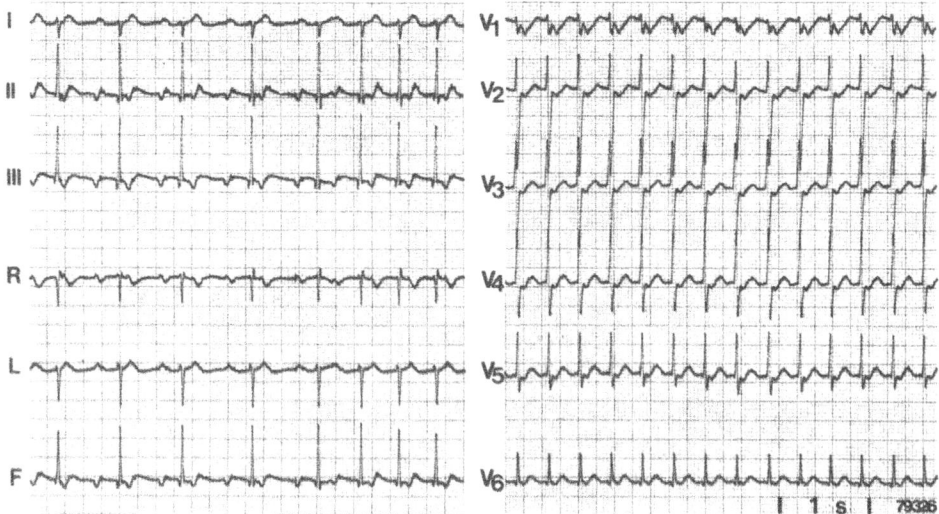

Incessant atrial tachycardia showing a change from 2 to 1 into 1 to 1 AV conduction. Frequently in patients with incessant tachycardia this change cannot be prevented by pharmacological means during exercise.

Figure 2.

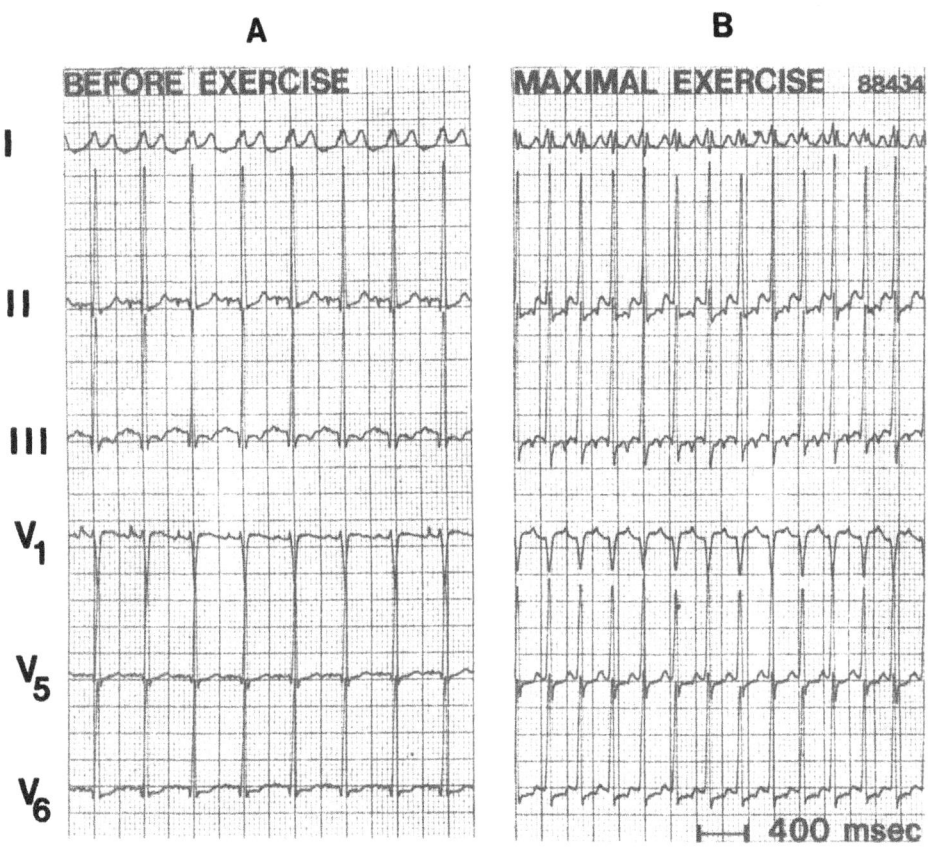

Effect of exercise in a patient with incessant atrial tachycardia. Note that heart rate increases from 150/minute (rest) to 240/minute (maximal exercise).

Figure 3.

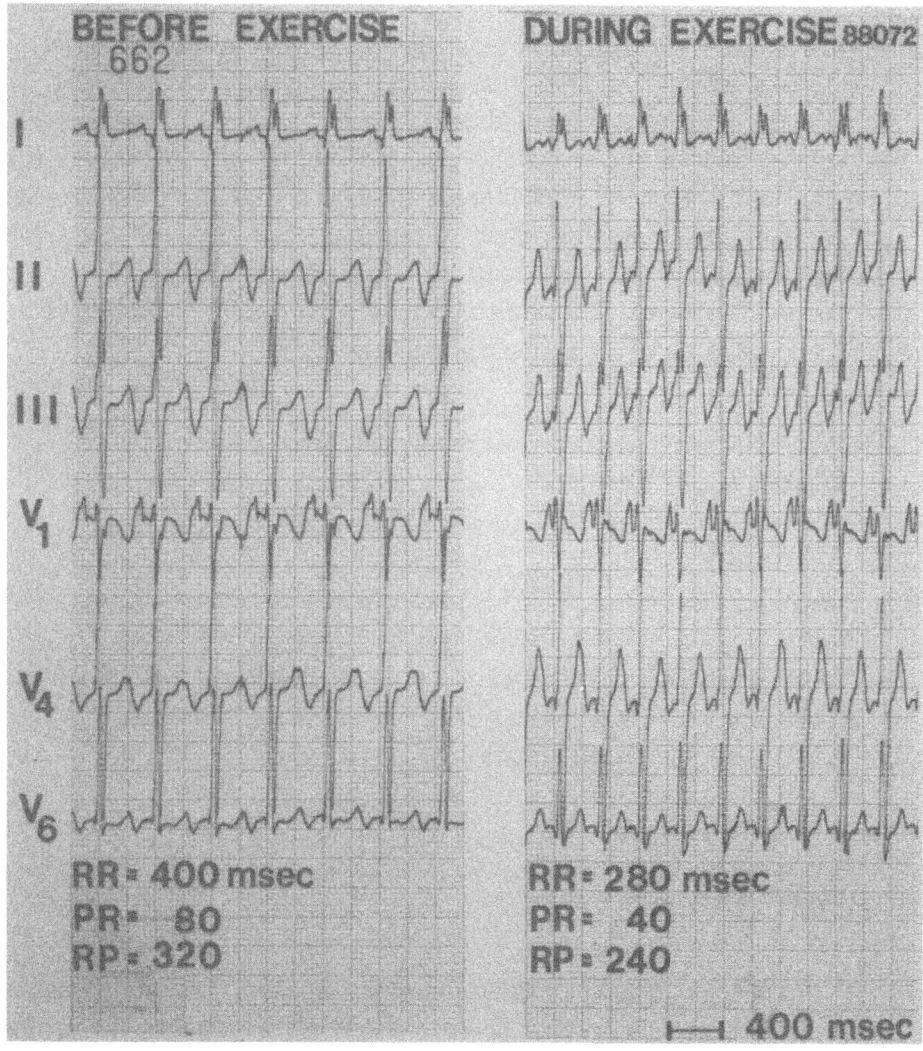

Effect of exercise in a patient with circus movement tachycardia using a slowly conducting accessory pathway for ventriculo-atrial conduction. In rest the heart rate measures 150/minute. During exercise heart rate increases to 215/minute because of shortening of both the PR and the RP interval.

reported on the reversibility of the tachycardia-induced cardiomyopathy by surgical interruption of the slowly conducting accessory atrio-ventricular pathway[8].

Table 3 gives information on our patients with circus movement tachycardia using a slowly conducting accessory atrio-ventricular pathway. As shown no differences were present in patients with or without cardiomyopathy in sex, age, duration of the arrhythmia and tachycardia rate. We cannot rule out however that differences were present in tachycardia rate during exercise (Figure 3). Table 4 shows the effect of surgical interruption of the slowly conducting accessory atrio-ventricular pathway on left heart function and dimensions in 10 patients with cardiomyopathy. One patient is scheduled for radiofrequency ablation of his accessory pathway.

Table 4. **Incessant circus movement tachycardia using a slowly conducting accessory pathway**

| | *Effect of surgery in pts with CMP (10 pts)* | | | |
	before		after	P
LVEF (%)	24-45	(39±6)	42-70 (53±9)	<0,0001
LA size (mm)	34-50	(40±5)	34-46 (39±4)	NS
LVESD (mm)	32-52	(42±7)	27-40 (34±4)	<0,005
LVEDD (mm)	42-64	(56±7)	42-60 (49±6)	<0,05

LA = left atrium; LVEF = left ventricular ejection fraction; LVEDD = left ventricular end diastolic diameter; LVESD = left ventricular systolic diameter. Mean values within brackets.

C. *Primary or idiopathic atrial fibrillation.* Recently we retrospectively analyzed 30 patients with primary or idiopathic atrial fibrillation in whom the atrio-ventricular conduction system was interrupted because of failure to control the ventricular rate pharmacologically[13]. Twelve of the 30 patients had left ventricular ejection fractions equal to or less than 50%. As shown in Table 5 there were no differences in age, sex, type of atrial fibrillation (paroxysmal or chronic) and type of ablation procedure in patients with a left ventricular ejection fraction above or below 50%. Only the duration of atrial fibrillation differed significantly between the two groups of patients. As shown in Table 6 patients with a lowered left ventricular ejection fraction showed significant improvement in left sided heart function after ablation. These observations suggest that also primary atrial fibrillation in the absence of concommitant heart disease, may eventually lead to a tachycardiomyopathy. Interestingly many patients had paroxysmal atrial fibrillation, with the arrhythmia occurring frequently without appropriate control of the ventricular rate in spite of pharmacological treatment. The true incidence of the development of a tachycardiomyopathy in patients with primary atrial fibrillation is not known. Our patients were obviously selected ones, being those having frequent and long lasting complaints and inability of arrhythmia control by pharmacological means.

Table 5. **Characteristics of patients with primary or idiopathic atrial fibrillation having a left ventricular ejection fraction of more or less than 50%**

	LVEF ≤50%	LVEF >50%
Nb	12	18
Sex (M/F)	9/3	11/7
Age (yrs)	46-78, mean 62	36-70, mean 56
Type AF (par/chr)	9/3	18/0
Type AV Ablation		
DC shock	7	9
Alcohol	3	4
Surgery	1	5
RF	1	
Duration AF (yrs)	8-28, mean 11	2-14, mean 5,4
	⌊———— $p < 0,05$ ————⌋	

AF = atrial fibrillation; AV = atrioventricular; DC = direct current;
F = female; LVEF = left ventricular ejection fraction; RF = radiofrequency.

Table 6. **Echocardiographic findings (mean values) before and after ablation of AV nodal conduction in patients with primary atrial fibrillation**

		LVEF < 50% (12 pts)			LVEF > 50% (18 pts)		
		before	after	P	before	after	P
LVEF		43±8	54±7	<0.001	59±3	59±4	NS
LVESD	(mm)	40±5	34±5	<0.003	31±3	31±4	NS
LVEDD	(mm)	54±5	50±5	<0.02	49±4	48±5	NS
LAS	(mm)	54±6	50±6	<0.002	46±6	47±5	NS

after = after ablation; before = before ablation; LAS = left atrium size; LVEDD = left ventricular end diastolic diameter; LVEF = left ventricular ejection fraction; LVESD = left ventricular end systolic diameter.

PRACTICAL IMPLICATIONS

Frequently occurring episodes of supraventricular tachycardia may lead to cardiac dilatation and impaired cardiac function. Our observations indicate that although the occurrence of this complication is relatively rare, awareness of that possibility is of importance because cure of the arrhythmia will usually lead to normalization of cardiac function.

The cardiologist should know that especially three types of supraventricular tachycardia (incessant atrial tachycardia, incessant circus movement tachycardia using a slowly conducting accessory atrio-ventricular pathway, and primary atrial fibrillation) may eventually lead to a tachycardiomyopathy. Frequent echocardiographic measurements in patients with these types of arrhythmias is therefore necessary to recognize the development of cardiac dilatation. Most of our patients with tachycardiomyopathy were cured by surgery. Current developments in radiofrequency ablation make it likely that that approach will increasingly be used in the future. Its value in the treatment of incessant atrial tachycardia deserves further evaluation.

References

[1]   Morgan CL, Nadas AS. Chronic ectopic tachycardia of infancy and childhood. Am Heart J 1964;67:617-627.

[2]   Scheinman MM, Basu D, Holenberg M. Electrophysiologic studies in patients with persistent atrial tachycardia. Circulation 1974;50:266-273.

[3]   Gillette PC, Garson A. Electrophysiological and pharmocologic characteristics of automatic ectopic atrial tachycardia. Circulation 1977;56:571-584.

[4]   Engel TR, Bush CA, Schaal SF. Tachycardia aggravated heart disease. Ann Int Med 1974;80:384-388.

[5]   McLaren CJ, Gersh BT, Sugrue DD, Hammil SC, Seward JB, Holmes DR. Tachycardia induced myocardial dysfunction, a reversible phenomenon? Br Heart J 1985;53:323-327.

[6]   Packer DL, Bardy GH, Worly SJ, Smith MS, Cobb FR, Coleman RE, Gallagher JJ, German LD. Tachycardia induced cardiomyopathy: a reversible form of the left ventricular dysfunction. Am J Cardiol 1986;57:563-570.

[7]   Damiano RJ, Tripp HF, Asano T, Small KW, Jones RH, Lowe JE. Left ventricular dysfunction and dilatation resulting from chronic supraventricular tachycardia. J Thorac Cardiovasc Surg 1987;94:135-143.

[8]   Cruz FES, Cheriex EC, Smeets JLRM, Atie J, Peres AK, Penn OCKM, Brugada P, Wellens HJJ. Reversibility of tachycardia induced cardiomyopathy after cure of incessant supraventricular tachycardia. J Am Coll Cardiol 1990;16:739-744.

[9]   Rabbani L, Wang PL, Couper GL, Friedman PL. Time course of improvement in ventricular function after ablation of incessant automatic atrial tachycardia. Am Heart J 1991;121:816-819.

[10]   Spinale FG, Crawford FA, Hewitt KW, Carabello BA. Ventricular failure and cellular remodeling with chronic supraventricular tachycardia. J Th Cardiovasc Surg 1991;102:874-882.

[11]   Tomita M, Spinale FG, Crawford FA, Zile MR. Changes in left ventricular volume, mass and function during the development and regression of supraventricular tachycardia induced cardiomyopathy. Circulation 1991;83:635-644.

[12]   Wellens HJJ, Brugada P. Mechanisms of supraventricular tachycardia. Am J Cardiol 1988;62:10D-15D.

[13]   Rodriguez LM, Smeets JLRM, Xie Bayan, De Chillou C, Cheriex EC, Pieters F, Metzger J, Den Dulk K, Wellens HJJ. Improvement in left heart function by ablation of AV nodal conduction in selected patients with primary atrial fibrillation. Circulation: in press.

Chapter 12

SINUS RHYTHM, THE AUTONOMIC NERVOUS SYSTEM,

AND QUALITY OF LIFE

Francis D. Murgatroyd

A. John Camm

Department of Cardiological Sciences
St George's Hospital Medical School
London SW17 0RE
United Kingdom

J. H. Kingma et al. (eds.), Atrial fibrillation, a treatable disease?, 195–210.

INTRODUCTION _____

Much of our knowledge of the nature of atrial fibrillation (AF), and in particular the pattern of electrical activation in the atrium during AF, is derived from the testing of theory in animal models. Thus our current understanding of AF is based on Moe's "multiple wavelet" hypothesis[1], developed from computer simulations, and the work of Allessie and Bonke, originally in a canine model of atrial flutter, demonstrating that re-entry can occur around a zone of functional block[2,3]. Mapping of atrial activation during AF, using multiplexed recordings from large arrays of electrodes, has only recently been performed in humans[4,5]. Although our theoretical understanding has benefitted greatly from such studies of induced AF in animals and chronic AF in humans, they do not tell us directly what causes AF in patients. Unfortunately, the presence of the arrhythmia itself renders conventional investigations of electrophysiology impossible during AF. However, valuable insights can be gained from patients with paroxysmal atrial fibrillation (PAF). In particular, observations regarding the timing of attacks in such patients have highlighted the possible aetiological role of the autonomic nervous system. Furthermore, comparisons can be made between PAF patients in sinus rhythm, and controls, indicating those electrophysiologic parameters which are associated with susceptibility to AF. In this chapter, we will discuss some of the lessons that can be learned about the nature and causes of clinical AF from observations made in patients during periods of sinus rhythm. Finally, we will address the important issues of quality of life in regard to paroxysmal arrhythmias, and their implications for treatment.

AUTONOMIC FACTORS _____

Recurrent PAF frequently occurs in individuals with no evidence of structural cardiac disease or metabolic abnormality. A clue to the aetiology of some cases of "lone" PAF has come from the description by Coumel et al. of a group of patients in whom arrhythmia appears to be associated with periods of enhanced vagal tone[6]. Attacks in these patients, who are typically men aged 30-50, occur at rest (usually in the evenings and at night), and can sometimes be aborted by exercise. In individual cases described by Coumel, the onset of AF is preceded by a progressive slowing of the heart rate, and a rise in the power of high frequency heart period variability (considered a marker of vagal tone) with a fall in low frequency power (which reflects sympathetic tone)[7,8]. It is known that the effects of vagal stimulation on atrial electrophysiology are to shorten the effective refractory period and slow conduction in a non-uniform manner:[9] both of these effects reduce the "wavelength" of the propagating impulse and thus facilitate fibrillation[10]. Indeed, vagal stimulation or cholinergic drugs have long been employed to produce experimental AF in animal models[11]. Thus it is tempting to suppose that, in Coumel's "vagotonic" PAF patients, the primary abnormality may be a pathological enhancement of the normal parasympathetic response. Indeed, anecdotal experience suggests that symptoms in this difficult group of patients tend to respond selectively to anticholinergic antiarrhythmic drugs such as disopyramide and quinidine, and can be worsened by digitalis, which has vagotonic electrophysiologic effects[12,13].

There is also a group of patients in whom, conversely, AF tends to occur in association with enhanced sympathetic tone - typically, during exercise and shortly after waking in the morning. These patients tend to be somewhat older than the "vagotonic" group, and (in our experience) are more likely to have minor associated cardiac abnormalities, such as mitral valve prolapse. AF is preceded by a progressive increase in heart rate and the power of low frequency heart period variability. Intense b-adrenoceptor blockade, for example with nadolol, may benefit these patients where other drugs have failed[14]. Again, it can be hypothesised that sympathetic activity may encourage the occurrence of AF: atrial refractoriness is shortened (although conduction is slowed, and the overall effect on wavelength is unknown in humans), and automaticity is increased: this may account for the atrial ectopic activity which appears to initiate AF in these patients.

The existence of Coumel's "vagotonic" and "adrenergic" groups of patients is supported by the experience of many clinicians. However, there is a lack of published data describing the frequencies of these patterns amongst the population of PAF patients. Furthermore, there have been no prospective controlled studies evaluating the effects of digitalis, vagolytic, and sympatholytic drugs in patients with PAF. The CRAFT (Controlled Randomized Atrial Fibrillation Trials) group was set up specifically to examine some of these issues. CRAFT-1 is a multi-centre, double-blind, placebo-controlled cross-over

trial of digoxin in PAF, using transtelephonic monitoring to document symptomatic arrhythmias. At time of writing, recruitment for this study is almost
complete. CRAFT-2 employs a similar design to investigate the effectiveness of
disopyramide (selected because it is the most anticholinergic antiarrhythmic
drug) and atenolol in PAF.

In order to examine the prevalence of Coumel's "vagotonic" and
"adrenergic" patterns of PAF, we have compiled a draft autonomic profile
questionnaire (Table 1). This aims to score each patient according to the
degree with which symptoms are associated with various activities, each
thought to be associated with increased vagal or adrenergic tone. As some
activities would seem to be stronger discriminators than others, scores were
calculated both with and without weighting for these activities. In fact, there
was a high degree of correlation between weighted and unweighted scores
(Fig.1), and weighting was therefore abandoned. When this questionnaire was
put to 38 consecutive PAF patients, it appeared that symptoms are more
commonly associated with factors causing increased vagal tone than

Table 1. **Proposed Autonomic Profile Questionnaire**

My attacks tend to start..."	Score (unweighted)*	Score (weighted)*
...shortly after waking	A	2A
...after meals	V	V
...after alcohol	A	A
...after tea or coffee	A	A
...during exercise	A	2A
...after exercise	V	V
...with twisting of the neck/shoulders	V	V
...resting or going off to sleep	V	2V
...during sleep	V	2V
...with emotional stress	A + V	A + V

"Never" = 0 points; "Rarely" = 1 point; "Sometimes" = 2 points; "Often" = 3
points; "Usually" = 4 points.

*A: points count toward adrenergic score; V: points count toward vagotonic
score; 2A: points are doubled before counting toward adrenergic score; 2V:
points are doubled before counting toward vagotonic score.

Figure 1. **Weighting of autonomic scores.** The weighted vagotonic score for each of 38 patients is plotted against the unweighted score. There is a high degree of correlation, and the use of weighting has therefore been abandoned.

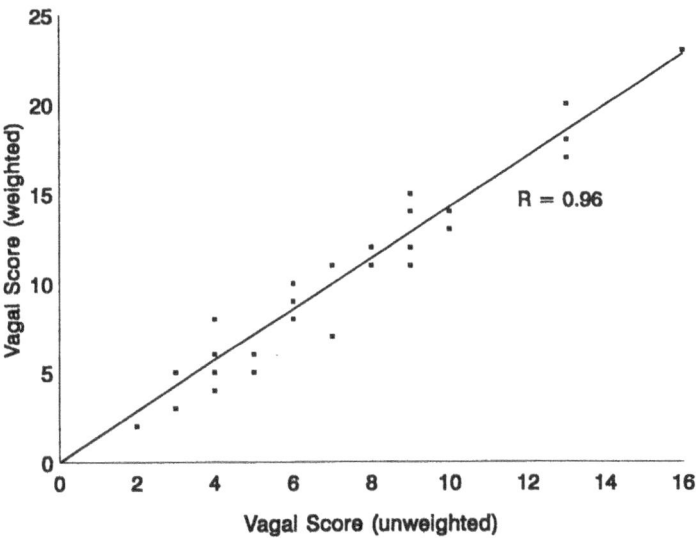

Figure 2. **Vagotonic versus adrenergic score.** For each of 28 lone PAF patients and 14 with cardiac disease, the adrenergic score is subtracted from the vagotonic score. In the majority of patients, the onset of symptoms appears to be more frequently associated with vagal than adrenergic tone. Disease = AF associated with underlying heart disease.

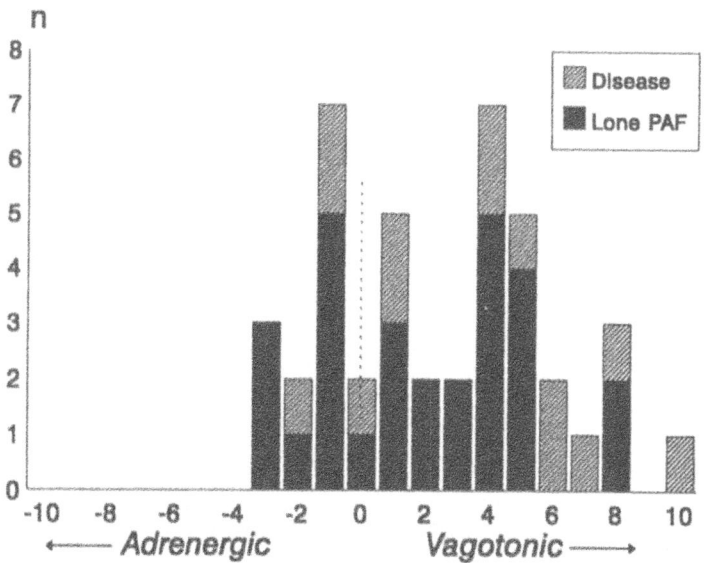

Figure 3. **Vagotonic score and associated disease.** No association is found between the presence of associated cardiac disease and vagal onset of symptoms.

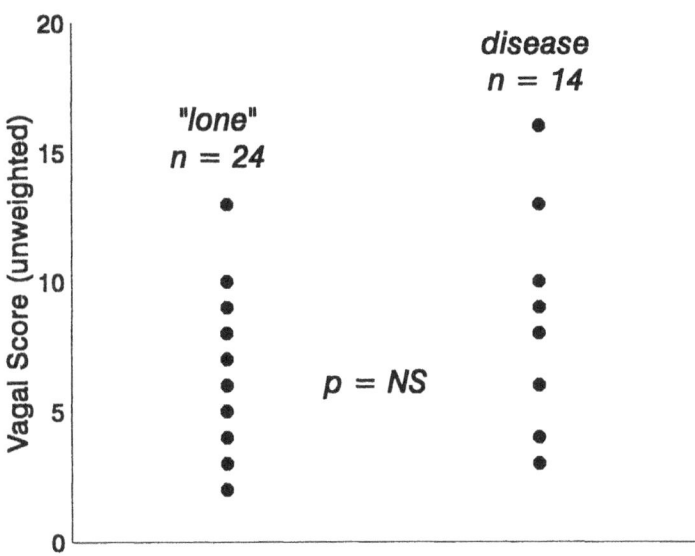

Figure 4. **Vagotonic score and baroreflex sensitivity.** Baroreflex sensitivity was assessed by phenylephrine bolus injection in 28 patients. No correlation was found with vagal score.

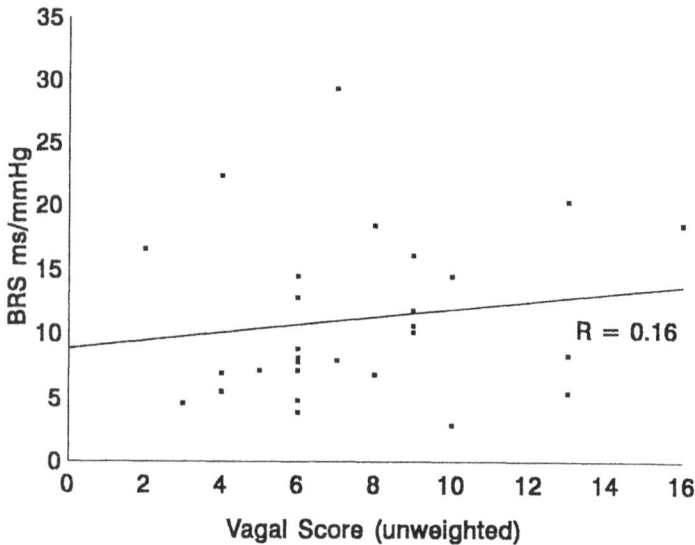

increased adrenergic tone (Fig.2). No significant difference was detected in vagal "score" between those patients with "lone" PAF and those with associated cardiac disease (Fig.3). It is hoped that the autonomic profile questionnaire can be refined and validated by comparison with Holter recordings.

If the autonomic nervous system is involved in the aetiology of PAF, the pathology could lie (i) within the nervous system itself, (ii) in an abnormal sinus node response to normal variations in efferent autonomic traffic, or (iii) in abnormal responses of the electrophysiologic substrate of the atrium itself. Orthodox tests of cardiac autonomic responses, such as those employing postural haemodynamic changes, and the Valsalva and baroreceptor reflexes, examine the integration of a variety of afferent limbs, manifested principally in changes in heart rate (i.e the modulation of sinus node activity by vagal and sympathetic efferents). We have performed baroreflex testing in 28 patients with PAF using the phenyloephrine bolus method of Smyth et al.[15] No relationship was found between vagal score and baroreflex sensitivity (Fig.4). Such a relationship might have been expected had increased vagal efferent traffic, or an enhanced sinus node response, been present in the patients with "vagal" PAF. If baroreflex sensitivity and other conventional tests of autonomic response prove not to differ between vagal PAF patients and controls, we may deduce that autonomic integration and sino-atrial function is normal. Indeed, these patients are distinct from those with the sick sinus syndrome,and do not generally exhibit excessive bradycardia even at times when high vagal tone appears to be provoking AF. We can speculate in this case that the abnormality must reside in the responses of the atrium itself. However, clinical techniques for the investigation of atrial autonomic responses are inadequately developed in humans.

ELECTROPHYSIOLOGY OF AF PATIENTS IN SR _____

The P wave. It has long been known that abnormalities in P wave morphology correlate with conditions affecting the atria and predisposing to AF. It is thought that, in "P mitrale", the bifid appearance of the P wave arises from delayed conduction of the cardiac impulse within the left atrium. This results in increased temporal separation between the surface manifestations of (normal, early) right atrial activation and (delayed) left atrial activation.

Conversely, in pulmonary disease, right atrial activation may be delayed sufficiently to coincide with left atrial activation; the resultant superimposition of electrical activity gives rise to the tall, narrow appearance of "P pulmonale". The advent of clinical cardiac electrophysiology has enabled direct measurements of inter- and intra-atrial conduction to be made, confirming that these changes in P wave morphology are a surface manifestation of conduction delays.

The low signal-to-noise ratio in the conventionally-recorded P wave limits the possibility of looking for small changes in its morphology or duration. In order to circumvent this problem, several investigators have recently applied signal-averaging techniques to the P wave. Engel, using R-wave triggered averaging, found no significant differences in high-frequency minus unfiltered P wave duration, or signal duration less than 10mV, between 17 patients with PAF and 35 controls[16]. Opolski, conversely, found significantly increased high-frequency P wave duration in 25 patients compared with 20 controls: a bifurcation value of 104ms gave a sensitivity of 76% and a specificity of 90%[17]. Fukunami examined 42 patients and 50 controls and found that the presence of atrial "late potentials" (defined as filtered P wave duration greater than 120ms and root mean square voltage of the terminal 20 ms of the P wave less than 3.5 mV) predicted PAF with a sensitivity of 91% and a specificity of 76%[18]. The disparity between findings almost certainly relates to methodology, which is a continued source of controversy in the field of signal averaging. A particular problem has been the alignment of P waves for averaging: if the succeeding QRS complex is used, beat-to beat variation in PR interval will reduce the accuracy of the technique. On the other hand, the P wave itself does not have a sharp enough onset to trigger the conventional algorithms used in QRS complex averaging.

These problems become even more acute when moving from the time domain to the frequency domain. Yamada used P-wave triggered averaging in 28 patients and 38 controls to analyse the frequency content of the terminal portion of the P wave[19]. Activity in the 20-30Hz region of the spectral curve, as estimated by either the area under the curve or the absolute magnitude at specific points on it, was significantly greater in patients with a history of AF. Interestingly this difference appeared to be specific to AF, as it was not seen between those with and without organic heart disease, but was maintained when the presence of heart disease was taken into account in the AF patients. Stafford used a sliding-template algorithm to average the P wave in 9 patients and 15 controls, and analysed the frequency content for the entire signal[20]. Along with a greater P wave duration, patients were found to have an increased high frequency content (greater than 30-40Hz). This difference was found to reside, not in the terminal portion of the P wave, but in its third quarter.

While it would appear that signal-averaging provides a method for detecting those patients at risk of atrial fibrillation, it is not yet clear what contribution the technique will make to our understanding of the pathophysiology of AF. It would seem that the abnormalities detected represent regional conduction delay, but such delays cannot yet be precisely located within the atrium. It is unlikely that current techniques for signal-averaging will be able to examine atrial repolarization, which is usually swamped by ventricular activation. Furthermore, beat-to beat variations in conduction are, of course, "ironed out" by the averaging process, which can therefore only detect fixed features of atrial activation.

Invasive studies. Several attempts have been made to use conventional invasive techniques to characterize the electrophysiological abnormalities associated with AF. Most of these studies have been conducted in patients with PAF, and have involved fairly simple parameters: the inducibility of repetitive atrial firing and AF itself, and the measurement of intra-atrial conduction times and refractory periods. Their findings are summarized in Table 2.

A common finding at electrophysiological study is repetitive atrial firing (RAF) induced by premature atrial extrastimuli. RAF probably represents local re-entry within the atrium, and usually only lasts for a few beats: it appears more frequently in patients with a history of AF than those without. However, it is a non-specific finding: the sensitivity and specificity of RAF as a marker for AF have been estimated, respectively, as 50% and 53% by Cosio[21], 75% and 32% by Ohe[22], and 62% and 74% by Hashiba[23]. In contrast, Buxton found the sensitivity and specificity of the inducibility of sustained AF to be 84% and 100%, respectively[24], and in a larger and more recent study Kuhlhamp has obtained figures of 82% and 80% [25].

Table 2. **Atrial Electrophysiology in PAF Patients**

Study	Atrial Conduction Times	Atrial Refractoriness
Simpson 1982 [26]	increased	normal AERP
Cosio 1983 [21]	increased	shortened AERP
Buxton 1984 [24]	increased	shortened AERP
Hashiba 1989 [23]	increased	
Kumagai* 1991 [27]	increased	shortened AERP
Kuhlkamp 1992 [25]	increased	normal AERP, shortened AFRP

AERP = atrial effective refractory period; AFRP = atrial functional refractory period. *Study performed in chronic AF patients shortly after direct current cardioversion .

Abnormalities of conduction within the atria have been a consistent finding in PAF. In 1982, Simpson compared 13 patients with P wave duration[3] 115ms, with 7 controls (P duration <115ms). In the first group, 3 patients had evidence of sino-atrial disease, and 6 had a history of atrial tachycardia or AF. There was an increased conduction time of early, though not late, extra-stimuli[26]. Cosio found longer delays in the conduction of extrastimuli, and a wider conduction delay zone (the range of intervals after which an extras-timulus causes delayed conduction) in patients compared with controls[21]: these findings have been reproduced by Buxton[24], Kuhlkamp[25], and Hashiba[23].

In contrast, authors have differed in their findings with respect to the atrial refractoriness in patients with PAF. Neither in Simpson's small, early study, nor in Kuhlkamp's larger group was a difference in atrial effective refractory period (ERP) detected between PAF patients and controls[25,26]. In the latter study, the right atrial functional refractory period was prolonged, but this is not surprising, as this propertly, unlike the ERP, is related to conduction in the atrium. On the other hand, both Cosio and Buxton found that, at a basic cycle length of 600ms, the atrial ERP in PAF patients was approximately 210ms, whereas that in controls or patients with atrial flutter was over 230ms.

Two recent studies are worthy of mention, as their methods have been somewhat different from the above. Kumagai compared the electrophysiology of 12 patients with *chronic* lone atrial fibrillation, immediately following direct current cardioversion, with that of patients without atrial arrhythmias[27]. The findings were similar to those in the studies of PAF patients: both the width of the conduction delay zone and the maximum conduction delay were greater, and the atrial ERP was shorter in patients. The P wave duration was longer in the chronic AF patients than the controls, and there was an increased incidence of sinus node dysfunction and inducibility of RAF. Asano has taken the unusual step of correlating properties of the atrial electrogram *during AF* with spontaneous reversion to sinus rhythm, in patients with AF inducible at electrophysiological study[28]. A "wavelength index" was obtained by dividing the interval between the fibrillation waves (taken to be a measure of local refractoriness) by their duration (fractionation, taken to be a measure of slowed conduction). AF spontaneously terminated in 20 of the 30 patients: in these patients, the wavelength index was higher at the outset and rose just prior to reversion to sinus rhythm. The methodology of this study is unusual, but the results are appealing and consistent with the wavelength model of susceptibility to AF[10].

Both slowed conduction and shortened atrial ERP are factors which reduce the wavelength of the atrial impulse and predispose to re-entry. While conduction delay is a universal finding, the discrepancy between studies of atrial refractoriness may reflect different methodologies. Furthermore, it is likely that refractoriness is a more dynamic variable, reflecting alterations in, for example, autonomic tone and metabolic changes, than conduction.

QUALITY OF LIFE _____

Finally, it is necessary to consider the issues affecting quality of life in patients with paroxysmal atrial fibrillation, which differ from those in other cardiac conditions in several important respects. For example, in the treatment of patients at risk of ventricular tachycardia and fibrillation, the risk of sudden cardiac death outweighs all other considerations. Similarly, in the treatment of cardiovascular risk factors such as hypertension and hyperlipidaemia, the goal of preventing myocardial infarction and cerebrovascular events (and the consequent drastic reduction in quality of life) is considered sufficiently important to outweigh non-life-threatening side-effects, such as those of beta-adrenergic blocking drugs and lipid-lowering agents. In chronic stable angina pectoris, aside from the long-term goal of preventing myocardial infarction, treatment is aimed at reducing the severity of symptoms which are usually relatively predictable and reproducible. These examples are illustrated in Figure 5.

For most patients, episodes of AF are not in themselves dangerous, as they do not give rise to severe angina or syncope. Furthermore, there is no clear evidence that episodes lasting for hours, or even days, constitute a thromboembolic risk, and this seems unlikely, other than in those patients whose AF is a marker of serious cardiac pathology. It therefore follows that, in the majority of patients, the treatment of PAF can be regarded entirely as a quality-of-life issue. However, this makes the goals of treatment, if anything, more difficult to determine (Fig.6). The simplest measure is the frequency of symptomatic attacks of AF, and this can now be documented using patient-activated monitors. This method, promoted by Pritchett, was used to evaluate flecainide in the treatment of PAF, and has since become the standard for such studies[29]. However, many patients may prefer a pattern of frequent, very mild, attacks of AF to one of rare but severe symptoms. It therefore becomes necessary to measure the severity of symptoms, such as dyspnoea, dizziness, palpitations, and chest pain, during episodes of AF. This is usually performed by interrogating patients during episodes or asking them to keep symptom diaries. Such subjective measures are really only valid within the context of double-blind studies. Another index of the severity of a paroxysm is the duration of symptoms. Again, this subjective measure is perhaps more important than the duration of AF itself, which may, if the ventricular rate falls during the course of an attack, continue without causing futher symptoms. Many patients experience profound after-effects following severe, but short-lived, episodes of AF. The mechanism for this phenomenon is not known, but may relate to the intense sympathetic discharge triggered by the attack. Again, this category of symptoms is difficult to measure. Finally, the quality of life *between* episodes of AF must be considered, as this constitutes the majority of most patients time. In addition to the side-effects of anti-arrhythmic agents, which can be limiting, the patients level of activity and mental state may be adversely affected by the fear of the next paroxysm, even if attacks are infrequent. This fear may be reduced by familiarity and understanding of the condition, but may nevertheless limit the patient's ability to undertake

Figure 5.

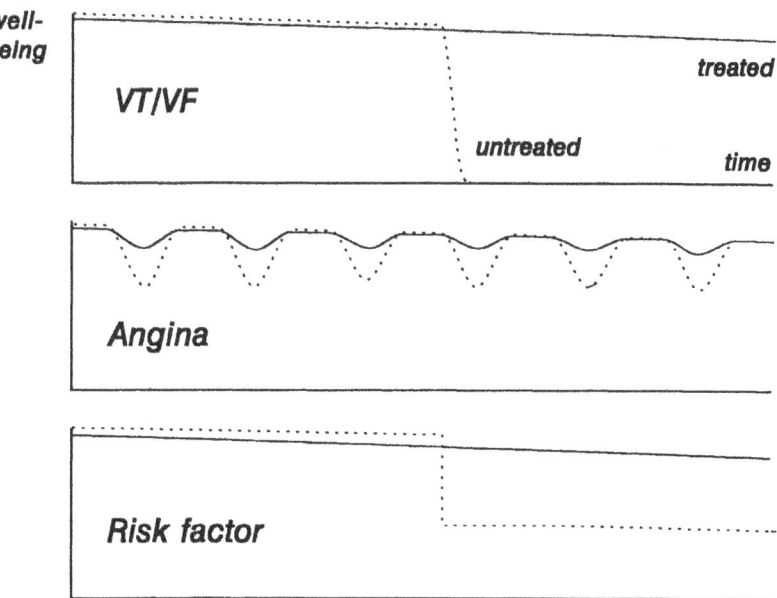

Figure 6.

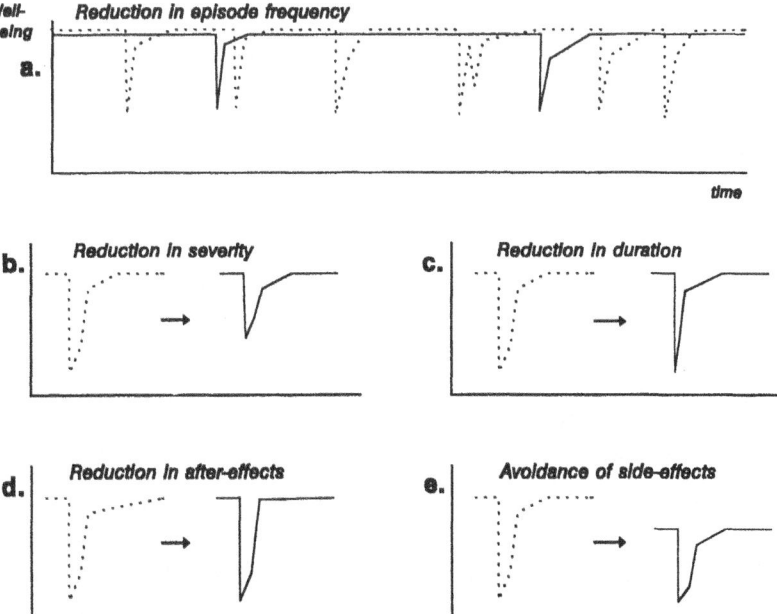

Figure 5. **Quality of life and cardiac disease.** Each graph is a representation of the aims of treatment in cardiovascular disease, with the vertical axis representing a scale of "well-being", and the horizontal axis representing time on an indeterminate scale: the dotted line represents the natural history of the condition, and the solid line the intended effect of treatment.

Top: in ventricular tachycardia and fibrillation, the end-point is death, and the aim of treatment must be the complete abolition of events.

Middle: in stable angina, one of the aims of treatment is the reduction in severity of a relatively predictable variable, which may be measured as chest pain, ST segment depression, exercise limitation, or nitrate consumption.

Bottom: in the treatment of risk factors, such as hypertension or hyperlipidaemia, a small reduction in quality of life (due to the side-effects of treatment) is often judged acceptable, when weighed against the larger reduction which would result from a myocardial infarction or stroke.

Figure 6. **Quality of life and paroxysmal atrial fibrillation.** Most studies to date have focussed on the frequency of symptomatic episodes of AF (a). Additionally, some have reported on the severity of symptoms as assessed by patients (b), and their duration (c). However, other end-points, which have not been addressed, include the after-effects of episodes (d) and the quality of life between episodes, which may be adversely affected by treatment side-effects and the fear of severe attacks.

activity likely to cause attacks (such as physical occupations), or activity during which attacks would be dangerous or embarrassing (such as piloting aircraft or giving lectures). This last issue is inadequately addressed by general psychological health questionnaires and those conventionally employed in cardiology. It is possible that, in terms of quality of life, the treatment of PAF bears more resemblance to that of epilepsy than other cardiac conditions.

CONCLUSIONS

Much can be learned from the study of AF patients during periods of sinus rhythm. Clinical patterns of the onset of PAF implicate the autonomic nervous system in its aetiology, and this may indicate a fruitful line for both research and treatment. However, the importance of autonomic factors is unknown, as are the mechanisms by which they may exert their effect. Signal-averaging of the P wave has shown abnormalities which probably reflect slowed atrial conduction. However, it is unlikely that this technique will be able to shed much light on the pathophysiology of PAF in the near future, and it is uncertain whether it will have any clinical role. Similarly, the finding of repetitive atrial firing at electrophysiological study is of limited value because of its lack of specificity. Slowed conduction within the atria is a constant finding in PAF patients, but the mechanism is not known, nor is the importance of shortened refractoriness established. Clinical studies of PAF patients in sinus rhythm are perhaps unlikely to yield substantially more information unless methods are improved to take account of temporal variations and physical dispersion of electrophysiological parameters within individuals. Because of the nature of the condition, the treatment of PAF must address all issues of quality of life, and not just the frequency of attacks. However, current measures are inadequately developed, especially in regard to patients' well-being between attacks.

References

[1]   Moe GK. On the multiple wavelet hypothesis of atrial fibrillation. Arch Int Pharmacodyn Ther 1962;140:183-188.

[2]   Allessie MA, Bonke FIM, Schopman FJG: Circus movement in rabbit atrial muscle as a mechanism of tachydardia. III. The 'leading circle' concept: a new model of circus movement in cardiac tissue without the involvement of an anatomical obstacle. Circ Res 1977;41:9-18.

[3]   Allessie MA, Lammers WJEP, Bonke FIM, Hollen JM: Experimental evaluation of Moe's multiple wavelet hypothesis of atrial fibrillation. In: Zipes DP, Jalife J (eds), Cardiac electrophysiology and arrhythmias. Orlando, Florida, Grune & Stratton, 1985, pp 265-275.

[4]   Allessie MA, Brugada J, Boersma L, et al. Mapping of atrial fibrillation in man. Eur Heart J 1990;11(suppl):5(Abstract).

[5]   Cox JL, Canavan TE, Schuessler RB, Cain ME, Lindsay BD, Stone C, Smith PK, Corr PB, Boineau JP. The surgical treatment of atrial fibrillation. II. Intraoperative electro-physiologic mapping and description of the electrophysiologic basis of atrial flutter and atrial fibrillation. J Thorac Cardiovasc Surg 1991;101:406-426.

[6]   Coumel P, Attuel P, Lavallée JP, Flammang D, Leclercq JF, Slama R. Syndrome d'arythmie auriculaire d'origine vagale. Arch Mal Coeur 1978;71:645-656.

[7]   Coumel P. Clinical approach to paroxysmal atrial fibrillation. Clin Cardiol 1990;13:209-212.

[8]   Coumel P. Role of the autonomic nervous system in paroxysmal atrial fibrillation, in Touboul P, Waldo AL (eds), Atrial arrhythmias. Current concepts and management. St Louis, Mosby-Year Book, 1990, pp 248-261.

[9]   Ninomiya I. Direct evidence of nonuniform distribution of vagal effects on dog atria. Circ Res 1966;19:576-583.

[10]   Smeets JLRM, Allessie MA, Lammers WJEP, Bonke FIM, Hollen JM. The wavelength of the cardiac impulse and reentrant arrhythmia in isolated rabbit atrium. Circ Res 1986;58:96-108.

[11]   Burn JH, Vaughan Williams EM, Walker JM. Effects of acetylcholine in heart-lung preparations including the production of auricular fibrillation. J Physiol 1955;128:277-293.

[12]   Coumel P, Leclercq J-F, Attuel P. Paroxysmal atrial fibrillation, in Kulbertus HE, Olsson SB, Schlepper M (eds), Atrial fibrillation. Mölndal, Sweden, AB Hässle, 1982, pp 158-175.

[13]   Hordof AJ, Spotnitz AJ, Mary Rabine L, Edie RN, Rosen MR. The cellular electroph-
        ysiologic effects of digitalis on human atrial fibers. Circulation 1978;57:223-229
[14]   Coumel P, Escoubet B, Attuel P. Beta-blocking therapy in atrial and ventricular
        tachyarrhythmias: experience with nadolol. Am Heart J 1984;108:1098-1108.
[15]   Smyth HS, Sleight P, Pickering GW. Reflex regulation of arterial pressure during sleep
        in man. Circ Res 1969;24:109-121.
[16]   Engel TR, Vallone N, Windle J. Signal-averaged electrocardiograms in patients with
        atrial fibrillation or flutter. Am Heart J 1988;115:592-597.
[17]   Opolski G, Stanislawska J, Slomka K, Kraska T. Value of the atrial signal-averaged
        electrocardiogram in identifying patients with paroxysmal atrial fibrillation. Int J Cardiol
        1991;30:315-319.
[18]   Fukunami M, Yamada T, Ohmori M, Kumagai K, Umemoto K, Sakai A, Kondoh N,
        Minamino T, Hoki N. Detection of patients at risk for paroxysmal atrial fibrillation
        during sinus rhythm by P wave-triggered signal-averaged electrocardiogram. Cir-
        culation 1991;83:162-169.
[19]   Yamada T, Fukunami M, Ohmori M, Kumagai K, Sakai A, Kondoh N, Minamino T, Hoki
        N. Characteristics of frequency content of atrial signal-averaged electrocardiograms
        during sinus rhythm in patients with paroxysmal atrial fibrillation. J Am Coll Cardiol
        1991;19:559-563.
[20]   Stafford PJ, Turner I, Vincent R. Quantitative analysis of signal-averaged P waves in
        idiopathic paroxysmal atrial fibrillation. Am J Cardiol 1991;68:751-755.
[21]   Cosio FG, Palacios J, Vidal JM, Cocina EG, Gomez-Sanchez MA, Tamargo L. Electro-
        physiologic studies in atrial fibrillation. Slow conduction of premature impulses: a
        possible manifestation of the background for reentry. Am J Cardiol 1983;51:122-130.
[22]   Ohe T, Matsuhisa M, Kamakura S, Yamada J, Sato I, Nakajima K, Shimomura K.
        Relation between the widening of the fragmented atrial activity zone and atrial fibril-
        lation. Am J Cardiol 1983;53:1219-1222.
[23]   Hashiba K, Tanigawa M, Fukatani M, Shimizu A, Konoe A, Kadena M, Mori M. Electro-
        physiologic properties of atrial muscle in paroxysmal atrial fibrillation. Am J Cardiol
        1989;64:20J-23J.
[24]   Buxton AE, Waxman HL, Marchlinski FE, Josephson ME. Atrial conduction; effects of
        extrastimuli with and without atrial dysrhythmias. Am J Cardiol 1984;54:755-761.
[25]   Kuhlkamp V, Haasis R, Seipel L. Atrial vulnerability and electrophysiology determined
        in patients with and without paroxysmal atrial fibrillation. PACE 1992;15:71-80.
[26]   Simpson RJJ, Foster JR, Gettes LS: Atrial excitability and conduction in patiens with
        interatrial conduction defects. Am J Cardiol 1982;50:1331-1337.
[27]   Kumagai K, Akimitsu S, Kawahira K, Kawanami F, Yamanouchi Y, Hiroki T, Arakawa K.
        Electrophysiological properties in chronic lone atrial fibrillation. Circulation 1991;84:
        1662-1668.
[28]   Asano Y, Saito J-I, Matsumoto K, Kaneko K, Yamamoto T, Uchida M. On the mecha-
        nism of termination and perpetuation of atrial fibrillation. Am J Cardiol 1992;69:1033-
        1038.
[29]   Anderson JL, Gilbert EM, Alpert BL, Henthorn RW, Waldo AL, Bhandari AK, Hawkin-
        son RW, Pritchett ELC. Prevention of symptomatic recurrences of paroxysmal atrial
        fibrillation in patients initially tolerating antiarrhythmic therapy. A multicenter, double-
        blind, crossover study of flecainide and placebo with transtelephonic monitoring.
        Flecainide Supraventricular Tachycardia Study Group. Circulation 1989;80:1557-1570.

Chapter 13

ATRIAL TACHYARRHYTHMIAS

FOLLOWING CORONARY BYPASS SURGERY:

SYMPATHETIC MECHANISMS

Jonathan M. Kalman

Muhammad Munawar

Anthony Yapanis

Laurence G. Howes

William J. Louis

Brian F. Buxton

Lawrence A. Doolan

Jane Tippett

Andrew M. Tonkin

Departments of
Cardiology, Clinical Pharmacology and Cardiac Surgery
Austin Hospital
Heidelberg
Melbourne, Australia

J. H. Kingma et al. (eds.), Atrial fibrillation, a treatable disease?, 211–225.
© 1992 *Kluwer Academic Publishers.*

INTRODUCTION _____

The development of atrial tachyarrhythmias following cardiothoracic surgery has long been recognised[1]. In an initial series published in 1943, of seventy-eight patients who underwent total pneumonectomy, five developed transient atrial fibrillation (AF) and two atrial flutter, most episodes occurring within two weeks of surgery[1]. None of these patients had organic heart disease and none subsequently developed a sustained atrial arrhythmia. Since then a number of larger series have shown that the incidence of atrial arrhythmias is higher in patients having larger operative procedures, with advancing age, pre-existing cardiovascular disease and with carcinoma of the lung particularly with pericardial involvement[2,3].

Studies of patients undergoing cardiac surgery have shown a wide variation in reported incidence of atrial arrhythmias of between 5-100%[4-6]. This variation reflects the different monitoring techniques and the definition of atrial arrhythmia used. In one series of forty-one patients undergoing coronary artery bypass surgery who were monitored continuously for seven days after surgery, all were found to have atrial arrhythmias during this period[6]. These included, in addition to atrial flutter and fibrillation of varying durations, episodes of atrial tachycardia including those of less than ten beats duration. In contrast, other studies which have reported a much lower incidence of atrial arrhythmias (of the order of 15-20%) and have relied on data derived from nursing staff observations of monitor screens and patients' reports of symptoms[7,8]. Such methods will usually detect only episodes of sustained and/or symptomatic atrial arrhythmias. In a review of sixteen studies published over the previous ten years Vecht et al.[9] found a mean incidence of 33.4% of atrial arrhythmias in patients who had undergone coronary surgery. Most have found that the peak time of onset is between 24-60 hours post-operatively and that AF occurs most commonly,with atrial flutter less frequent and atrial tachycardia unusual[4,5].

Numerous studies, many of which have been retrospective, have attempted to determine possible aetiologic factors in the pathogenesis of AF following coronary surgery[4,10-13]. Diverse variables have been examined including age, sex, pre-operative drug therapy, systemic hypertension, previous myocardial infarction, presence of unstable angina, poor left ventricular function, extent of coronary artery disease, number of bypass grafts, duration of aortic cross clamp time, electrolyte levels, left and right atrial pressures and arterial blood gas measurements. Of these the only two factors which have been related to the development of post-operative AF with any degree of consistency have been advanced age and pre-operative withdrawal of betablocker therapy[14,15]. Increasing sympathetic activity with advancing age has been well documented [16]. Several clinical studies have examined the role of betablockers in the pathogenesis of AF following coronary artery bypass surgery[6,10]. Many patients will have been receiving chronic betablocker therapy pre-operatively as treatment of angina. Withdrawal of such therapy has been associated with a number of adverse peri-operative events including atrial fibrillation. White et al.[6] and Salazar et al.[10] both found a 2-5 fold increase in incidence of AF in patients in whom betablockers were ceased when compared to those whose drugs were continued post-operatively. These observations may be due to the effects of betablocker withdrawal on adrenergic tone and beta-adrenergic receptor density[17,18]. It is also noteworthy that these arrhythmias occur 20-60 hours post-operatively at the time of maximal rebound effect from betablocker withdrawal[4,5]. Furthermore, a number of randomized controlled studies have found that betablockers given prophylactically significantly reduce the incidence of post-operative AF[6,19]. In contrast, prophylactic digoxin has met with mixed results and several studies have found post-operative AF relatively resistant to digoxin therapy[7,20,21].

However many of these studies have been retrospective and incomplete and the precise aetiology of post-operative atrial arrhythmias and the best means of prevention are still unclear. Therefore the aim of this study was to prospectively define risk factors for the development of atrial arrhythmias and in particular to determine whether the mechanism of AF following coronary surgery is related to excess sympathetic nervous activity. Knowledge of the relevant mechanisms has obvious implications for a more appropriate approach to prophylaxis.

METHODS _____

Subjects:

One hundred and fifty consecutive patients undergoing coronary bypass surgery were studied. Excluded were patients undergoing concomitant cardiac procedures such as valve repair or replacement, resection of a left ventricular aneurysm, or repair of a septal defect. Patients who were found to be in AF pre-operatively, with a past history of AF or taking amiodarone or other anti-arrhythmic agents were also excluded. In those patients taking betablocking drugs, these were stopped on the day prior to operation and were not recommenced. No patient received drugs as prophylactic therapy for AF.

Technique of Anaesthesia and Cardioplegia. Anaesthesia was by medium dose fentanyl for induction followed by an intermittent inhalational agent (halothane or enflurane). Two stage right atrial venous cannulation was used. All patients received warm blood cardioplegia for induction and reperfusion.

Holter Monitoring and Definitions. All patients were monitored using a two channel electrocardiography monitor (Cardiodata) connected in the immmediate post-operative period and continued for up to 80 hours. All tapes were analysed manually by freezing the monitor when an arrhythmia was detected during tape scanning and details of the arrhythmia were noted by review of a hard copy electrocardiography print out.

Atrial fibrillation was considered non-sustained if it lasted between ten beats and ten minutes, and sustained if it persisted for more than ten minutes. Criteria for the diagnosis of ectopic atrial tachycardia included an atrial rate in excess of 120 bpm, and a P wave morphology distinctly different from that of the sinus P wave. After the third post-operative day all patients had daily 12-lead electrocardiograms until discharge in order to detect late sustained AF. Nursing notes and clinical observations were also used to detect AF during this period.

Assessment of Left Ventricular function and Echocardiography. Left ventricular end-diastolic pressure was measured at the time of cardiac catheterisation and ejection fraction was digitised from the left ventriculogram. In all patients angiography had been undertaken within 3 months preoperatively. Left atrial size was assessed within twenty-four hours post-operatively and prior to onset of atrial fibrillation using the parasternal long axis view.

Noradrenaline Sampling. Right atrial plasma noradrenaline (N.A.) levels were measured prior to institution of cardiopulmonary bypass and post-operatively at four hourly intervals for 48 hours. Samples were drawn from the proximal port of the Swan-Ganz catheter with the patient resting at 45 degrees. Analysis of noradrenaline levels was by high performance liquid chromatography with electrochemical detection.

Statistical analysis. Students unpaired t-test, chi-square analysis, or Fishers exact test were used where appropriate to analyse the following variables in patients with and without AF: pre-operative noradrenaline level, post-operative N.A. levels at each sampling interval, age at operation, pre-operative usage of betablocker, pre- and post-operative magnesium levels, left atrial size, and ejection fraction. Multiple stepwise logistic regression was also performed on these variables and mean post-operative N.A. levels.

RESULTS

Of the 150 patients undergoing coronary artery bypass surgery who were studied, in 19 patients data collection was incomplete. These patients were excluded from analysis. Of the remaining 131 patients there were 109 males and 22 females with a mean age of 66.4± 7.5 years.

Arryhthmias. Atrial fibrillation or flutter developed in 70 patients (53%) within 80 hours post-operatively. In 54 (41%) the arrhythmia was classified as sustained (duration > 10 minutes) and in 16 (12%) as nonsustained (duration 10 beats-10 minutes). Forty-nine patients (37%) required treatment for AF as determined by the managing physician. The mean time of onset post-operatively in those patients with a sustained arrhythmia was 42.7± 219.7 hours, the distribution of time of onset being shown in Figure 1. There was no diurnal variation in time of onset throughout a 24 hour period (Fig. 2).

Ectopic atrial tachycardia developed in 15 of the 131 (11%) patients and was nonsustained (duration 10 beats-10 minutes) in 14. Thirteen of these 15 patients subsequently developed AF.

Figure 1.

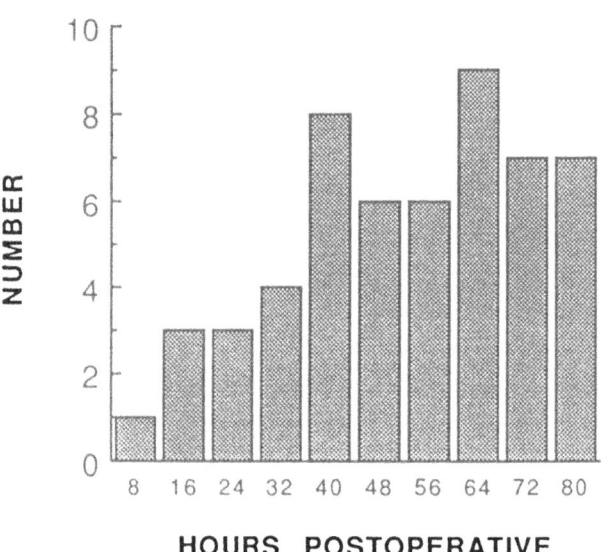

TIME OF ONSET OF A.F.

Figure 2.

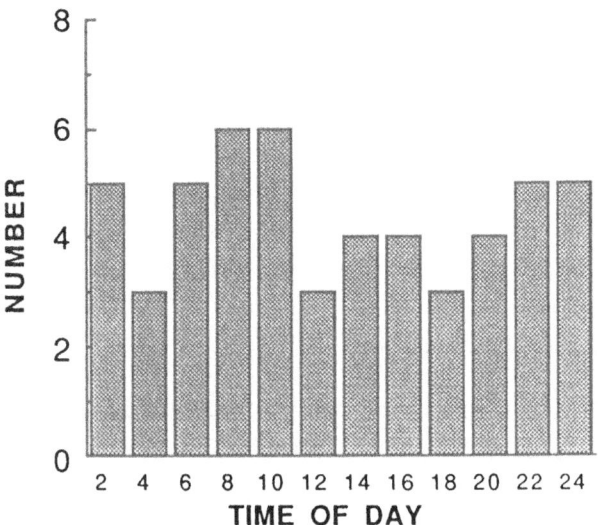

DISTRIBUTION OF A.F. ONSET

The onset of atrial arrhythmia was preceded in most patients by a pattern of increasing sinus rate over 1-2 hours and frequently by a further increase in the 10 minutes immediately prior to AF. A typical mean heart rate trend analysis from a Holter monitor is shown in Figure 3. In addition there was a significant increase in the frequency of atrial ectopic activity in the period immediately preceding AF. Statistical analysis of this and heart rate trend is included in Table 1.

Figure 3.

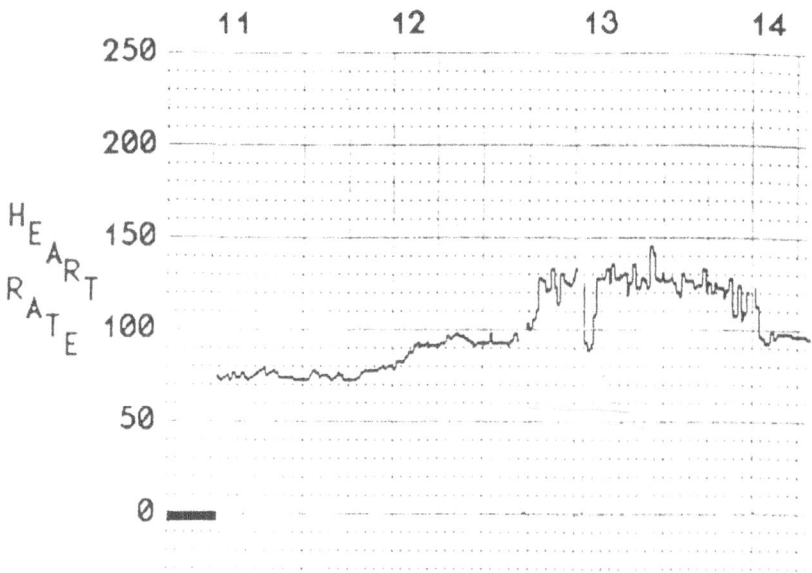

Table 1. Rhythm preceding onset of AF

	Mean during 3 minutes prior to AF onset	Mean during 3 hours prior to AF onset	Unpaired t-test
SINUS RATE (bpm)	96.4 ± 14.9	87.7 ± 9.1	p <0.05
ATRIAL ECTOPIC BEATS (n/3 mins)	11.7 ± 7.3	5.7 ± 5.6	p = 0.0001

Figure 4.

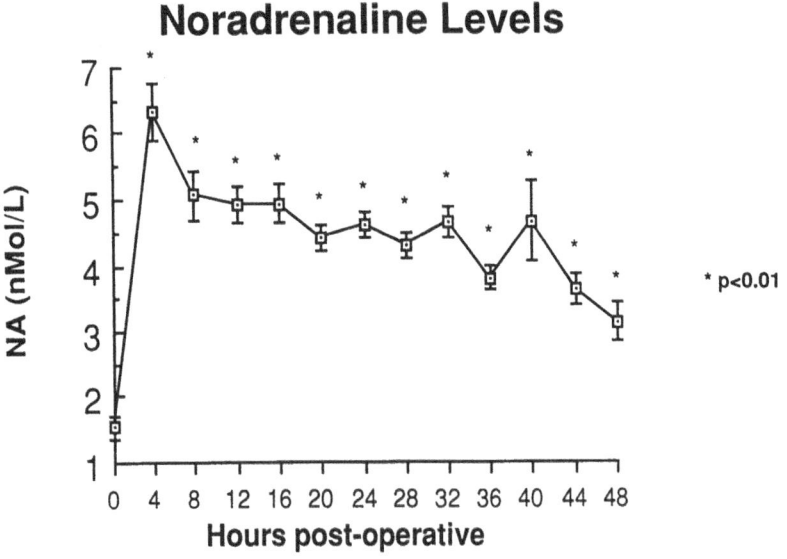

Figure 5.

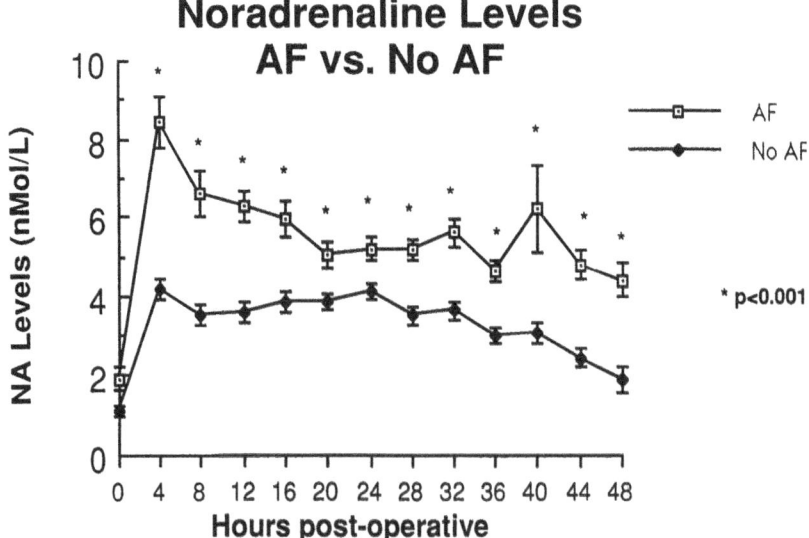

Noradrenaline analysis. There was a dramatic increase in plasma N.A. levels in the immediate post-operative period followed by a plateau and then a gradual decline after 40 hours (Figure 4). The plasma N.A. levels in patients who developed AF as opposed to those who did not are demonstrated in Figure 5. At every 4 hourly post-operative sampling interval there was a highly significant difference in right atrial N.A. levels with increased values in patients who developed AF ($p < 0.0001$). Both increased pre-operative N.A. levels and increased mean post-operative N.A. levels were on univariate analysis associated with AF ($p < 0.05$ and $p < 0.0001$, respectively).

Other variables. Table 2 shows other variables with a possible influence on development of AF. On univariate analysis, increasing age, low post-operative serum magnesium level and cessation of betablocker therapy pre-operatively were associated with the development of post-operative AF. Neither left atrial size nor left ventricular ejection fraction were found to be significant. Using multiple stepwise logistic regression, elevated mean post-operative N.A. levels, increased age and decreased post-operative serum magnesium were found to be independently associated with AF (Table 3).

Table 2. **Comparison of patients with post-operative atrial fibrillation and normal sinus rhythm**

VARIABLE	NO AF	AF	p value
Age (years)	64.1 ± 8.8	68.3 ± 5.6	p = 0.002
Preoperative betablockade	21/61 (34%)	40/70 (57%)	p = 0.01
Preoperative N.A. (nMol/L)	1.12 ± 1.0	1.92 ± 2.40	p = 0.03
Postoperative N.A. mean (nMol/L)	3.40 ± 1.17	5.96 ± 1.98	p = <0.0001
Postoperative Mg^{2+} (mMol/L)	0.83 ± 0.1	0.79 ± 0.09	p = 0.016
L.A. size (cm)	3.7 ± 0.4	3.9 ± 0.4	p = ns
L.V.E.F. (%)	56.9 ± 16.3	60.6 ± 14.0	p = ns

Table 3. Multivariate analysis

VARIABLE	ß	S.E.	Odds Ratio (C.I.)	p
Postoperative N.A. mean (nMol/L)	0.6308	0.1491	1.88 (1.40-2.52)	0.0001
Age (years)	0.0716	0.0334	1.07 (1.01-1.14)	0.0320
Postoperative Mg^{2+} (mMol/L)	-6.1788	2.8518	0.002 (0.0001-0.56)	0.0303
Constant	-2.4085	2.9108	—	0.4080

DISCUSSION

The mechanism of AF has generated much interest. In addition to structural heart disease, the autonomic nervous system has been implicated in both its initiation and perpetuation.

Initiation of AF depends on a change in electrophysiological properties in the atrium with a shortening of average refractory period and an inhomogeneity between different cells[22]. This will be more likely to occur with structural heart disease such as that associated with rheumatic and other valvular disease, the most common situation underlying AF. However, the refractory period of the atrium may be shortened by both vagal and sympathetic influences, and the inhomogeneity be due either to a non-uniformity of neural distribution or to a non-uniform disease process within the atria. Furthermore, it has been demonstrated that fibrillation may start with a period of rapid extrasystolic activity[23]. Early experimental preparations demonstrated that atrial fibrillation could be generated by single and multiple rapidly firing automatic foci. Aconitine induced AF was first demonstrated by Scherf et al. and subsequently by others[23,24]. Atrial fibrillation induced in this manner was dependent for perpetuation on the site where aconitine was applied and isolating that site from the rest of the atrium successfully terminated the fibrillation. The presumed mechanism was the development of a single ectopic focus whose frequency of impulse discharge was so rapid that uniform excitation of the atrium was no longer possible. Similarly, high frequency atrial stimulation produces a very fast automatic focus and conduction disturbance which rapidly degenerates into AF.

These findings are easily reproduced in humans in the electrophysiology laboratory by rapid atrial pacing or by a critically timed atrial extra stimulus and these techniques are routinely used by clinical electrophysiologists to examine the electrical properties of the human atrium. The spontaneous development of a rapidly firing focus may be caused by re-entry, by discharge of an automatic focus or by triggered activity due to afterpotentials. In the setting of increased sympathetic activity or excess catecholamines, the latter two may constitute the mechanisms which trigger the fibrillation process. These two mechanisms may also be responsible for atrial ectopic activity and atrial tachycardia.

The phenomena that initiate AF are not necessarily the same as those which maintain it and in the experimental undiseased atrium, AF terminates as soon as the manoeuvres provoking a shortening of refractory period and non-uniformity are discontinued.

Most evidence now suggests that AF is re-entrant in origin. Moe et al. first proposed the multiple wavelet hypothesis and used computer modelling to demonstrate multiple circulating excitation wavefronts[25]. This hypothesis has since been confirmed both in a canine model and subsequently in humans [26,27]. In the computer model the persistence of fibrillation depends upon the number of wavelets present[28]. Multiple wavelets are favoured not only by a short atrial refractory period and an inhomogeneity of refractoriness but also by a larger mass of tissue (atrial size) and slowing of conduction velocity. The latter two conditions are also produced by structural disease of the atrium. While both limbs of the autonomic nervous system have the same effect of shortening the action potential, they do not modify intra-atrial conduction in the same way and only vagal stimulation slows conduction. In most cases, AF which develops for the first time in the period immediately following coronary surgery is shortlived suggesting that the provocative stimulus has discontinued[4].

Corresponding to this experimental data relating to autonomic effects, Coumel et al. have described two separate clinical syndromes of paroxysmal AF in patients with structurally normal hearts, the more common being vagally mediated and the other occurring at times of high sympathetic tone[29,30].

Those patients with no underlying structural heart disease who tend to have episodes of paroxysmal AF at times of increased sympathetic activity typically have this during the day time and in association with exercise or emotional stress. Patterns on Holter monitoring in this group contrast sharply with those of vagally-induced atrial arrhythmia. Atrial fibrillation usually has its onset in the morning and is preceded by an increasing sinus rate. With increasing heart rate there are increasingly frequent atrial premature beats with short coupling interval. Frequently, there are runs of ectopic atrial tachycardia alternating with sinus rhythm but without atrial flutter. Atrial fibrillation may be precipitated in these patients at electrophysiology study by administration of isoprenaline. Our observations in this study of the pattern of atrial arrhythmias and premonitory changes on Holter monitor were typical of an adrenergic mechanism.

This is corroborated by our observations relating to plasma N.A. levels. Some discussion of the method of estimation of sympathetic activation is appropriate. The predominant sources of circulating N.A. in humans are sympathetic nerve endings and the adrenal medulla[31]. The adrenomedullary contribution is usually very small and has been estimated at between 2-7.5% at rest. However during stress, it is possible that the relative contribution of adrenomedullary secretion to circulating N.A. is increased. Thus circulating N.A. probably derives largely from sympathetic nerve endings and in particular from the sympathetic innervation to vascular walls especially to small arteries and arterioles.

Sympathetic outflow to the various vascular beds is not uniform[31]. The relative contribution of a particular organ to peripheral venous N.A. depends both on the amount of N.A. released and on the regional blood flow to that particular organ. Thus, while sampling N.A. from a peripheral vein may predominantly reflect N.A. release in peripheral musculature, central mixed venous N.A. levels are more likely to provide an accurate picture of "overall sympathetic activity". While it may be argued that coronary sinus levels would most accurately reflect cardiac sympathetic activity, from a practical viewpoint, in most patients following coronary surgery, right atrial sampling may be the method of choice.

A marked elevation in N.A. levels following coronary bypass surgery has been well demonstrated[32,33]. Several studies have found that in patients with post-operative hypertension N.A. levels increased from the pre-operative baseline whereas there was little change from the pre- to post-operative periods in patients who remained normotensive[33,34].

To our knowledge only one study[35] has attempted to correlate post-operative plasma N.A. levels with the development of arrhythmias. This examined only nineteen patients and these included both patients undergoing coronary revascularization and those having valve replacement or repair. The investigators found no correlation between post-operative N.A. levels and the development of cardiac arrhythmias which were analysed as a group and included both supraventricular and ventricular arrhythmias. Noradrenaline levels in this study were sampled at twenty-four hourly intervals from a peripheral vein.

The only other variables shown in our study to be significantly associated with development of post-operative atrial arrhythmias were increasing age and decrease in serum magnesium. Both of these may be operative at least in part by an effect mediated by or reflecting increase in N.A. levels[36].

In summary, we have demonstrated a very significant and independent difference in right atrial N.A. levels in patients who developed atrial arrhythmias compared with those who did not. This difference was maintained throughout the 48 hours of sampling, and was independent of left ventricular function. The results provide very strong evidence that AF post coronary artery surgery is mediated by the sympathetic nervous system. Furthermore the development of an increase in sinus rate prior to the onset of AF coupled with increasingly frequent atrial extrasystoles and episodes of atrial tachycardia is further evidence of sympathetic activation. In addition, the finding of a low serum magnesium on the third postoperative day was an independent predictor of AF.

These findings suggest that the most logical approach to prevention of AF in patients following coronary artery bypass surgery would be by methods which blunt sympathetic activation and/or effects.

Acknowledgements:
This study was performed during tenure by Dr. Kalman of a Postgraduate Medical Research Scholarship of the National Health and Medical Research Council of Australia.

References

[1]   Bailey CC, Betts RH: Cardiac arrhythmias following pneumonectomy. N Engl J Med 1943;
        229:356-359.
[2]   Ghosh P, Pakrashi BC: Cardiac dysrhythmias after thoracotamy. Br Heart J 1972;34:
        374-376.
[3]   Beck-Nielsen J, Rahbek Sorensen H, Alstrup P. Atrial fibrillation following thoracotomy for
        non-cardiac diseases, in particular cancer of the lung. Acta Med Scand 1973;193:425-429.
[4]   Lauer MS, Eagle KA, Buckley MJ, DeSanctis RW. Atrial fibrillation following coronary artery
        bypass surgery. Prog Cardiovasc Dis 1989;31:367-378.
[5]   Groves PH, Hall RJC: Atrial tachyarrhythmias after cardiac surgery. Eur Heart J 1991;
        12:458-463.
[6]   White HD, Antman GM, Glynn MA, et al. Efficacy and safety of timolol for prevention of
        supraventricular tachyarrhythmias after coronary artery bypass surgery. Circulation 1984;
        70:479-784.
[7]   Tyras DH, Stothert JC Jr, Kaiser GC, et al. Supra-ventricular tachyarrhythmias after
        myocardial revascularization: A randomized trial of prophylactic digitilization. J Thorac
        Cardiovasc Surg 1979;77:-310-314.
[8]   Silverman NA, Wright R, Levitsky S. Efficacy of low-dose propranolol in preventing
        postoperative supraventricular tachyarrhythmias: A prospective, randomized study. Ann
        Surg 1982;196:194-97.
[9]   Vecht RJ, Nicolaides EP, Ikweuke JK, et al. Incidence and prevention of supraventricular
        tachyarrhythmias after coronary bypass surgery. Int J Cardiol 1986;13:124-134.
[10]   Salazar C, Frishman W, Friedman S, et al. Beta-blockade therapy for supraventricular
        tachyarrhythmias after coronary surgery: A propranolol withdrawal syndrome? Angiology
        1979;30:816-891.
[11]   Chee TP, Prakash NS, Desser KB, et al. Postoperative supraventricular arrhythmias and
        the role of prophylactic digoxin in cardiac surgery. Am Heart J 1982;104:974-977.
[12]   Crosby LH, Pifalo WB, Woll KR, Burkholder JA. Risk factors for atrial fibrillation after
        coronary artery bypass grafting. Am Heart J 1990;66:1520-1522.
[13]   Leitch JW, Thomson D, Baird DK, Harris PJ. The importance of age as a predictor of atrial
        fibrillation and flutter after coronary artery bypass grafting. J Thorac Cardiovasc Surg
        1990;100:338-342.
[14]   Boudalas H, Snyder GL, Lewis RP, et al. Safety and rationale for continuation of
        propranolol therapy during coronary bypass operation. Ann Thorac Surg 1978;26:222-229.
[15]   Fuller JA, Adams GG, Buxton B. Atrial fibrillation after coronary artery bypass surgery. Is
        it a disorder of the elderly? J Thorac Cardiovasc Surg 1989;97:821-825.
[16]   Hoeldtke RD, Cilmi KM. Effects of aging on catecholamine metabolism. J Clin End and
        Metab 1985;60:479-484.
[17]   Boudalas H, Lewis RP, Kates RE, et al. Hypersensitivity to adrenergic stimulation after
        propranolol withdrawal in normal subjects. Ann Int Med 1977;87:433-436.
[18]   Aarons RD, Nies AS, Gal J, et al. Elevation of beta-adrenergic receptor density in human
        lymphocytes after propranolol administration. J Clin Invest 1980;65:949-957.
[19]   Matangi MF, Neutze JM, Graham IC, et al. Arrhythmia prophylaxis after aorta-coronary
        bypass: The effect of minidose propranolol. J Thorac Cardiovasc Surg 1985;89:439-443.
[20]   Johnson LW, Dickstein RA, Freuhan CT, et al. Prophylactic digitilization for coronary artery
        bypass surgery. Circulation 1976;53:819-822.
[21]   Csicsko JF, Schatzlein MH, King RD. Immediate post-operative digitilization in the
        prophylaxis of supraventricular arrhythmias following coronary artery bypass. J Thorac
        Cardiovasc Surg 1981;81:419-422.

[22]   Waldo AL. Mechanisms of atrial fibrillation, atrial flutter and ectopic atrial tachycardia: a brief review. Circulation 1987;5:III-37.

[23]   Scherf D. Studies on auricular tachycardia caused by aconitine administration. Proc Exp Biol Med 1947;64:233.

[24]   Brown BB, Acheson GH. Aconitine induced auricular arrhythmias and their relation to circus movement flutter. Circulation 1952;6:529.

[25]   Moe GK, Rheinholdt WC, Abildskov J.A. A computer model of atrial fibrillation. Am Heart J 1964;67:200-220.

[26]   Allessie M, Lammers WJEP, Bonke FI, Hollen J. Experimental evaluation of Moe's multiple wavelet hypothesis of atrial fibrillation. In: Zipes D, Jalife J (eds), Cardiac electrophysiology and arrhythmias. New York, Grune & Stratton 1985, pp 265-275.

[27]   Cox JL, Canavan TE, Schuessler RB, et al. The surgical treatment of atrial fibrillation: II. Intraoperative electrophysiologic mapping and description of the electrophysiologic basis of atrial flutter and fibrillation. J Thorac Cardiovasc Surg 1991;101:406-426.

[28]   Moe GK. On the multiple wavelet hypothesis of atrial fibrillation. Arch Int Pharmacodyn Ther 1962;140:183-188.

[29]   Coumel P, Leclercq JF, Attuel P. Paroxysmal atrial fibrillation. In: Kulbertus HE, Olsson SB, Schlepper M (eds), Atrial fibrillation. Kiruna, Sweden, 1981, pp 158-175.

[30]   Coumel P, Leclercq JF, Attuel P, Lavalee JP, Flammang D. Autonomic influences in the genesis of atrial arrhythmias: atrial flutter and fibrillation of vagal origin. In: Narula OS (ed), Cardiac arrhythmias electrophysiology, diagnosis and management. Baltimore, London, Williams and Wilkins, 1979, pp 243-255.

[31]   Goldstein DS, McCarty R, Polinsky RJ, Kopin IJ. Relationship between plasma norepinephrine and sympathetic neural activity. Hypertension 1983;5:522-559.

[32]   Reed HL, Chernow B, Lake CR, Zaloga GP, Stoiko MA, Beardsly D, Cruess D, Lee C, Smallridge RC. Alterations in sympathetic nervous system activity with intraoperative hypothermia during coronary artery bypass surgery. Chest 1989;95:616-622.

[33]   de Leeuw PW, van der Starre JA, Harinck-de Weerdt JE, de Bos R, Tchang PT, Birkenhager WH. Humoral changes during and following coronary bypass surgery: relationship to postoperative blood pressure. Journal of Hypertension 1983;1 (suppl 2):52-54.

[34]   Goldstein DS. Plasma norepinephrine as an indicator of sympathetic neural activity in clinical cardiology. Am J Cardiol 1981;48:1147-1154.

[35]   Engleman RM, Haag B, Lemeshow S, Angelo A, Rousou JH. Mechanism of plasma catecholamine increases during coronary artery bypass and valve procedures. J Thorac Cardiovasc Surg 1983;86:608-615.

[36]   Reves JF, Karp RB, Buttner EE, et al. Neuronal and adrenomedullary catecholamine release in response to cardiopulmonary bypass in man. Circulation 1982;66:49-55.

Chapter 14

MANAGEMENT OF PAROXYSMAL ATRIAL FIBRILLATION AND ATRIAL FLUTTER SHORTLY AFTER CORONARY ARTERY BYPASS GRAFT SURGERY

Maarten J. Suttorp

J. Herre Kingma

Norbert M. van Hemel

Jo A.M. Defauw

Freddy E.E. Vermeulen

Sjef M.P.G. Ernst

Departments of Cardiology and Cardiothoracic Surgery
St Antonius Hospital
Nieuwegein
The Netherlands

J. H. Kingma et al. (eds.), Atrial fibrillation, a treatable disease?, 227–236.

INTRODUCTION _____

Supraventricular tachyarrhythmias are very common in patients shortly after cardiac surgery, frequently as atrial fibrillation, less often as atrial flutter and seldom as atrial tachycardia[1]. These transient postoperative supraventricular tachyarrhythmias are considered a form of paroxysmal atrial arrhythmia of recent onset. Atrial tachyarrhythmias commonly complicate the early postoperative course after cardiac surgery. Atrial arrhythmias occurring immediately after operation can jeopardize hemodynamic stability or lead to intolerable symptoms. These arrhythmias are usually benign, but could require additional drug therapy, cardiac pacing or even electrical cardioversion.

Coronary artery bypass graft surgery.

As shown in Table 1, the spectrum of incidence of postoperative supra-ventricular tachyarrhythmias reported in the literature in patients shortly after bypass surgery varies between 11.4% and 100% (mean incidence 27.5%), with a peak incidence of the arrhythmia within the first 3 days after coronary artery bypass graft surgery. Our results confirm these data and show an incidence of 32.7% in patients treated with placebo shortly after coronary artery bypass graft surgery[2-4].

The extreme variation shown in Table 1 can be explained in part by the methods used in detecting these postoperative arrhythmias, i.e. whether continuous electrocardiographic monitoring was used or not[5,6]. Further-more, multiple additional factors may be involved in an increased occurrence of atrial tachyarrhythmias. These include metabolic, fluid and temperature changes, high circulating catecholamine levels, surgical trauma to atrial tissue, the lack of adequate atrial cardioplegia, the occurrence of pericarditis, and the use of various anesthetic agents.

Valvular surgery.

Supraventricular tachyarrhythmias after valvular surgery have been less well studied. The incidence of these tachyarrhythmias is higher in patients who underwent valvular surgery than after coronary artery bypass graft surgery. The reported incidence varies between 32% and 60%[5,7-9]. Smith and co-workers reported that supraventricular tachyarrhythmias were more frequently observed after mitral valve replacement than after aortic valve replacement[7].

Table 1. **Incidence of Supraventricular Tachyarrhythmias in Untreated Patients Shortly after Coronary Artery Bypass Graft Operations**

First author [references]			No. of Pts	Incidence of SVT (%)
Tyras	1979	[21]	79	11.4
Silverman	1982	[22]	50	28.0
Csicsko	1981	[34]	270	15.0
Mills	1983	[11]	90	30.0
Parker	1983	[35]	56	21.4
Ivey	1983	[23]	56	16.1
White	1984	[6]	20	100.0
Matangi	1985	[36]	82	23.0
Janssen	1986	[24]	50	36.0
Daudon	1986	[17]	50	40.0
Vecht	1986	[26]	66	19.7
Rubin	1987	[18]	40	37.5
Khuri	1987	[25]	74	42.0
Lamb	1988	[27]	30	37.0
Suttorp	1991	[3]	<u>150</u>	<u>32.7</u>
			1120	27.5
				(range 11.4-100)

SVT = supraventricular tachyarrhythmias.

CARDIOVASCULAR RISK FACTOR ANALYSIS FOR DEVELOPING POSTOPERATIVE SUPRAVENTRICULAR TACHYARRHYTHMIAS

Studies to analyse cardiovascular risk factors for the development of supraventricular tachyarrhythmias early after coronary artery bypass graft surgery are still very limited. In previous studies it has been suggested that older age[10-14], male gender[13], previous cardiac surgery[7], history of myocardial infarction[8], left atrial enlargement[12], cardiomegaly[12], hypertension[15], preoperative use of ß-blockers[16,17], number of anasto-moses[10], and longer aortic crossclamp or bypass time[10] were associated with a higher prevalence of atrial fibrillation or atrial flutter. A randomized prospective study by Rubin and co-workers demonstrated that no pre-, intra- or post-operative characteristics can predict patients who have an increased risk of postoperative atrial fibrillation[18]. As shown in Table 2, by using multivariate analysis, Suttorp and co-workers found that male gender and older age, as well as one- or two-vessel coronary artery disease were independent risk factors for developing supraventricular tachyarrhythmias[3]. In contrast to several other reports, it was striking that the preoperative use of ß-blocking agents did not increase the risk of postoperative arrhythmias.

Table 2. **Multivariate Analysis of Patient Variables for the Risk of Post-operative Supraventricular Tachyarrhythmias by Means of Stepwise Logistic Regression***

Variables	OR	95%-CI
Treatment with Sotalol	0.3	(0.2-0.6)
Male sex	2.3	(1.1-5.0)
1- or 2-vessel CAD	2.0	(1.1-3.9)
Age (years)	1.1	(1.0-1.1)[#]

* The odds ratios and 95% confidence intervals are given for those varia-bles with independent influence on the occurrence of postoperative supraventricular tachyarrhythmia.
# Odds ratio per year of age.
CAD = coronary artery disease; CI = confidence interval; OR = odds ratio.

PREVENTION OF SUPRAVENTRICULAR TACHYARRHYTHMIAS AFTER CARDIAC SURGERY _____

Inconsistent data have been reported regarding the effectiveness and safety of various drugs in preventing atrial fibrillation or atrial flutter early after operation. The data inconsistency could be partly explained by the many variables introduced during and after cardiac surgery. These variables differ from institution to institution but they could also be due to patient selection, differences in electrocardiographic monitoring and suboptimal study designs such as open randomization. The reported success rates for preventing atrial fibrillation or atrial flutter with various drugs range from 100% in patients treated with acebutolol started at 36 hours after coronary artery bypass operation to 0% in patients treated with digoxin starting immediately postope-rative[10,17].

Digoxin. A few studies evaluating results of digoxin before and after coronary artery bypass graft surgery have suggested beneficial effects from this drug. In a randomized, controlled trial Johnson and co-workers showed a reduction of 26% in the control group compared with 6% in the patients given digoxin for 2 to 3 days preoperatively and continued postoperatively[19]. Selzer and colleagues warned against the routine use of digoxin because it increases myocardial sensitivity and thus increases the danger of toxicity[20]. Other studies have failed to demonstrate any benefit during the prophylactic administration of digoxin. Tyras and co-workers showed that prophylactic usage of digoxin yielded no benefit in preventing supraventricular tachy-arrhythmias shortly after coronary artery bypass graft surgery and may even predispose patients to these postoperative arrhythmias[21]. According to the available data digoxin is not beneficial as a prophylactic agent and should not be recommended for prevention following coronary artery bypass graft surgery.

ß-adrenoceptor blocking agents.

ß-adrenoceptor blocking drugs are reported to be effective in reducing the incidence of postoperative atrial tachyarrhythmias. However, in various studies conflicting data have been reported regarding the efficacy and safety of various ß-blocking agents for prevention of these arrhythmias shortly after coronary artery bypass graft surgery.

Propranolol. Several studies with various designs have demonstrated the efficacy of both low-dose propranolol (10 mg every 6 hours) and high-dose propranolol (20 mg every 6 hours) for preventing supraventricular tachy-arrhythmias[2,15,16,22]. In our study we found an incidence of 18.8% in patients treated with low-dose propranolol[2]. In contrast to our study, Silverman and colleagues reported a reduction in frequency of supraventricular tachyarrhythmias from 28% to 6% in patients with low-dose propranolol, although their treatment was started at 24 hours after operation[22]. Salazar and colleagues showed a reduction in supraventricular tachyarrhythmias from 50% to 25% in patients treated with low-dose propranolol, with treatment starting immediately after surgery[16]. Mohr and colleagues reported that both low- and high-dose propranolol, started at 6 hours after surgery, was very effective in reducing supraventricular tachyarrhythmias early after coronary artery bypass graft surgery[15]. Ivey and co-workers reported an incidence of 13.2% in patients treated with high-dose propranolol versus an incidence of 13.7% in our study; however, in their study, treatment was started 24 hours after operation and they noted that high-dose propranolol was ineffective in reducing the incidence of these arrhythmias[2,23]. In contrast, Rubin and colleagues noted an incidence of 16.2% in patients treated with high-dose propranolol versus 37.5% in untreated patients. Thus, they concluded that propranolol prophylaxis was effective compared with untreated patients in whom the incidence of atrial tachyarrhythmia was 37.5%[18].

Sotalol. Only three reports have described the preventive effect of sotalol after coronary artery bypass graft operation[2,3,24].

Janssen and coworkers observed a reduction in atrial tachyarrhythmias after surgery from 36% to as low as 2.4%. However, this open-label study suffered from a suboptimal design and a limited number of patients[24]. Their patients received sotalol intravenously during the first hour following coronary artery bypass graft operation and thereafter orally at a dose of 80 mg every 8 hours beginning after 24 hours. The authors attribute this effect to the additional class III antiarrhythmic properties of sotalol. In their study there were no adverse effects requiring discontinuation of the drug. Our findings are in disagreement with their study.

In an open trial performed by our group, we found an incidence of supraventricular tachyarrhythmia of 13.9% using low-dose sotalol (40 mg every 8 hours) versus 10.9% using high-dose sotalol (80 mg every 8 hours). Adverse effects possibly related to the treatment and necessitating discontinuation of the drug were less prominent in patients receiving low-dose sotalol (2.8%) compared with patients receiving high-dose sotalol (10.5%)[2]. In another randomized, double-blind, placebo controlled study, our group reported a reduction in the incidence of supraventricular tachyarrhythmia from 32.7% in the control group to 16% in patients who were treated with low-dose sotalol (40 mg every 6 hours). Almost no adverse effects were observed requiring discontinuation of the drug[3].

Other ß-blocking agents.

Other studies report that acebutolol, nadolol, timolol, metropolol and atenolol have been found to be effective in preventing supraventricular tachyarrhythmias after cardiac surgery. In a randomized controlled study Daudon and co-workers reported 100% success in preventing atrial tachyarrhythmias in a small number of patients treated with acebutolol, even though this treatment was started 36 hours after coronary artery bypass graft surgery[17]. In a double-blind placebo-controlled study Khuri and colleagues showed that 42% of the placebo group but only 9% of patients treated with nadolol experienced sustained supraventricular tachycardia requiring clinical intervention[25]. In another double-blind placebo-controlled study Vecht and co-workers reported a significant reduction of postoperative arrhythmias from 19.7% in patients receiving placebo to 7.5% in those receiving timolol[26]. White and colleagues reported that prophylactic use of timolol after coronary artery bypass graft surgery was effective and safe in both decreasing the frequency and severity of supraventricular tachyarrhythmias[6]. Janssen and colleagues reported a reduction in atrial tachyarrhythmias shortly after coronary artery bypass graft surgery from 36% in a control group to 15.3% in patients treated with metropolol compared with 2.4% in patients treated with sotalol[24]. Lamb and co-workers gave atenolol and they demonstrated a reduction in atrial tachyarrhythmias from 37% in the control group to 3% in their study group[27]. It should be stated that in most of these studies only small numbers of patients were studied.

Combination of digoxin with ß-adrenoceptor blocking agents.

In a non-randomized trial, Roffman and colleagues reported that the combination of postoperative digoxin shortly after operation together with propranolol beginning at 48 hours after surgery reduced the prevalence of supraventricular tachyarrhythmias from 28.2% in the control group and 28.9% in the digoxin group to 2.2% in the combined digoxin/propranolol group[10]. Interestingly, comparable results from a randomized study were also shown by Mills and co-workers who reported a reduction from 30% down to 3.4% in those receiving a combination of digoxin and oral propranolol therapy, started at 6 hours after surgery[11].

Other antiarrhythmic agents.

Verapamil does not seem to be very effective in preventing supraventricular tachyarrhythmias shortly after cardiac surgery[28,29].

Up to now, in contrast to the large number of reports requiring immediate pharmacological conversion of supraventricular tachyarrhythmias shortly after cardiac surgery, no data is available on the prophylactic use of newer antiarrhythmic drugs such as flecainide, propafenone or amiodarone for maintaining sinus rhythm shortly after coronary artery bypass graft surgery.

Pharmacological conversion.

As already discussed elsewhere in this volume, the reported success rate for acute pharmacological reversion of postoperative supraventricular tachyarrhythmias varies from up to 43% in patients treated with intravenous propafenone or amiodarone[9,30] to even 89% in patients treated with intravenous sotalol, flecainide or digoxin/disopyramide combination[31-33].

CONCLUSIONS _____

Supraventricular tachyarrhythmias often complicate the early postoperative period and they continue to present a significant cause of early postoperative morbidity after cardiac surgery. However, these atrial arrhythmias are often paroxysmal and self-limiting in the early postoperative period. Prophylactic treatment with various ß-blocking agents remains a controversial subject, although more recent studies do recommend ß-blocking therapy for the prevention of these arrhythmias shortly after coronary artery bypass graft surgery. The prophylactic use of digoxin or verapamil as single therapy has shown to be of no benefit for patients early after myocardial revascularization. However, a combination therapy of propranolol with digoxin is more effective and should therefore be considered.

An alternative is to consider starting antiarrhythmic therapy at the onset of atrial tachyarrhythmia. These atrial arrhythmias can be managed by controlling ventricular heart rate using digoxin, verapamil, ß-blockers or to restore sinus rhythm by using quinidine, disopyramide, flecainide, propafenone, sotalol or amiodarone. Direct current cardioversion is only recommended in the early postoperative period if supraventricular tachyarrhythmias are accompanied by hemodynamic deterioration or if the atrial arrhythmia proves to be resistant to therapy with various antiarrhythmic drugs.

References

[1]   Mohr R, Smolinsky A, Goor DA. Prevention of supraventricular tachyarrhythmias with low-dose propranolol after coronary bypass. J Thorac Cardiovasc Surg 1981;81:840-845.

[2]   Suttorp MJ, Kingma JH, Tjon Joe Gin RM, Koomen EM, Defauw JAM, van Hemel NM, Adan T, Ernst JMPG. Low and high dose sotalol versus propranolol in prevention of supraventricular tachyarrhythmias early after coronary artery bypass surgery. J Thorac Cardiovasc Surg 1990;100:921-926.

[3]   Suttorp MJ, Kingma JH, Peels JOJ, Koomen EM, Tijssen JGP, van Hemel NM, Defauw JAM, Ernst JMPG. Effectiviness of sotalol in preventing supraventricular tachy-arrhythmias shortly after coronary artery bypass grafting. Am J Card 1991;68:1163-1169.

[4]   Suttorp MJ. Paroxysmal atrial fibrillation and atrial flutter: current concepts and new strategies. Thesis. University of Groningen, The Netherlands, 1992.

[5]   Michelson EL, Morganroth J, MacVaugh H. Postoperative arrhythmias after coronary artery and cardiac valvular surgery detected by long-term electrocardiographic monitoring. Am Heart J 1979;97:442-448.

[6]   White HD, Antman EM, Glynn MA, Collins JJ, Cohn LH, Shemin RJ, Friedman PL. Efficacy and safety of timolol for prevention of supraventricular tachyarrhythmias after coronary artery bypass surgery. Circulation 1984;70:479-484.

[7]   Smith R, Glassman E, Spencer FC. Arrhythmias following cardiac valve replacement. Circulation 1972;1018-1023.

[8]   Chee TP, Sri Prakash N, Desser KB, Benchimol A. Postoperative supraventricular arrhythmias and the role of of prophylactic digoxin in cardiac surgery. Am Heart J 1982;104:974-977.

[9]   McAlister HF, Luke RA, Whitlock RM, Smith WM. Intravenous amiodarone bolus versus oral quinidine for atrial flutter and fibrillation after cardiac operations. J Thorac Cardiovasc Surg 1990;99:911-918.

[10]   Roffman JA, Fieldman A. Digoxin and propranolol in the prophylaxis of supraventricular tachydysrhythmias after coronary artery bypass graft surgery. Ann Thorac Surg 1981;31:496-501.

[11]   Mills SA, Poole GV Jr, Breyer RH, Holliday RH, Lavender II SW, Blanton KR, Hudspeth AS, Johnston FR, Cordell R. Digoxin and propranolol in the profylaxis of dysrhythmias after coronary artery bypass grafting. Circulation; 1983:68:suppl II:222-225.

[12]   Dixon FE, Genton E, Vacek JL, Moore CB, Landry J. Factors predisposing to supraventricular tachyarrhytmias after coronary artery bypass grafting. Am J Cardiol 1986;58:476-478.

[13]   Fuller JA, Adams GG, Buxton B. Atrial fibrillation after coronary artery bypass grafting. J Thorac Cardiovasc Surg 1989;97:821-825.

[14]   Leitch JW, Thomson D, Baird DK, Harris PJ. The importance of age as a predictor of atrial fibrillation and flutter after coronary artery bypass grafting. J Thorac Cardiovasc Surg 1990;100:338-342.

[15]   Mohr R, Smolinsky A, Goor DA. Prevention of supraventricular tachyarrhythmias with low-dose propranolol after coronary bypass. J Thorac Cardiovasc Surg 1981;81:840-845.

[16]   Salazar C, Frishman W, Friedman S, Patel J, Lin YT, Oka Y, Frater RWM, Becker RM. Beta-blockade therapy for supraventricular tachyarrhythmias after coronary artery surgery: a propranolol withdrawal syndrome? Angiology 1979;30:816-819.

[17]   Daudon P, Corcos T, Gandjbakhch I, Levasseur JP, Cabrol A, Cabrol C. Prevention of

atrial fibrillation or flutter by acebutolol after coronary bypass grafting. Am J Cardiol 1986;58:933-936.

[18]   Rubin DA, Nieminski KE, Reed GE, Herman MV. Predictors, prevention, and long-term prognosis of atrial fibrillation after coronary artery bypass graft operation. J Thorac Cardiovasc Surg 1987;94:331-335.

[19]   Johnson LW, Dickstein RA, Fruehan CT, Kane P, Potts JL, Smulyan H, Webb WR, Eich RH. Prophylactic digitalization for coronary artery bypass. Circulation 1976;53:819-822.

[20]   Selzer A, Kelly JJ Jr, Gerbode F, Kerth WJ, Osborn JJ, Ropper RW. Case against routine use of digitalis in patients undergoing cardiac surgery. JAMA 1966;195:141-144.

[21]   Tyras DH, Stothert JC, Kaiser GC, Barner HB, Codd JE, Willman VL. Supraventricular tachyarrhytmias after myocardial revascularization: A randomized trial of prophylactic digitalization. J Thorac Cardiovasc Surg 1979;77:310-314.

[22]   Silverman NA, Wright R, Levitsky S. Efficacy of low-dose propranolol in preventing postoperative supraventricular tachyarrhytmias. Ann Surg 1982;196:194-197.

[23]   Ivey MF, Ivey TD, Bailey WW, Williams DB, Hessel EA, Miller DW. Influence of propranolol on supraventricular tachycardia early after coronary artery revascularization. J Thorac Cardiovasc Surg 1983;85:214-218.

[24]   Janssen J, Loomans L, Harink J, Taams M, Brunninkhuis L, van der Starre P, Kootstra G. Prevention and treatment of supraventricular tachycardia shortly after coronary bypass grafting: A randomized open trial. Angiology 1986;37:601-609.

[25]   Khuri SF, Okike OS, Josa M, Vander Salm TJ, Assoussa S, Leone L, Silverman A, Siouffi S, Olukotun AY. Efficacy of nadolol in preventing supraventricular tachycardia after coronary artery bypass grafting. Am J Cardiol 1987;60:51D-58D.

[26]   Vecht RJ, Nicolaides EP, Ikweuke JK, Liassides C, Cleary J, Cooper WB. Incidence and prevention of supraventricular tachyarrhthmias after coronary bypass surgery. Int J Card 1986;13:125-134.

[27]   Lamb RK, Prabhakar G, Thorpe JAC, Smith S, Norton R, Dyde JA. The use of atenolol in prevention of supraventricular arrhythmias following coronary artery surgery. Eur Heart J 1988;9:32-36.

[28]   Smith EE, Shore DF, Monro JL, Ross JK. Oral verapamil fails to prevent supraventricular tachycardia following coronary bypass surgery. Int J Cardiol 1985; 9:37-44.

[29]   Williams DB, Misbach GA, Kruse AP, Ivey TD. Oral verapamil for prophylaxis of supraventricular tachycardia after myocardial revascularization. J Thorac Cardiovasc Surg 1985;90:592-596.

[30]   Connolly SJ, Mulji AS, Hoffert DL, Davis C, Shragge BW. Randomized placebo-controlled trial of propafenone for treatment of atrial tachyarrhythmias after cardiac surgery. J Am Coll Cardiol 1987;10:1145-1148.

[31]   Campbell JJ, Gavaghan TP, Morgan JJ. Intravenous sotalol for the treatment of atrial fibrillation and flutter after cardiopulmonary bypass. Comparison with disopyramide and digoxin in a randomized trial. Br Heart J 1985;54:86-90.

[32]   Gavaghan TP, Feneley MP, Campbell TJ, Morgan JJ. Atrial tachyarrhythmias after cardiac surgery: results of disopyramide therapy. Aust NZ J Med 1985;15:27-32.

[33]   Gavaghan TP, Keogh AM, Kelly RP, Campbell TJ, Thorburg C, Morgan JJ. Flecainide compared with a combination of digoxin and disopyramide for acute arrhythmias after cardiopulmonary bypass. Br Heart J 1988;60:497-501.

[34]   Csicsko JF, Schatzlein MH, King RD. Immediate post-operative digitalization in the prophylaxis of supraventricular arrhythmias following coronary artery bypass. J Thorac Cardiovasc Surg 1981;81:419-422.

[35]   Parker F, Greiner-Hayes C, Bove EL, Marvasti M, Johnson LW, Eich RH. Supraventricular arrhythmias following coronary artery bypass. J Thorac Cardiovasc Surg 1983;86:594-600.

[36]   Matangi MF, Neutze JM, Graham KJ, Hill DG, Kerr AR, Barratt-Boyes BG. Arrhythmia prophylaxis after aorta-coronary bypass. J Thorac Cardiovasc Surg 1985;89:439-43.

Chapter 15

RISK AND PREVENTION OF EMBOLISM

IN ATRIAL FIBRILLATION

A.T. Marcel Gosselink

Harry J.G.M. Crijns

Kong I. Lie

Department of Cardiology
Thoraxcenter
University Hospital Groningen
The Netherlands

J. H. Kingma et al. (eds.), Atrial fibrillation, a treatable disease?, 237–257.
© 1992 *Kluwer Academic Publishers.*

INTRODUCTION _____

The risk of embolic stroke and other systemic embolism among patients with atrial fibrillation and rheumatic heart disease has long been recognized. Although no randomized controlled trials evaluating this treatment have ever been performed in this group of patients, there has been a long-standing consensus that anticoagulant prophylaxis is justified in these patients. More recently there is a heightened awareness that nonrheumatic atrial fibrillation is also associated with an increased risk for embolization. This is especially important since nonrheumatic atrial fibrillation is present in 50-80% of all atrial fibrillation patients, whereas the incidence of rheumatic atrial fibrillation is decreasing[1-5]. To evaluate the efficacy and safety of antithrombotic therapy in nonrheumatic atrial fibrillation, several randomized trials have been initiated in recent years. Some of these trials have now been completed[6,8,9,10]. The results of these studies and an approach to the application of antithrombotic therapy based on pathogenesis will be discussed.

PREVALENCE AND INCIDENCE OF
ATRIAL FIBRILLATION _____

Epidemiological studies have reported wide variations in the prevalence of atrial fibrillation depending on the age and general health of the population. In young, healthy populations the prevalence appears to be very low, ranging from 0.004% to 0.4% [1,11,12], whereas it is relatively high in those over 60 years old, reaching 2% to 4% [13,14]. The Framingham study has clearly shown the age dependence of atrial fibrillation incidence and prevalence: The arrhythmia developed in 0.22% of men 25-34 years old and 3.79% of those 55-64 years old[1]. This increase in the prevalence of atrial fibrillation with age is associated with an increasing prevalence of underlying heart disease, although an independent direct effect of aging on atrial tissue cannot be excluded.

UNDERLYING HEART DISEASE _____

The vast majority of patients with atrial fibrillation have coexisting heart disease. Approximately 90% of cases are associated with structural heart disease. In the Framingham study cardiac failure and rheumatic heart disease were the strongest predictors of atrial fibrillation, whereas hypertensive heart disease, which is frequently associated with atrial fibrillation, was present in many controls and is therefore only weakly predictive[1]. Coronary artery disease is usually associated with atrial fibrillation only when left ventricular failure is present[15]. Atrial fibrillation in the absence of structural heart disease ("lone atrial fibrillation") accounts for a relatively low percentage of atrial fibrillation patients[2,3].

ATRIAL FIBRILLATION AND STROKE

Cerebrovascular embolism is by far the most important tromboembolic event associated with atrial fibrillation. Visceral and limb arterial embolism are both less frequent. At least 15% of all ischemic strokes and more than one third of ischemic strokes in the elderly are associated with atrial fibrillation[16-[16-21]. About one in three people with atrial fibrillation will experience a stroke during their lifetime if not treated with anticoagulants[2,17,22-24].

Several studies have reported the incidence of stroke among patients with atrial fibrillation and have clarified the relative risks among patients with rheumatic and nonrheumatic heart disease. The Framingham study[1] demonstrated that among patients who developed chronic atrial fibrillation during 24 years of follow-up, the risk of stroke was significantly increased compared with those who did not. The risk ratio for stroke was 17.56 for those with rheumatic heart disease and 5.6 for those with nonrheumatic atrial fibrillation. The absolute annual rate of stroke was approximately 4% in both groups. In an analysis of the data after 30 years of follow-up [18] including only nonrheumatic atrial fibrillation, the annual incidence of stroke was 3.8%; in comparison to controls matched for multiple risk factors, the relative risk was approximately 4.

More recent data on stroke incidence among patients with nonrheumatic atrial fibrillation are provided by follow-up of the placebo groups in recently completed trials. In the Copenhagen Atrial Fibrillation Trial (AFASAK) study[6], the annual incidence of stroke among the 336 placebo patients was 4.9%. In the Stroke Prevention in Atrial Fibrillation (SPAF) study[8] (528 placebo patients) and the Canadian Atrial Fibrillation Anticoagulation (CAFA) Study[10] the annual stroke incidences were 5.7% and 5.2% respectively, whereas in the Boston Area Anticoagulation Trial for Atrial Fibrillation (BAATAF) study[9] this figure was just under 3%. In the latter, however, patients were allowed to take aspirin and 46% did so.

In addition to these clinical strokes, atrial fibrillation has been associated with an undue risk of subclinical, "silent" strokes[25,26]. Silent infarcts detected by computed tomography (CT) have been found in 35% of nonrheumatic atrial fibrillation patients without a history of stroke[25]. While these infarcts are labelled "silent", it is likely that they take a subtle, but cumulative toll on cognition in elderly people[27].

Although atrial fibrillation is the most common cardiac disorder associated with stroke, this does not necessarily mean that there is a causal relation between atrial fibrillation and stroke; other causes also exist, especially in elderly patients. Atrial fibrillation, often being an expression of underlying (heart) disease may be a risk marker for stroke rather than a cause. The latter is also suggested by the fact that strictly defined "lone atrial fibrillation" (that which occurs in the absence of cardiopulmonary disease or a history of hypertension and before the age of 60) is associated with a very low risk of stroke[28] (<0,5% per year versus 2-4% in the general nonanticoagulated atrial fibrillation population). Although there is a tendency to attribute stroke to cardioembolic sources when atrial fibrillation is present, the fraction of atrial fibrillation-associated strokes due to cardiogenic embolism versus embolism in the setting of coexistent cerebrovascular disease is uncertain. Clinical estimates of the cardioembolic fraction vary widely, from 19% to 75% [19,20,27]. An inability to diagnose cardioembolic mechanisms with certainty, even at autopsy, clouds this issue, but it is likely that a substantial fraction of strokes associated with atrial fibrillation is cardioembolic in origin. In the SPAF study[7,8], using sophisticated techniques including CT-scanning, the cardioembolic fraction of stroke was restudied among atrial fibrillation patients. In this study, predetermined criteria for diagnosing type of stroke were used. More than 50% of all strokes were cardioembolic and only a minor fraction of strokes could not be determined.

The incidence of cardioembolic origin of stroke in a study population will depend on the number and type of investigations used and their sensitivity in detecting intracardiac thrombi. In this respect the role of echocardiography in detecting cardiac derived embolism should be noted. Whereas conventional transthoracic echocardiography is not very accurate, transesophageal echocardiography has shown to detect atrial thrombi, particularly appendage thrombi, with much greater sensitivity[30,31].

Of the total population with atrial fibrillation several distinct subgroups can be identified readily, some of which may be at relatively high or low risk of stroke.

Lone atrial fibrillation. Lone atrial fibrillation is only found in a relatively small percentage of patients with atrial fibrillation. The natural history of lone atrial fibrillation was addressed by the Framingham investigators[32] who followed 30 of these patients (mean age, 70 years) for more than 10 years and found a fourfold increase in the incidence of stroke as compared with matched controls, with an annual risk of stroke of 2.5%. The majority of patients with a stroke had chronic atrial fibrillation. Aside from the small sample size, other limitations of the analysis were the fact that patients with hypertensive heart disease and diabetes mellitus were not excluded from the study. In a retrospective study Kopecky[28] analysed 97 patients (mean age, 44 years) with strictly defined lone atrial fibrillation i.e. atrial fibrillation in the absence of cardiopulmonary disease (including hypertension) and diabetes. The annual yearly risk of a thromboembolic event was 0,55%. Notably, there was no difference in the risk of stroke in the subgroups with chronic and paroxysmal atrial fibrillation. However, the small proportion (9%) of patients with chronic atrial fibrillation and the relatively low mean age limit the generalizability of these data to all lone atrial fibrillation patients. Although the risk of stroke in younger patients with lone atrial fibrillation, and particularly in those with paroxysmal atrial fibrillation seems to be low, the risk may be more substantial in older patients with chronic atrial fibrillation.

Paroxysmal atrial fibrillation. The role paroxysmal atrial fibrillation plays in the development of thromboembolic complications has been examined retrospectively by several studies. In a study by Takahashi[33] of 94 patients with paroxysmal atrial fibrillation, only 6.4% experienced embolism during a 10-year follow-up period, but further details on etiology, and the duration of paroxysmal atrial fibrillation as related to embolism are unknown. In another retrospective study by Petersen and Godtfredsen[34] 426 consecutive patients with paroxysmal atrial fibrillation were analysed. It was concluded that par-oxysmal atrial fibrillation was a lesser risk factor for stroke, because the mean yearly incidence of systemic emboli was 2.0% before transition to chronic atrial fibrillation and 5.1% afterward. However, because progression to chronic atrial fibrillation depended on etiology (rheumatic heart disease) an indirect interaction between etiology and occurrence of embolic complication is implied. In a retrospective study of 115 patients with nonvalvular atrial fibrillation, Wiener[35] reported that the only significant independent predictor of embolism was the chronicity of atrial fibrillation. Seventy-six percent of patients who had an embolic event had chronic atrial fibrillation compared with only 40% of those without embolism. The Framingham study[15] on patients with coronary artery disease also demonstrated that among men with chronic atrial fibrillation, the annual stroke rate was 5.4% and the relative risk was 4.7, whereas with transient atrial fibrillation, the annual stroke rate was only 1.3% and the relative risk was 0. In women the differences were less marked. On the other hand, the SPAF study[8] in which 452 patients with paroxysmal atrial fibrillation were included, the majority associated with underlying heart disease, could not demonstrate a difference in the risk of stroke between patients with chronic and paroxysmal atrial fibrillation. Although none of the studies is conclusive, paroxysmal atrial fibrillation seems to be associated with a lower risk of stroke than chronic atrial fibrillation.

Previous embolism. In atrial fibrillation patients who suffered an embolism in the past, the recurrence rate appears to be considerable. In atrial fibrillation associated with rheumatic heart disease overall embolic recurrence rate has been reported to range from 30% to 75% [36] Nonrheumatic atrial fibrillation patients with a previous clinical stroke also have a substantial risk of subsequent stroke[24,37,38], with a recurrence rate of 15-20%. In the Framingham study[37] there was a distinct clustering of recurrent stroke events in the early months following the initial stroke in patients with nonrheumatic atrial fibrillation. Kelly[39] reported a recurrence rate of stroke in 33% of 36 patients with atrial fibrillation during a mean follow-up of 2.5 months. In a report by Darling[40] 20% of 148 patients with rheumatic and nonrheumatic atrial fibrillation experienced a recurrent embolism within 14 days. Half of all recurrent thromboembolisms during the first 2 years occurred within the first 2 weeks after the initial embolic event. In contrast, Sage[38] describing the natural history of a population of 140 patients with nonrheumatic atrial fibrillation who presented with a stroke, reported that the risk of recurrent emboli was 17% in the first year but remained at or above this level for at least the subsequent nine years. Thus, there appears to be an increased risk of recurrent stroke after the initial stroke, although it is unclear whether this high risk is limited to the initial weeks or persists indefinitely.

MECHANISMS OF EMBOLISM

To derive a rational approach to the application of antithrombotic therapy in atrial fibrillation it is important to consider the pathogenesis of embolism in this patient group. The mechanisms of ischemic stroke are probably diverse[41-43]. The causes include emboli due to 1) stasis-related left atrial thrombi (associated with altered atrial blood-flow patterns, enlarged atria, mitral regurgitation, and thrombi in the atrial appendages), 2) stasis-related left ventricular thrombi (associated with left ventricular enlargement), 3) structural abnormalities of the mitral valve (including myxomatous or thickened valvular leaflets or mitral annular calcification), and 4) cerebrovascular disease (intracranial or extracranial) or 5) atherosclerotic disease of the ascending aorta.

Stasis, due to impaired effective mechanical atrial activity, appears to play a predominant pathogenetic role in atrial thrombus formation in atrial fibrillation. Transesophageal echocardiography in patients with atrial fibrillation has shown spontaneous echoes within the left atrium highly suggestive of sluggish flow[31]. These stasis-related causes of stroke would be expected to be prevented by anticoagulation with warfarin but not by platelet inhibition, since fibrin formation may predominate over platelet activation[43]. Causes of stroke chiefly due to structural abnormalities of the mitral valve may be related to turbulent flow, with activation of platelets and some formation of fibrin, and may therefore be prevented by aspirin or anticoagulation with warfarin. In cerebrovascular and ascending aortic atherosclerotic disease, often associated with atrial fibrillation, the sources of emboli may be platelet-fibrin thrombi or lipid "gruel"; therefore, platelet inhibition or anticoagulation with warfarin may be only of partial benefit. Apart from arterial embolism, reduced cerebral blood flow during atrial fibrillation[44] as compared to sinus rhythm may also be a contributing factor to the development of cerebrovascular complications i.e. ischemic stroke in patients with atrial fibrillation.

PREVENTION OF EMBOLISM - ANTITHROMBOTIC THERAPY _____

Although there are two basic strategies for stroke prevention in atrial fibrillation, i.e. restoration of sinus rhythm by cardioversion and antithrombotic therapy, only the latter will be discussed here.

Rheumatic atrial fibrillation. Several nonrandomized retrospective studies[45-47] of short- and long-term anticoagulation in atrial fibrillation patients with rheumatic heart disease have reported a beneficial effect of this treatment. However, no properly controlled trials of antithrombotic therapy for the prevention of embolism in this patient group have been reported. Nevertheless, anticoagulant therapy is generally considered to be effective and warranted in these patients. In a retrospective study by Szekely[45] of 30 atrial fibrillation patients without prior embolism, the incidence of systemic emboliza-tion was 63% of control when patients received anticoagulant therapy. Adams [46] followed a group of 84 patients for a total of 209 patient-years and found an increased risk for fatal embolism in the untreated group compared with patients receiving warfarin. Cosgriff[47] reported 103 embolic episodes among 28 patients during 275 patient-months of follow-up before anticoagulation coagulation and 13 embolic episodes during 625 months after anticoagulation. Although methodologically weak, the available data suggest a beneficial effect of anticoagulant therapy in patients with atrial fibrillation associated with rheumatic heart disease.

Secondary Prevention. Studies evaluating the usefulness of antithrombo-tics in atrial fibrillation patients who had a stroke, indicate that anticoagulant treatment may be beneficial in preventing the recurrence of embolic events in this patient group. There have been extensive reviews of non-randomised studies of anticoagulants in patients with stroke that was presumed to be due to embolism from the heart, and some of the reviews have come out very strongly in favour of the use of anticoagulants, with a 65-90% reduction in the number of embolic events[24,48-50]. But, non-randomised studies do not in general yield reliable data and should be interpreted with caution. In addition, many of the studies were done before CT scanning and transesophageal echocardiography were available and included a high proportion of cases with rheumatic heart disease. In a recent, controlled, but non-randomised study [51], the benefits of long-term anticoagulant treatment of patients with nonrheumatic atrial fibrillation and cerebral infarction were studied by comparing two series of patients with stroke from centres with different policies on anticoagulant treatment. There appeared to be no difference in either the rate of survival or the rate of recurrent stroke between patients receiving anticoagulants and those who did not. Because of the sample size (120 patients) and the wide confidence intervals, however, the results are compatible with the hypothesis that long-term anticoagulant treatment halves or doubles the risk of recurrent stroke or death. At this moment, a large, randomised, controlled trial assessing the value of anticoagulating stroke patients in atrial fibrillation is ongoing (European Atrial Fibrillation Trial). Until then the use of prophylactic anticoagulants for secondary prevention seems to be warranted.

Nonrheumatic atrial fibrillation. Nowadays nonrheumatic heart disease is the most common cause of atrial fibrillation. The question whether or not to use antithrombotic agents in these patients has aroused much controversy [1-4,52,53]. Data from the Framingham study[18,22] indicated that nonrheumatic atrial fibrillation is associated with a more than fivefold increase in the risk of stroke and it appears to account for 7 to 31% of all strokes in persons over the age of 60.

Several prospective randomised clinical trials assessing efficacy and safety of prophylactic antithrombotic medication in patients with nonrheumatic atrial fibrillation are ongoing in Europe and North America[54]. Some of them have recently been completed[6,8,9]. Study characteristics and final results are shown in Table 1-3.

In the Copenhagen AFASAK study[6], 1007 patients with chronic atrial fibrillation were randomly assigned to receive warfarin (given openly, dose adjusted to create a prothrombine-time ratio of 1.5 to 1.9; international normalized ratio [INR], 2.8 to 4.2), aspirin (75 mg per day), or placebo. The median age was 74 years and more than half had a history of heart failure. The follow-up time was 2 years for each patient. Primary endpoint was a thromboembolic complication (transient cerebral ischemic attack, stroke, and systemic embolism). A relatively large number of the patients assigned to warfarin (38%) were withdrawn from the study, mostly because of the

Table 1. Randomized Trials of Antithrombotics in Atrial Fibrillation

	AFASAK [6]	SPAF [8]	BAATAF [9]	CAFA [10]
N	1007	1330	420	383
groups	warfarine aspirine placebo	warfarine aspirine placebo	warfarine controle	warfarine placebo
aspirin mg/day	75	325		
INR	2.8-4.2	2.0-3.5	1.5-2.7	2.0-3.0
1° events	S,E,T,H	S,E	S,E	S,E,H,F
F.U. (yr)	2	1.3	2.3	1.3
age (yr)	74	67	68	68
PAF	none	34%	48%	7%

AFASAK, Copenhagen Atrial Fibrillation Trial; SPAF, Stroke Prevention in Atrial Fibrillation Trial; BAATAF, Boston Area Anticoagulation Trial in Atrial Fibrillation; CAFA, Canadian Atrial Fibrillation Anticoagulation Study; INR, International Normalized Ratio; S, stroke; E, non-central nervous embolism; T, transient cerebral ischemic attack; H, intracerebral hemorrhage; F, fatal hemorrhage; F.U., duration of follow-up; PAF, paroxysmal atrial fibrillation.

inconvenience of frequent blood sampling and the side effects of treatment (7%, mostly minor bleeding complications). In comparison, aspirin and placebo treatments resulted in fewer withdrawals (13% and 15%, respectively) and side effects (2% in each group). The yearly incidence of thromboembolic complications was 2.0% on warfarin and 5.5% on aspirin and placebo. Intention-to-treat analysis showed a benefit of warfarin in preventing thromboembolic complications, but no benefit of aspirin.

In the SPAF study[7,8], 1330 patients (34% of whom had paroxysmal atrial fibrillation) were randomly assigned to one of two groups. The patients in group 1, who were eligible for warfarin, took warfarin (dose adjusted to create a prothrombin-time ratio between 1.3 and 1.8 times control; INR between 2.0 and 3.5), aspirin (325 mg per day), or placebo; those in group 2, who were not eligible for warfarin (including patients >75 years of age and patients with lone atrial fibrillation), took aspirin or placebo in a double-blind fashion. Primary endpoints were ischemic stroke or systemic embolism. The patients were followed for a mean period of 1.3 years. Mean age was 67 years; only 19% of the patients had a history of heart failure. The assignment to placebo of patients eligible for warfarin was terminated, because each active agent in group 1 was superior to placebo (combined event rates, 1.6% and 8.3% per year, respectively; risk reduction, 81%). Among the group 1 patients, by comparison with placebo, the rate of primary outcomes among the warfarine-treated patients was reduced from 7.4% to 2.3% per year (absolute reduction, 5.1% per year; risk reduction 67%). Considering only disabling ischemic strokes or vascular deaths, patients assigned to warfarin had a 54% reduction compared with placebo. In all patients (group 1 and 2 combined) given aspirin, the primary-event rate was 3.6% per year, as compared with 6.3% in those given placebo (risk reduction 42%). Disabling ischemic stroke or vascular death was reduced by 22% in patients assigned to aspirin relative to placebo therapy. There was no benefit from aspirin in the patients over the age of 75. Withdrawals from therapy for reasons other than study outcome were rather uncommon, occurring in only 11.2%, 5% and 6.6% of patients assigned to warfarin, aspirin and placebo, respectively. The major bleeding complications on warfarine were remarkably few (1.5% per year total and 0.4% per year with residua); by comparison with placebo an absolute decrease of 0.1% per year for all major bleeding and an increase of 0.4% per year for bleeding with residua. Thus, the risk/benefit ratio is clearly in favor of warfarin therapy. By comparison with placebo, with aspirin there was an absolute decrease of major bleeding of about 0.5% per year and an absolute increase of 0.5% per year for bleeds with residua. Although the risk/benefit ratio favors the use of aspirin, the benefit is much less marked than that for warfarin.

In the BAATAF study[9] 420 patients (17% of whom had paroxysmal atrial fibrillation) were randomly assigned to the group taking warfarin (prothrombine-time ratio, 1.2 to 1.5; INR, 1.5 to 2.7) or the control group (no therapy, but aspirin was allowed and taken by 46% of these patients) and followed for 2.3 years. End points were ischemic stroke and systemic embolism. The mean age was 68 years; 26% of the patients had a history of heart failure and 48% had lone atrial fibrillation. The incidence of stroke was markedly reduced in the warfarin group as compared with control (0.41% vs 3.0% per year; risk reduction, 86%). For unexplained reasons the death rate was significantly lower in the warfarin group than in the control group (2.3% vs 5.4% per year), especially the noncardiac death rate. Ten percent of the patients assigned to warfarin discontinued the medication. Major bleeding from warfarin was not significantly increased in this study.

Recently the results of the CAFA study[10] were published. This study was terminated preliminary after publication of the reports of the AFASAK and SPAF study. In the CAFA study 383 patients were randomly assigned to warfarin (given blinded, INR, 2.0-3.0) or placebo. Duration of follow-up was 15 months. Primary outcome events were any ischemic stroke except lacunar, other systemic embolism and intracranial or fatal hemorrhage. The annual rate of the primary outcome event cluster in patients receiving warfarin or placebo was 3.5% and 5.2% respectively (risk reduction 45%, 95% confidence limits - 64%, 76%). The annual rate of fatal or major hemorrhage was 2.5% in those receiving warfarin and 0.5% in those receiving placebo.

The results of these studies were confirmed by the recently reported interim analysis of the Veterans Co-operative Study, Stroke Prevention in Nonrheumatic Atrial Fibrillation (SPINAF)[55]. In this study, including 538 male with chronic atrial fibrillation, low dose coumadin (given blinded, target prothrombin-time ratio between 1.2 and 1.5 times control) was compared with placebo. The primary endpoint was stroke, secondary endpoints were cerebral hemorrhage and death. Interim analysis showed a 73% risk reduction of stroke in the coumadin treated group. Major bleeding complications were equally divided between the two groups. This benefit of coumadin was seen with advancing age, including patients between 70 and 80. Based on these results,

Table 2. **Results of Randomized Trials of Antithrombotic Therapy in Atrial Fibrillation: Embolic Complications in Different Treatment Groups**

	AFASAK [6]	SPAF [8]	BAATAF [9]	CAFA [10]
placebo/control[*]	5.5%	6.3-7.4%	3 %	5.2%
warfarin	2.0%	2.3 %	0.4%	3.5%
aspirin	5.5%	3.6 %		

AFASAK, Copenhagen Atrial Fibrillation Trial; SPAF, Stroke Prevention in Atrial Fibrillation Trial; BAATAF, Boston Area Anticoagulation in Atrial Fibrillation Trial; CAFA, Canadian Atrial Fibrillation Anticoagulation Study.
[*]in BAATAF study.

Table 3. **Results of Randomized Trials of Antithrombotic Therapy in Atrial Fibrillation: Risk Reduction of Embolism with Warfarin and Aspirin**

RISK REDUCTION

	Warfarine		Aspirin	
	Observed	95% CI	Observed	95% CI
AFASAK [6]	60%	11%, 81%	14%	-53%, 60%
SPAF [8]	67%	27%, 85%	42%	9%, 63%
BAATAF [9]	86%	51%, 96%	not studied	
CAFA [10]	45%	-50%, 80%	not studied	

AFASAK, Copenhagen Atrial Fibrillation Trial; SPAF, Stroke Prevention in Atrial Fibrillation Trial; BAATAF, Boston Area Anticoagulation in Atrial Fibrillation Trial; CAFA, Canadian Atrial Fibrillation Anticoagulation Trial. minimum by the use of a low dose (INR, 1.5 to 3.0) which has been shown to be effective. However, the optimal therapeutic range for warfarin may vary depending on the underlying cause of atrial fibrillation.

the study was terminated early.

Despite differences between the studies (Table 1), they are very consistent with regard to the risk reduction seen with warfarin (Table 2 and 3). The evidence that anticoagulant therapy in patients with nonrheumatic atrial fibrillation prevents systemic embolism with an acceptable risk of hemorrhage is very compelling. Therefore, patients with nonrheumatic atrial fibrillation should be seriously considered for anticoagulant therapy. The number of serious bleeding complications due to warfarin therapy may be limited to a minimum by the use of a low dose (INR, 1.5 to 3.0) which has been shown to be effective. However, the optimal therapeutic range for warfarin may vary depending on the underlying cause of atrial fibrillation.

The AFASAK[6] and SPAF[7,8] study also evaluated aspirin, with one reporting no effect and the other reporting a clinically significant effect. If both studies are analyzed based on the intention-to-treat principle, and if only stroke and other systemic embolism are included as events, the 95% confidence intervals of the estimates of risk reduction of aspirin of the two studies overlap, indicating that the results are, at least statistically, consistent with one another[56]. Several explanations may be offered for the difference between these results. The dose of aspirin in the AFASAK study was 75 mg, as compared with 325 mg in the SPAF trial. In addition, the AFASAK study involved older patients. Also, the fact that in the AFASAK study the incidence of heart failure (probably related to a higher prevalence of stasis-related thrombi) was more than 3 times as high as in the SPAF trial, may explain the difference in response to aspirin.

The evidence for the efficacy of aspirin against stroke in atrial fibrillation is less compelling than the evidence supporting warfarin therapy. Future studies are necessary to find out whether aspirin and warfarin are equally effective in preventing thromboembolism. This aspect is now studied in the SPAF II study. Until then warfarin appears to be the first choice for antithrombotic prophylaxis in patients with atrial fibrillation.

Risk stratification. The present studies on antithrombotic therapy in patients with nonrheumatic atrial fibrillation do not allow for risk stratification in order to further identify subgroups of patients who may benefit from this treatment, and those who may not. As stated before, several factors, like underlying heart disease and type of the arrhythmia (chronic versus paroxysmal) may influence the risk of embolic stroke, and thus the potential benefit of antithrombotics. In addition, age may also be an important parameter to estimate a patient's risk/benefit ratio with respect to antithrombotic treatment. Previous studies have shown that the elderly (i.e. patients older than 75 years) are at particularly high risk for serious bleeding complications of anticoagulants. Although these patients were included in the present studies, their numbers were rather small; mean age was considerably younger in all of them, except perhaps the AFASAK trial. Thus, although antithrombotic therapy was superior to placebo in the overall group, it may not be justified to simply extrapolate these results to patients of high age; the benefits of antithrombotic treatment may not outweigh its side effects. The persisting hemorrhagic risk necessitates prudent institution of this therapy.

ANTITHROMBOTICS IN CARDIOVERSION
OF ATRIAL FIBRILLATION _____

It has been appreciated since long that restoration of sinus rhythm with normal atrial contraction might itself be associated with embolization of poorly adherent thrombi. Estimates on the thromboembolic event rate in patients undergoing electrical cardioversion and not receiving anticoagulants, range from 1.1% to 7.0% [3,57-61]. However, these studies were uncontrolled and the numbers of patients were relatively small. In a controlled study, Bjerkelund and Orning[62] reported on 572 attempted cardioversions in 437 patients and observed a 0.8% incidence of embolization in long-term anticoagulated patients compared with a 5.3% incidence in unanticoagulated patients. The emboli were noted 1 to 6 days following cardioversion. Shortcomings of this study included lack of randomization, no evaluation of short-term therapy and inclusion of arrhythmias such as atrial flutter and atrial tachycardia. In an unpublished study at our institution, involving 246 patients with chronic atrial fibrillation undergoing electrical cardioversion, only 1 patient (0.4%) had a cardioversion related embolic event, occurring 5 days after restoration of sinus rhythm. All patients had been on long-term anticoagulation therapy.

Emboli related to cardioversion may occur up till several days after cardioversion. A physiologic basis for this phenomenon lies in the observation that resumption of atrial contractility may be delayed for days after cardioversion even though the ECG shows the immediate onset of sinus P waves [63,64]. Therefore anticoagulant therapy should be continued for some weeks following cardioversion. This treatment will reduce the formation of a new clot in a noncontractile atrium if mechanical resumption of atrial activity should be delayed. From our own experience, continuation of anticoagulation therapy for a period 4 weeks following cardioversion appears to be safe; in a group of 83 patients no thromboembolic complications were seen after discontinuation of warfarin after this period. Long-term anticoagulation beyond the first four weeks after cardioversion is indicated only if atrial fibrillation recurs or recurrence may be expected, or if other considerations such as rheumatic mitral valve disease or previous embolism are present.

The minimum time for thrombi to form in the fibrillating atria is unknown. Usually patients certain to have had the onset of atrial fibrillation within the preceding one or two days, are not given anticoagulation therapy. The implicit assumption in such cases is that thrombus formation in the atria in the presence of atrial fibrillation takes at least several days. There are, however, no reliable data to support this assumption. Lown's group[65] has recommended that it is safe to perform cardioversion without prior anticoagulation, if atrial fibrillation has been present for a week or less, if there is no other reason to suspect atrial thrombus.

In summary, despite the ubiquitous nature of atrial fibrillation and the numerous studies available in the literature, the value of short-term anticoagulation prior to cardioversion is still not precisely defined. Based on the information available a reasonable approach might be to anticoagulate patients with atrial fibrillation, regardless of etiology, some weeks prior to and after elective cardioversion even in cases of relatively recent onset of this arrhythmia [66,67]. This short-term anticoagulation appears to be a beneficial prophylactic manoeuvre, with little risk of significant hemorrhagic sequelae as compared to long-term anticoagulation[68].

SUMMARY AND RECOMMENDATION _____

Atrial fibrillation is a common arrhythmia. Its incidence increases with age, reaching 2-4% in those over 65 years of age. Furthermore, atrial fibrillation is the most common underlying cardiac disorder predisposing to systemic embolism, a potentially devastating complication with an annual incidence of stroke of 4-5% regardless of whether there is associated rheumatic heart disease. The relative risk is approximately 4 in patients with nonrheumatic heart disease, and 17 in patients with rheumatic heart disease. The risks appears to be lower with lone or paroxysmal atrial fibrillation. Patients at highest risk are those with a history of systemic embolism: in this group the embolic risk approaches 10% to 20% a year. Although no prospective randomized trials are available, the current recommendation in these patients is long term anticoagulant therapy aiming at a prothrombin-time ratio 1.5-2.0 times control (INR, 3.0-4.5).

Patients at a lower but nevertheless substantial risk of embolism are those with atrial fibrillation associated with rheumatic heart disease, especially mitral stenosis. Based on known embolic risk and on the results of clinical trials, chronic anticoagulation to prolong prothrombin-time to 1.3-1.5 times control (INR, 2.0-3.0) is recommended for these patients.

At the lower end of the spectrum of embolic risk in patients with atrial fibrillation are those without evidence of associated organic heart disease i.e. lone atrial fibrillation. The hazards of chronic anticoagulation may not outweigh its potential benefits. Aspirin however, having fewer side effects than warfarin, may be a reasonable alternative in these patients. It seems also justified not to prescribe any antithrombotic therapy at all in this group of low risk patients.

Between these two poles exists a large group of patients with an intermediate but incompletely defined risk of embolism: those with nonrheumatic atrial fibrillation associated with various forms of cardiovascular disease. The embolic risk in these patients lies between 4% and 6% per year[6,8,67]. As recent studies[6-10] have shown, preventive therapy is the only rational approach in this patient group. Prolongation of prothrombin time to 1.2-1.5 time control (INR, 2.0-3.0) may be sufficient to avoid embolization[9,68]. With these regimens of anticoagulant dosage, major bleeding and cerebral hemorrhage are uncommon. In patients of high age however, who are particularly prone to serious complications of antithrombotics, the relative and absolute benefit of this treatment remains uncertain. The differentiation of subgroups in the broad category of nonrheumatic atrial fibrillation that stand to gain most from anticoagulation remains to be established. The role of aspirin is still somewhat uncertain. In certain subgroups of patients this compound may also be effective[8]. This holds especially for patients with platelet-rich thrombi due to structural abnormalities of the mitral valve or to the rupture of an arterial plaque with associated mural thrombus in cerebrovascular or ascending aortic atherosclerotic disease. Finally, an active diagnostic approach, aiming at visualization of the left atrium and appendage by transesophageal echocardiography, may prove helpful in identifying patients at risk for thromboembolic complications. Recent studies have shown that spontaneous contrast and left atrial appendage peak flow velocities may be used to identify atrial fibrillation patients prone to systemic embolism[69,70].

It is recommended that anticoagulation therapy should be given at least four weeks before electrical cardioversion and be continued until sinus rhythm has been maintained for at least four weeks.

References

[1] Kannel WB, Abbott RD, Savage DD, McNamara PM. Epidemiological features of chronic atrial fibrillation. N Engl J Med 1982;306:1018-1022.
[2] Hinton RC, Kistler JP, Fallon JT, Friedlich AL, Fisher CM. Influence of etiology of atrial fibrillation on incidence of systemic embolism. Am J Cardiol 1977;40:509.
[3] Hurst JW, Paulk EA Jr, Proctor HD, Schlant RC. Management of patients with atrial fibrillation. Am J Cardiol 1964;37:728.
[4] Aberg H. Atrial fibrillation. A study of atrial thrombosis and systemic embolism in a necropsy material. Acta Med Scand 1969;185:373.
[5] Gajewski J, Singer RB. Mortality in an insured population with atrial fibrillation. JAMA 1981;245:1540-1544.
[6] Petersen P, Boysen G, Godtfredsen J, Andersen ED, Andersen B. Placebo controlled, randomised trial of warfarin and aspirin for prevention of thromboembolic complications in chronic atrial fibrillation: the Copenhagen AFASAK study. Lancet 1989;1:175-179.
[7] Stroke Prevention in Atrial Fibrillation Study Group Investigators. Preliminary report of the Stroke Prevention in Atrial Fibrillation Study. N Engl J Med 1990;322:863-868.
[8] Stroke Prevention in Atrial Fibrillation Investigators. Stroke Prevention in Atrial Fibrillation Study (final results). Circulation 1991;84:527-539.
[9] The Boston Area Anticoagulation Trial for Atrial Fibrillation Investigators. The effect of low-dose warfarin on the risk of stroke in patients with nonrheumatic atrial fibrillation. N Engl J Med 1990;323:1505-1511.
[10] Connolly SJ, Laupacis A, Gent M, Roberts RS, Cairns JA, Joyner C, for the CAFA Study Coinvestigators. Canadian Atrial Fibrillation Anticoagulation (CAFA) Study. J Am Coll Cardiol 1991;18:349-355
[11] Ostrander LD, et al. Electrocardiographic findings among the adult population of a total natural community, Tecumseh, Michigan. Circulation 1965;31:888-897.
[12] Hiss RG, Lamb LE. Electrocardiographic findings in 122,043 individuals. Circulation 1962;25:947-961.
[13] Hill JD, Mottram EM, Killeen PD. Study of the prevalence of atrial fibrillation in general practice patients over 65 years of age. J Roy Coll Gen Pract 1987;37:172-173.
[14] Kitchen AH, Milne JS. Longitudinal survey of ischaemic heart disease in randomly selected sample of older population. Br Heart J 1977;39:889-893.
[15] Kannel WB, Abbott RD, Savage DD, McNamara PM. Coronary heart disease and atrial fibrillation: The Framingham study. Am Heart J 1983;106:389-396.
[16] Warlow C, Wade D, Sandercock P, et al. The epidemiology of stroke and transient ischaemic attack. In: Fry F, Sandler G, eds. Strokes. Ch 1. London: MTP Press, 1987.
[17] Treseder AS, Sastry BSD, Thomas TPL, Yates MA, Pathy MSJ. Atrial fibrillation and stroke in elderly hospitalized patients. Age aging 1986;15:89-92.
[18] Wolf PA, Abbott RD, Kannel WB. Atrial fibrillation: a major contribution to stroke in the elderly. Arch Intern Med 1987;147:1561-1564.
[19] Britton M, Gustafson C. Nonrheumatic atrial fibrillation as a risk factor for stroke. Stroke 1985;16:182-188.
[20] Olsen TS, Skriver EB, Herning M. Cause of cerebral infarction in the carotid artery. Its relation to the size and the location of the infarct and to the underlying vascular lesions. Stroke 1985;16:459-465.
[21] Kelley RE, Berger JR, Alter M, Kovacs AG. Cerebral ischemia and atrial fibrillation: Prospective study. Neurology 1984;34:1285-1291.

[22] Wolf PA, Dawber TR, Thomas HE, Kannel WB. Epidemiologic assessment of chronic atrial fibrillation and risk of stroke: The Framingham study. Neurology 1978;28:973-977.
[23] Fisher CM. Reducing risks of cerebral embolism. Geriatrics 1979;34:59-66.
[24] Sherman DG, Goldman L, Whiting RB, Jurgensen K, Kaste M, Easton JD. Risk of thromboembolism in patients with atrial fibrillation. Arch Neur 1984;41:708-710.
[25] Petersen P, Madsen EB, Brun B, Pedersen F, Gyldensted C, Boysen G. Silent cerebral infarction in chronic atrial fibrillation. Stroke 1987;18:1098-1100.
[26] Kempster PA, Gerraty RP, Gates PC. Asymptomatic cerebral infarction in patients with chronic atrial fibrillation. Stroke 1988;19:955-957.
[27] Ratecliffe PJ, Wilcock GK. Cerebrovascular disease in dementia: The importance of atrial fibrillation. Postgrad Med J 1985;61:201-204.
[28] Kopecky SL, Gersh BJ, McGoon MD, et al. The natural history of lone atrial fibrillation: a population based study over three decades. N Engl J Med 1987;317:669-674.
[29] Hart RG, Coull BM, Hart D. Early recurrent embolism associated with nonvalvular atrial fibrillation: A retrospective study. Stroke 1983;14:688-693.
[30] Aschenberg W, Schluter M, Kremer P, Schroder E, Siglow V, Bleifeld W. Transesophageal two-dimensional echocardiography for the detection of left atrial appendage thrombus. J Am Coll Cardiol 1986;7:163-166.
[31] Daniel WG, Nikutta P, Schroder E, Nellessen U. Transesophageal echocardiography detection of left atrial appendage thrombi in patients with unexplained arterial embolism (abstract). Circulation 1986;74 (suppl II):II-391.
[32] Brand FN, Abbott RD, Kannel WB, Wolf PA. Characteristics and prognosis of lone atrial fibrillation: 30-year follow-up in the Framingham study. JAMA 1985;254:3449-3453.
[33] Takahashi N, Seki A, Imataka K, Fujii J. Clinical features of paroxysmal atrial fibrillation. An observation of 94 patients. Jpn Heart J 1981;22:143-149.
[34] Petersen P, Godtfredsen J. Embolic complications in paroxysmal atrial fibrillation. Stroke 1986;17:622-626.
[35] Wiener I, Hafner R, Nicolai M, Lyons H. Clinical and echocardiographic correlates of systemic embolization in nonrheumatic atrial fibrillation. Am J Cardiol 1987;59:177-179.
[36] Easton JD, Sherman DG. Managements of cerebral embolism of cardiac origin. Stroke 1980;11:433-442.
[37] Wolf PA, Kannel WB, McGee DL, Meeks SL, Bharucha NE, McNamara PM. Duration of atrial fibrillation and the imminence of stroke: The Framingham study. Stroke 1983;14:664-667.
[38] Sage JI, Van Uitert RL. Risk of recurrent stroke in patients with atrial fibrillation and non-valvular heart disease. Stroke 1983;14:537-540.
[39] Kelly RE, Berger JR, Alter M, Kovacs AG. Cerebral ischemia and atrial fibrillation: Prospective study. Neurology 1984;34:1285-1291.
[40] Darling RC, Austen WG, Linton RR. Arterial embolism. Surg Gynecol Obstet 1987;124:106-114.
[41] Halperin JL, Hart RG. Atrial fibrillation and stroke: new ideas, persisting dilemmas. Stroke 1988;19:937-941.
[42] Cerebral Embolism Task Force. Cardiogenic brain embolism: the second report of the Cerebral Embolism Task Force. Arch Neurol 1989;46:727-743.
[43] Stein B, Fuster V, Halperin JL, Chesebro JH. Antithrombotic therapy in cardiac disease: an emerging approach based on pathogenesis and risk. Circulation 1989;80:1501-1513.
[44] Petersen P, Kastrup J, Videbaek R, Boysen G. Cerebral bloodflow before and after cardioversion of atrial fibrillation. J Cereb Blood Flow Metab 1989;9:422-425.
[45] Szekely P. Systemic embolism and anticoagulant prophylaxis in rheumatic heart disease. Br Med J 1964;1:1209.

[46] Adams GF, Merrett JD, Hutchinson WM, Pollock AM. Cerebral embolism and mitral stenosis: survival with and without anticoagulants. J Neurol Neurosurg Psychiatry 1974;37:378-383.
[47] Cosgriff SW. Chronic anticoagulant therapy in recurrent embolism of cardiac embolism. Ann Intern Med 1953;38:278-287.
[48] Genton E, Barnett HJM, Fields JS, Gent M, Hoak JC. XIV Cerebral ischaemia; the role of thrombosis and antithrombotic therapy. Stroke 1977;8:150-175.
[49] Yatsu F, Mohr JP. Anticoagulant therapy for cardiogenic emboli to brain. Neurology 1982;32:274-275.
[50] Mohr JP, Fisher CM, Adams RD. Cerebrovascular Disease. In: Isselbacher KJ, Adams RD, Braunwald E, Petersdorf RG, Wilson JD, eds. Harrison's principles of internal medicine (9th edn), New York: mcgraw-Hill, 1980:1932.
[51] Lodder J, Dennis MS, Van Raak L, Jones LN, Warlow CP. Cooperative study on the value of long term anticoagulation in patients with stroke and nonrheumatic atrial fibrillation. Br Med J 1988;43:362-365.
[52] Evans W, Swann P. Lone auricular fibrillation. Br Heart J 1954;16:189.
[53] Beer DT, Ghitman B. Embolization from the atria in arteriosclerotic heart disease. JAMA 1961;177:287.
[54] Walker MD. Atrial fibrillation and antithrombotic prophylaxis: A prospective meta-analysis. Lancet 1989;1:325-326.
[55] Ezekowitz MD, Bridgers SL, James KE, and SPINAF Investigators. Interim analysis of VA Co-operative Study, Stroke Prevention in Non Rheumatic Atrial Fibrillation (SPINAF). Circulation 1991;84 (Suppl):II-450.
[56] Cairns JA, Connolly SJ. Nonrheumatic atrial fibrillation: Risk of stroke and role of antithrombotic therapy. Circulation 1991;84:469-481.
[57] Goldman MJ. The management of chronic atrial fibrillation: Indications for and method of conversion to sinus rhythm. Prog Cardiovasc Dis 1960;2:465.
[58] Morris JJ Jr, Kong Y, North WC, McIntosh HD. Experience with "cardioversion" of atrial fibrillation and flutter. Am J Cardiol 1964;14:94.
[59] Morris JJ Jr, Peter RH, McIntosh HD. Electrical conversion of atrial fibrillation: Immediate and long-term results and selection of patients. Ann Intern Med 1966;65:216.
[60] Selzer A, Kelly JJ Jr, Johnsson RB, Kerth WJ. Immediate and long-term results of electrical conversion of arrhythmias. Prog Cardiovasc Dis 1966;9:90.
[61] Weinberg DM and Mancini GBJ. Anticoagulation for cardioversion of atrial fibrillation. Am J Cardiol 1989;63:745-746.
[62] Bjerkelund CJ, Orning OM. The efficacy of anticoagulant therapy in preventing embolism related to DC electrical conversion of atrial fibrillation. Am J Cardiol 1969;23:208.
[63] Ikram H, Nixon PGF, Arcan T. Left atrial function after electrical conversion of sinus rhythm. Br Heart J 1968;30:80.
[64] Rowlands DJ, Logan WFWE, Howitt E, Holmes AM. Atrial function after cardioversion. Am Heart J 1967;74:149.
[65] De Silva RA, Graboys TB, Podrid PJ, Lown B. Cardioversion and defibrillation. Am Heart J 1980;100:881.
[66] Mancini GBJ and Goldberger AL. Cardioversion of atrial fibrillation: Consideration of embolization, anticoagulation, prophylactic pacemaker, and long-term succes. Am Heart J 1982;104:617-621.
[67] Dunn M, Alexander J, De Silva R, Hildner F. Antithrombotic therapy in atrial fibrillation. Chest 1989;95:Suppl:118S-127S.
[68] Roy D, Marchand E, Gagne P, Chabot M, Cartier R. Usefulness of anticoagulant therapy in the prevention of embolic complications of atrial fibrillation. Am Heart J 1986;112:1039-1043.

[69] Kamp O, Van Huizem MA, Verhorst MJ, Visser CA. Left atrial flow velocity in patients with atrial fibrillation and systemic embolism. Circulation 1991;84 (Suppl II):II-411.

[70] Fisher EA, Stahl JA, Budd JA, Goldman RA. Left atrial "smoke" is a major risk factor for thrombus formation. Circulation 1991;84 (Suppl II):II-692.

Chapter 16

VALUE OF LEFT ATRIAL APPENDAGE FLOW VELOCITIES

IN PATIENTS WITH NONRHEUMATIC ATRIAL FIBRILLATION

AND SYSTEMIC EMBOLISM

Otto Kamp

Patrick M.J. Verhorst

Cees A. Visser

Department of Cardiology
Free University Hospital
Amsterdam
The Netherlands

and

Interuniversity Cardiology Institute
Utrecht
The Netherlands

J. H. Kingma et al. (eds.), Atrial fibrillation, a treatable disease?, 259–269.

INTRODUCTION

The occurrence of systemic embolism is a well-known potential risk in patients with atrial fibrillation[1,2,3,4,6]. Reliable identification of patient subgroups with atrial fibrillation with high risk for systemic embolism may importantly influence decisions regarding therapy (anticoagulant or antiplatelet therapy). Emboli may occur from thrombi forming within the left atrium and particularly in the left atrial appendage[1,4,5]. Stasis of blood flow is an important factor in the pathogenesis[7].

Transesophageal echocardiography (TEE) has proven to be a superior technique in imaging the left atrium and left atrial appendage because of its excellent resolution[8,9]. Therefore, TEE is increasingly being used to assess underlying cardiac sources of embolism.

We performed TEE to identify patients with nonrheumatic atrial fibrillation at risk for systemic embolism, by evaluating the presence of left atrial (appendage) thrombus, the presence of left atrial spontaneous contrast, left atrial size, and peak velocities of left pulmonary vein and left atrial appendage in patients with, and in a control group of patients without documented systemic embolism.

METHODS

Study patients. In a 10-month period, 54 consecutive patients with nonrheumatic atrial fibrillation were studied. Patients were assigned to one of the two groups depending on the presence or absence of a recent systemic embolic event. Group I consisted of 16 patients admitted because of recent proven systemic embolism; 14 patients with ischemic stroke and 2 patients with peripheral embolism, documented by CT-scan and/or angiography. Group II was composed of 38 patients without previous systemic embolism, who were first seen in our Heart Emergency Room with complaints of palpitations or chest discomfort. All patients had electrocardiographically documented atrial fibrillation on admission. Patients with atrial fibrillation due to mitral stenosis or those with prosthetic heart valves were excluded.

Transesophageal echocardiography study. TEE was performed with a Hewlett Packard ultrasonograph (HP 77020 AC) with a 5 MHz phased array transesophageal transducer. All patients fasted for at least 4 hours. Premedication was not given and a local anaesthetic (10% lignocaine) was sprayed into the patients hypopharynx. The transducer was introduced into the esophagus with patients lying in the left lateral decubitus position.

All TEE studies were performed within a time window of one week from admission.

Parameters evaluated by TEE were the presence of left atrial (appendage) thrombus, presence of left atrial spontaneous contrast, left atrial size (length and width), systolic and diastolic peak velocities of left pulmonary vein, and forward and backward peak velocities of left atrial appendage.

The left atrial cavity and left atrial appendage were adequately visualized by TEE, and two independent observers evaluated the presence of a left atrial (appendage) thrombus and/or left atrial spontaneous contrast.

Atrial length and width were measured and analyzed using the 4-chamber view in end-systole[8].

Velocities of pulmonary venous flow[10] and left atrial appendage flow were obtained using pulsed Doppler with the lowest possible filter setting (5 or 10 cm/sec). Measurements were performed in the direction of the flow within an angle of 30 degrees with the transducer; optimal alignment was thus assessed using simultaneous color flow imaging. Pulmonary venous flow velocity measurements were obtained with the sample volume placed in the left upper pulmonary vein at least 5 mm from the origin of the pulmonary vein into the left atrium. The sample volume was placed in the left atrial appendage, just below the basis of the appendage, to obtain left atrial appendage flow velocity measurements. In sinus rhythm, a biphasic flow pattern followed the P-wave on the electrocardiogram (Figure 1). In atrial fibrillation, a flow with a saw-tooth appearance was observed throughout the cardiac cycle (Figure 2).

Measurements of left pulmonary venous flow velocity and left atrial appendage flow velocity were recorded on a strip chart recorder. Mean values of the peak systolic and diastolic velocities of the left pulmonary vein flow, and peak forward and backward velocities of the left atrial appendage flow were obtained in 3 consecutive cardiac cycles during quiet respiration in patients with sinus rhythm and 10 cardiac cycles in patients with atrial fibrillation at the time of TEE.

Figure 1.
Doppler echocardiogram in the left atrial appendage in a patient with sinus rhythm.
Biphasic flow corresponds with contraction and relaxation of the left atrial appendage following the P-wave on the electrocardiogram.

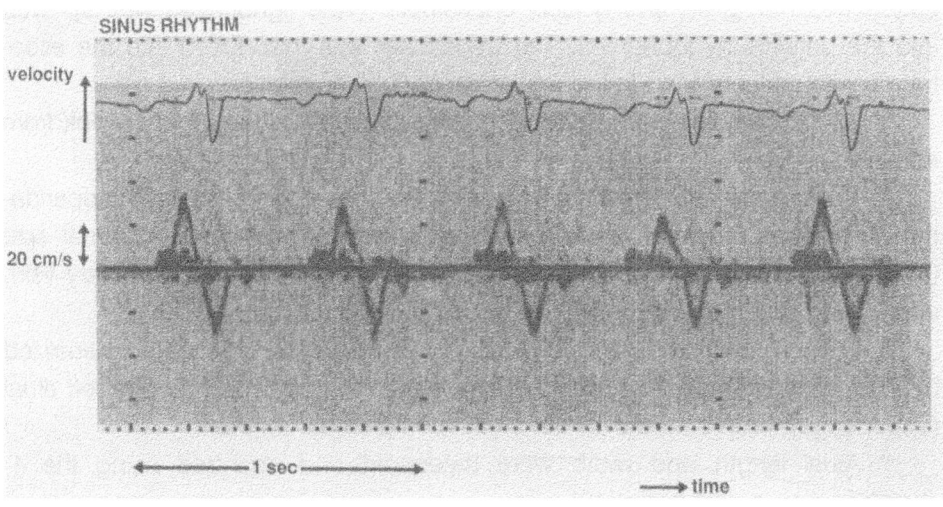

Figure 2.
Doppler echocardiogram in the left atrial appendage in a patient with atrial fibrillation. The flow signal displays a saw-tooth appearance, and the peak flow velocity is reduced, compared with that of sinus rhythm.

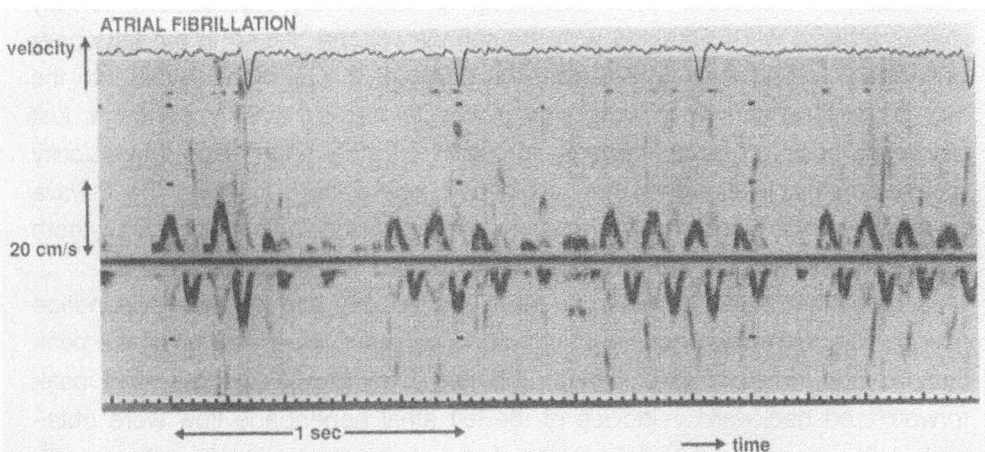

STATISTICS _____

Statistical analysis was performed by the Student t-test (p-values) for continuous variables and the Chi-square test to compare groups on the basis of categorical variables.

RESULTS _____

Patient characteristics. Baseline clinical characteristics including age, gender, duration, etiology of atrial fibrillation and prior aspirin or anticoagulant therapy were similar in both groups (Table 1).

Transesophageal echocardiography. At the time of TEE examination, 31 patients had atrial fibrillation and 23 patients had sinus rhythm. Sinus rhythm was observed in 5 of 16 patients of group I and 18 of 38 patients of group II at the time of TEE (p = not significant). The TEE findings are presented in Table 2. No difference in the presence of left atrial thrombus between the two groups was observed. Only in one patient of the embolism group (6%) a thrombus was found in the left atrial appendage. However, the occurrence of left atrial spontaneous contrast was significantly higher in the embolism group (38%) than in the non-embolism group (5%; p=0.01). Left atrial size, measured by atrial length (4.96 ± 0.84 cm vs 4.79 ± 1.38 cm) and atrial width (4.50 ± 0.96 cm vs 4.31 ± 1.24 cm), was not significant different in both groups. No significant difference in systolic peak velocity of the left pulmonary vein (0.39 ± 0.22 m/s vs 0.44 ± 0.22 m/s) was found, and only a trend for higher diastolic peak velocity of the left pulmonary vein (0.50 ± 0.17 m/s vs 0.42 ± 0.15 m/s;p=0.08) was observed in the embolism group.
Particularly worthy is our observation that left atrial appendage peak flow velocities (forward peak velocity: 0.25 ± 0.19 m/s vs 0.39 ± 0.23 m/s; backward peak velocity: 0.23 ± 0.15 m/s vs 0.33 ± 0.16 m/s) were significantly (p<0.05) lower in patients with nonrheumatic atrial fibrillation and systemic embolism compared to the non-embolism group.

Table 1. **Patient characteristics**

Demographics	Group I embolism + (n = 16)	Group II embolism - (n = 38)	p value
Age mean (years)	69	61	ns
Gender (male)	8	24	ns
CAD	7	9	ns
Hypertension	6	6	ns
Valvular disease	6	12	ns
Hyperthyroidism	0	3	ns
Others	3	8	ns
Lone AF	3	16	ns
Duration AF (months)	25	21	ns
Paroxysmal AF	12	26	ns
Prior aspirin use	1	0	ns
Prior anticoagulant use	3	4	ns

AF = atrial fibrillation, CAD = coronary artery disease, ns = not significant.

Table 2. **Outcome of transesophageal echocardiography**

Variables	Group I embolism + (n = 16)	Group II embolism - (n = 38)	p value
LA-thrombus	1 (6%)	0	ns
LA-SC	6 (38%)	2 (5%)	p=0.01
LA-length	4.96 ± 0.84	4.79 ± 1.38	ns
LA-width	4.50 ± 0.96	4.31 ± 1.24	ns
PV-S	0.39 ± 0.22	0.44 ± 0.22	ns
PV-D	0.50 ± 0.17	0.42 ± 0.15	p=0.08
LAA-F	0.25 ± 0.19	0.39 ± 0.23	p<0.05
LAA-B	0.23 ± 0.15	0.33 ± 0.16	p<0.05

B = backward peak velocity (m/sec); D = diastolic peak velocity (m/sec);
F = forward peak velocity (m/sec); LA = left atrium; LAA = left atrial
appendage; ns = not significant; PV = pulmonary vein; S = systolic peak
velocity (m/sec); SC = spontaneous contrast.

DISCUSSION

Atrial fibrillation is associated with a relative high risk of systemic embolism[1,2]. The annual incidence of systemic embolism in atrial fibrillation is about 5%[11]. Of all ischemic strokes, 15% are caused by an embolism of cardiac origin, for which nonrheumatic atrial fibrillation is in almost 50% of the cases responsible[5]. The risk of embolism per patient year is the highest during the first months after onset of atrial fibrillation. Fewer embolic complications are observed during the course of chronic atrial fibrillation[3,12]. Paroxysmal atrial fibrillation and lone atrial fibrillation carry a relatively low risk of embolism, as compared with chronic atrial fibrillation[6]. Patients with an initial embolus have a subsequent high risk of recurrence[9]. Apart from the often dramatic morbidity and mortality, systemic embolism has a great impact on social and economic aspects of our society. With a growing elderly population the incidence of systemic embolism will increase correspondingly, making it a matter of urgent concern in the near future.

Before the results of recent studies, there was the dilemma of antithrombotic treatment, weighing the reduced risk of embolism against the increased risk of bleeding. Now there is enough evidence that patients with atrial fibrillation benefit from antithrombotic treatment (anticoagulant or antiplatelet therapy) by significantly reducing the risk of systemic embolism with only few bleeding complications[13,14,15,16]. So far, anticoagulant therapy seems preferable over antiplatelet therapy in high risk patients, despite the low but still persistent risk of bleeding. However, in patients at low risk for systemic embolism the dangers associated with anticoagulant therapy may outweigh its benefit. Therefore, an objective and measurable test to predict patients with low or high risk of systemic embolism with nonrheumatic atrial fibrillation is desirable to identify patients who more likely benefit anticoagulant therapy because of a high likelihood of a cardiac source of embolism. Echocardiography, and especially the transesophageal technique, might provide such a test.

Naturally, the presence of a left atrial (appendage) thrombus found by echocardiography in patients with atrial fibrillation and systemic embolism increases the likelihood of a cardiac origin. In one study of 11 patients with nonrheumatic atrial fibrillation and a systemic embolus, a left atrial thrombus was found in 4 patients (36%)[17]. We observed a low incidence of only 1 left atrial thrombus (6%) in a group of 16 patients. This can be explained by the high incidence of paroxysmal atrial fibrillation and the exclusion of patients with mitral stenosis and mitral prosthesis.

Often, when a left atrial thrombus is not present, left atrial spontaneous contrast, the dynamic "smoke-like" echoes, can be seen with TEE. This phenomenon is experimentally and clinically related to low flow rates[9]. A recent study demonstrated that left atrial spontaneous contrast is an independent predictor of thromboembolic risk in patients with non-valvular atrial fibrillation[18]. In the present study, significantly more cases of left atrial spontaneous contrast in the group of patients with embolism were observed (38% vs 5%; p=0.01).

Left atrial enlargement is associated with atrial fibrillation by the fact that atrial fibrillation probably contributes to left atrial enlargement rather than being caused by it[6,12]. Studies regarding the predictive value of left atrial enlargement for embolism are not conclusive[11,19]. Left atrial size by itself does not affect the probability of systemic embolism. In the present study, we also could not find a significant difference in atrial size between patients with and without systemic embolism.

Pulmonary venous flow velocity is a reflection of the pressure gradient between the pulmonary veins and the left atrium. Atrial relaxation is one of the factors responsible for systolic forward flow. Diastolic forward flow reflects the transmitral filling pattern. In the absence of atrial contraction, as in atrial fibrillation, forward flow is still present, although of lower velocity than diastolic forward flow[10]. Velocity measurement of pulmonary venous flow, especially systolic peak velocity, might be able to predict mean left atrial pressure[20]. We found no difference in systolic peak velocity, but we did observe a trend for higher diastolic peak velocity in the embolism group.

Interrogation of the outlet of the left atrial appendage with pulsed Doppler provided information about emptying (forward peak velocity) and filling (backward peak velocity) of the left atrial appendage. In sinus rhythm, a biphasic flow pattern representing left atrial appendage contraction and relaxation followed the P-wave on the electrocardiogram (Figure 1). In atrial fibrillation, a saw-tooth appearance was observed throughout the cardiac cycle with lower forward and backward velocities (Figure 2). In the present study, we demonstrated the significance of left atrial appendage flow velocities. Thus, significantly lower forward and backward peak flow velocities in the left atrial appendage in patients with nonrheumatic atrial fibrillation and systemic embolism were observed, as compared with patients without embolism. A recent study assessing left atrial appendage function found that left atrial appendage thrombus formation is associated with both left atrial appendage contraction and left atrial appendage dilatation[21].

LIMITATIONS OF THE PRESENT STUDY _____

A major problem with studying the origin of systemic embolism is the fact that the diagnosis itself is notoriously difficult. First, emboli may originate from noncardiac sources. Second, echocardiography will not demonstrate a cardiac lesion that has entirely embolized. Furthermore, no cardiac source might be detected when a peripheral vascular cause is present. This explains the rather large standard deviation in our study due to inclusion of patients with systemic embolism of noncardiac origin.

Regarding left atrial spontaneous contrast, its value is limited by the fact of its unknown day-to-day occurrence and because the accuracy of the diagnosis is influenced by transducer gain setting and interobserver variability[18].

When measuring velocity in the left pulmonary vein and left atrial appendage respectively, it is important to obtain true parallel interrogation. In all our measurements this technical difficulty was overcome as much as possible by placing the sample volume in an angle of less than 30 degrees with the flow.

Another limitation is the fact that the study group was too small to perform multivariant analysis in order to look at independent predictive parameters. Studies with a larger group size will probably provide that information.

CLINICAL IMPLICATIONS _____

Atrial fibrillation is a common disease associated with high risk of embolism which can significantly be reduced by antithrombotic treatment, especially anticoagulant therapy. Identifying the nature of embolism and knowing what precipitates it has important implications for the treatment and prevention of embolism. Such identification would make it possible to define patient subgroups at high risk, needing more aggressive therapy (e.g. anticoagulant therapy), and patient subgroups at low risk, needing less aggressive therapy (e.g. antiplatelet therapy).

Left atrial spontaneous contrast, and more particularly the objective and measurable left atrial appendage peak flow velocity can be used to identify patients with atrial fibrillation prone to systemic embolism. Using these parameters high and low risk subgroups can be defined. A prospective randomized study for treatment with anticoagulant therapy versus antiplatelet therapy, using TEE findings as a risk marker, is warranted.

References

[1]   Britton M, Gustafsson C. Non-rheumatic atrial fibrillation as a risk factor for stroke. Stroke 1985;16:182-188.
[2]   Brand FN, Abbott RD, Kannel WB, Wolf PA. Characteristics and prognosis of lone atrial fibrillation. JAMA 1985;254:3449-3453.
[3]   Petersen P, Godtfredsen J. Embolic complications in paroxysmal atrial fibrillation. Stroke 1986;17:622-626.
[4]   Sherman DG.Cardiac embolism: The neurologist's perspective. Am J Cardiol 1990;65: 32-37c.
[5]   Come PC, Riley MF, Bivas NK. Roles of echocardiography and arrhythmia monitoring in the evaluation of patients with suspected systemic embolism. Ann Neurology 1983; 13:527-531.
[6]   Petersen P. Thromboembolic complications of atrial fibrillation and their prevention: A review. Am J Cardiol 1990;65:24-28c.
[7]   Fuster V, Stein B, Halperin JL, Chesebro JH. Antithrombotic therapy in cardiac disease: An approach based on pathogenesis and risk stratification. Am J Cardiol 1990;65:38-44c.
[8]   Drexler M, Erbel R, Muller U, Wittlich N, Mohr-Kahaly S, Meyer J. Measurements of intracardiac dimensions and structures in normal young adult subjects by transesophageal echocardiography. Am Journal of Cardiol 1990;65:1491-1496.
[9]   Pearson AC, Labovitz AJ, Tatineni S, Gomez C. Superiority of transesophageal echocardiography in detecting cardiac source of embolism in patients with cerebral ischemia of uncertain etiology. J Am Coll Cardiol 1991;17:66-72.
[10]   Nishimura RA, Abel MD, Hatle LK, Tajik AJ. Relation of pulmonary vein to mitral flow velocities by transesophageal Doppler echocardiography. Circulation 1990;81:1488-97.
[11]   Cairns JA, Connolly SJ. Nonrheumatic atrial fibrillation. Risk of stroke and role of antithrombotic therapy. Circulation 1991;84:469-481.
[12]   Henry WL, Morganroth J, Pearlman AS, Clark CE, Redwood DR, Itscoitz SB, Epstein SE. Relation between echocardiographically determined left atrial size and atrial fibrillation. Circulation 1976;53:273-279.
[13]   Roy D, Marchand E, Gagne B, Chabot M, Cartier R. Usefulness of anticoagulant therapy in the prevention of embolic complications of atrial fibrillation. Am Heart J 1986;112:1-039-1043.

[14] Petersen P, Boysen G, Andersen ED, Andersen B. Placebo-controlled, randomised trial of warfarin and aspirin for prevention of thromboembolic complications in chronic atrial fibrillation: The Copenhagen AFASAK Study. Lancet 1989;1:175-179.

[15] Stroke Prevention in Atrial Fibrillation Study. Circulation 1991;84:527-539.

[16] Connolly SJ. Canadian Atrial Fibrillation Anticoagulant (CAFA) study. J Am Coll Cardiol 1991;18:349-355.

[17] Malone SA, Palac RT, Imus RL, Andrilenas KK, McDonald RW, Giraud GD. Prevalence of left atrial thrombi in symptomatic versus asymptomatic patients with nonvalvular atrial fibrillation (abstract). Circulation 1989;80:II-1.

[18] Black IW. Left atrial spontaneous echo contrast: a clinical and echocardiographic analysis. J Am Coll Cardiol 1991;18:398-404.

[19] Cabin HS, Clubbs KS, Hall C, Perlmutter RA, Feinstein AR. Risk for systemic embolization of atrial fibrillation without mitral stenosis. Am J of Cardiology 1990;65:1112-1116.

[20] Kuecherer HF, Muhiudeen IA, Kusumoto FM, Lee E, Moulinier LE, Cahalan MK, Schiller NB. Estimation of mean left atrial pressure from transesophageal pulsed Doppler echocardiography of pulmonary venous flow. Circulation 1990;82:1127-1139.

[21] Pollick CP, Taylor D. Assessment of left atrial appendage function by transesophageal echocardiography. Circulation 1991;84:223-231.

Chapter 17

MANAGEMENT OF ATRIAL FIBRILLATION:

FROM PALLIATION TO INTERVENTION

J. Herre Kingma

Maarten J. Suttorp

Willem P. Beukema

Department of Cardiology
St Antonius Hospital
Nieuwegein
The Netherlands

J. H. Kingma et al. (eds.), Atrial fibrillation, a treatable disease?, 271–284.

INTRODUCTION _____

Next to premature beats atrial fibrillation is the most common arrhythmia in man and has even been designated the grandfather of all arrhythmias[1]. Atrial fibrillation occurs only sporadically in younger people. It is a condition more prevalent in the older age group. Prevalence in the general population is 0.4%. However, in patients over 70 years of age this may increase to 10% to 25%, which figure even increases to up to 40% in those with congestive heart failure[2,3]. The prognosis of patients with atrial fibrillation is strongly determined by the risk of stroke. Data from the Framingham study indicate a 4.8 fold increase risk of stroke, which increases with age[4]. The outcome of recent trials indicates that this risk may be reduced by oral anticoagulant therapy and aspirin treatment[5,6,7].

Consequently, the management of atrial fibrillation is not restricted to the cardiologist. General practitioners, internists and neurologists have many patients with these arrhythmias in their practices. There is much confusion about terminology, as to the definition of paroxysmal and chronic atrial fibrillation. This is also reflected in the clinical approach, which may differ widely. Some consider atrial fibrillation a phenomenon of aging which does not require aggressive treatment but rather conservative treatment by heart rate control with digitalis. Others will be more aggressive and do not accept frequent paroxysms or chronic atrial fibrillation until failure of frequent attempts of DC cardioversion. Although the wide spread use of digitalis may be considered adequate treatment in many cases, at present more tailored treatments are possible directed to restoration and maintenance of sinus rhythm or aggressive rate control by catheter ablation of the AV junction (AVJ). In this chapter we will discuss how to select the proper approach to the individual patient with atrial fibrillation.

GENERAL APPROACH TO ATRIAL FIBRILLATION _____

At present a number of questions are pertinent to the selection of treatment in atrial fibrillation:

1. What is the type and duration of atrial fibrillation?
2. Is immediate treatment necessary?

3. Are there identifiable triggers and conditions, and can these be eliminated or prevented?
4. Is there a structural heart disease, and if so, is this accompanied with left ventricular dysfunction and symptomatic heart failure?
5. Is therapy directed to either restoration of sinus rhythm or rate control?
6. How are safety and efficacy balanced in the individual patient?

Type and duration? Atrial fibrillation and flutter can be divided into 3 different types according to duration and type of trigger (Table 1). The incidence of attacks should also be taken into consideration (Table 2).

Table 1. **Different types of atrial fibrillation**

Types	Mode of Onset and Duration
Paroxysmal AF Recent onset Long-standing	Sporadic, recurrent or frequent lasting ≤48 hours lasting >48 hours - <6 months
Transient AF	Acute, during intercurrent trigger/disease
Chronic AF	Sustained, frequently permanent lasting >6 months

AF = atrial fibrillation

(Adopted from reference 23, with permission of the author)

Table 2. **Number of attacks in patients with paroxysmal atrial fibrillation**

Frequency of attacks in AF	
Sporadic (infrequent)	Monthly or less
Recurrent	Weekly
Frequent	Almost daily, up to weekly
Incessant	Daily, covering >12 hours/day

AF = atrial fibrillation

(Adopted from reference 23, with permission of the author)

Paroxysmal atrial fibrillation may be defined as an arrhythmia with sporadic, recurrent or frequent episodes lasting from a few seconds to several months. By definition, this type of arrhythmia has to convert spontaneously or it should be possible to restore sinus rhythm either by using pharmacological intervention or DC cardioversion. When paroxysmal atrial fibrillation occurs daily, with attacks covering more than 12 hours per day, this is defined as incessant paroxysmal atrial fibrillation. Furthermore, paroxysmal atrial fibrillation should be subdivided into recent onset or longstanding atrial fibrillation. We define recent onset atrial fibrillation as an arrhythmia lasting shorter than 48 hours, and longstanding if the arrhythmia lasts more than 48 hours but less than 6 months. Transient atrial fibrillation is a type of paroxysmal atrial fibrillation which arises from a clearly identifiable intercurrent pathophysiologic trigger or condition such as myocardial infarction, exacerbation of congestive heart failure, pulmonary embolism, etc. It is usually reverted following resolution of these conditions and triggers.

In contrast, chronic atrial fibrillation by definition lasts longer than 6 months, without recurrent sinus rhythm, and very often cannot be converted to long-term sustained sinus rhythm. Although, there is considerable overlap in these conditions, distinction between paroxysmal and chronic atrial fibrillation is of great importance because of the different therapeutic strategies in these conditions.

Is immediate treatment necessary? The need for immediate treatment depends on the severity of symptoms, hemodynamic compromise, ventricular rate and the type of anti-arrhythmic drugs currently being used by the patient. Ideally, atrial fibrillation should be reverted to sinus rhythm as soon as possible since the success rate in conversion to sinus rhythm decreases with time, especially when using pharmacologic conversion. The decreasing efficacy of pharmacologic intervention with time has been shown in several studies usually showing a high efficacy when therapy is initiated within 24 to 48 hours[8,9]. This is supported by experimental data from Allessie et al. discussed earlier in this issue[10]. However, acute conversion either pharmacologically or electrically is not always possible. Contraindications are longstanding atrial fibrillation i.e. longer than 48 hours in the presence of an enlarged left atrium, or clinical triggers ad conditions which may sustain the attack of atrial fibrillation.

Triggers and conditions? Several conditions and triggers can lead to atrial fibrillation and flutter (Table 3). Very important are left atrial size and its early and

Table 3. **Conditions and triggers associated with atrial fibrillation**

Cardiac related

Coronary heart disease

- Acute myocardial ischemia and infarction
- Congestive heart failure

Valvular heart disease

Hypertensive heart disease

Cardiomyopathy

Inflammatory or infiltrative disease

- Myocarditis
- Amyloidosis
- Sarcoidosis
- Metastasis
- Hemochromatosis

Congenital heart disease

- Atrial septal defect

Sinus and AV-node dysfunction

- Bradycardia-tachycardia syndrome

Pre-excitation

Intracardiac tumours

- Myxoma
- Thrombi
- Metastatic tumours

Cardiothoracic surgery

Miscellaneous

- Atrial fibrosis
- Pericarditis
- Atrial hypertrophy

Non-cardiac related

Vagal origin

- Resting and digesting, alcohol

Adrenergic origin

- Exercise and emotional stress
- Hyperthyroidism, pheochromocytoma

Toxic and metabolic conditions

- Alcohol, caffeine, drugs
- Hyperthyroidism
- Infections
- Others

Pulmonary disease

- Chronic obstructive disease
- Pulmonary hypertension
- Pulmonary emboli

Post surgery and general anaesthesia

No apparent cardiac conditions or triggers

Absence of underlying disease

- Idiopathic or 'Lone'

(Modified from reference 23)

late electrophysiologic sequelae. Changes in autonomic tone may also precipitate atrial fibrillation, although atrial fibrillation itself is frequently accompanied by arousal of the autonomic system. Management of a number of these conditions and triggers will eventually lead to restoration of sinus rhythm. In particular, atrial fibrillation in congestive heart failure should rather be approached by treatment of heart failure than the administration of antiarrhythmic drugs. This also applies to metabolic conditions such as alcohol abuse, drugs and hyperthyroidism. In a large quantity of patients no etiology can be found. This form is called idiopathic or lone atrial fibrillation. In these patients treatment can only be directed to the arrhythmia itself.

Structural heart disease?   Presence of structural heart disease may constitute a trigger or condition which deserves special attention of the attending physician. Use of antiarrhythmic drugs in these patients may further worsen left ventricular dysfunction or even precipitate serious ventricular arrhythmias. The CAST investigators[11] have shown that the use of Class Ic drugs in patients following myocardial infarction may be associated with an excess risk of sudden death. Therefore, we advocate an approach which at each decision level stratifies patients for the presence of left ventricular dysfunction. This will be discussed in detail later.

Sinus rhythm or rate control?   The question whether restoration of sinus rhythm or rate control should be the goal of therapy is dependent on many of the previously mentioned conditions. Although, restoration of sinus rhythm may considerably improve quality of life, it also implies the long-term use of antiarrhythmic drugs with its associated risks, such as life threatening adverse reactions and proarrhythmic effects. Furthermore, the negative inotrope effects of most antiarrhythmic drugs may increase symptoms of heart failure and possibly increase the risk of proarrhythmic effects. On the other hand, heart rate control applied in patients with structural heart disease and chronic atrial fibrillation, implies lifelong anticoagulant therapy and an increased risk of thromboembolic complications. Pro's and con's are summarized in Table 4.

Safety and efficacy?   Patients with atrial fibrillation constitute a wide spectrum of clinical conditions. While patient without any structural heart disease can be safely treated with an acceptable dose of antiarrhythmic drugs, the approach to the patient with structural heart disease and or congestive heart

Table 4. **Should atrial fibrillation be prevented?**

CON's	PRO's
Long-term use of antiarrhythmics:	
Suboptimal therapeutic effect	Conservation physiologic rate and rhythm
Side effects	Optimal hemodynamics
Proarrhythmic effects	Prevention of embolism
Frequent drug monitoring	
'Well being'	'Well being'

failure is rate control, which usually can be accomplished with digitalis and/or verapamil. In the middle of the this spectrum there is the patient with moderate congestive heart failure, frequent attacks of paroxysmal atrial fibrillation, in need of increasing doses of a combination of antiarrhythmic drugs. When the risks of drug therapy outbalance the benefits of sinus rhythm, one should resign to rate control rather than exposing the patient to an excessive risk of long term antiarrhythmic therapy.

CLINICAL MANAGEMENT

When selecting proper treatment for the individual patient, first the type of atrial fibrillation must be identified, as well as potential triggers, the presence of structural heart disease and the previous therapeutic history. In our approach (summarized in Figure 1), 4 main streams can be distinguished:
1. Intervention of acute attacks of atrial fibrillation.
2. Episodic treatment in patients with infrequent attacks.
3. Maintenance therapy directed to prevention in patients with frequent paroxysmal atrial fibrillation.
4. Rate control in chronic atrial fibrillation.

Acute intervention. Patients with an acute attack of atrial fibrillation are primarily stratified in patients with or without structural heart disease and or symptomatic or asymptomatic heart failure. Patients with recent onset atrial fibrillation i.e. less than 48 hours with normal ventricular function will usually be treated by intravenous drug administration. As discussed earlier in this issue[12], intravenous flecainide seems safe and highly effective in recent onset atrial fibrillation. The decreasing response to pharmacotherapy of long-standing atrial fibrillation with time may imply the need for as early as possible institution of anti-arrhythmic treatment, preferably within 24 hours, which is the usual approach to other supraventricular tachycardias such as AV nodal- and circus movement WPW tachycardia. Ideally, such an antiarrhythmic drug should exhibit a short duration of action, it should yield short-lasting high plasma levels, and even higher in atrial tissue, comparable to the properties of i.v verapamil in circus movement tachycardias using the AV node. If atrial fibrillation is long standing i.e. longer than 48 hours, intravenous treatment is less effective[8,9]. These patients should be treated by oral loading with an antiarrhythmic drug and if left atrial size is increased, concomitantly with anticoagulant drugs. DC cardioversion should be applied in patients with normal atrial size if sinus rhythm is not restored within 2 days of drug therapy. In patients with enlarged atria, DC cardioversion will not take place until 4 weeks of proper anti-coagulant therapy and longstanding atrial fibrillation. Patients with abnormal LV function are stratified again to those with overt signs of congestive heart failure and those without symptoms. If congestive heart failure is present, treatment should be directed to congestive heart failure itself. In our opinion antiarrhythmics are strongly contraindicated under these circumstances and should not be used until full recompensation of the patient has been accomplished. Subsequently these patients can be treated with quinidine or amiodarone probably in combination with digitalis. In these patients, one should avoid the Class Ic agents with their possible negative inotropic effect on the left ventricle.

Episodic treatment. Episodic treatment is defined as treatment given at the very onset of an attack or even during its prodromal symptoms. This mode of therapy may involve one drug or a cocktail of several compounds. Especially patients with infrequent but sustained attacks of atrial fibrillation may benefit from this approach. This form of therapy has been discussed extensively earlier in this issue[13]. Its use is surrounded by the same restrictions as discussed for acute interventional therapy. Therefore, episodic therapy should be limited to the patient with short lived attacks of atrial fibrillation and a normal left ventricular function. Preferably, the administration of these drug formulations should have been tested in hospital before prescribing them on an outpatient basis.

From a theoretical point of view, several drugs may be useful in episodic treatment. Since formal controlled trials are not yet available this therapy is still in the area of try and error. Use of fast oral loading with quinidine may convert patients to sinus rhythm in 40-80% of cases[14,15], as compared to 67%-86% for intravenous flecainide, depending on the duration of the attack. However, adverse effects were seen in 40% after administration of quinidine. Oral flecainide may be used in tablets up to 200 mg in one dose, which can be repeated after 1 to 2 hours. In our experience, about 60% of patients may convert to sinus rhythm after oral loading with flecainide [unpublished data]. More promising is the cocktail described by Lie-A-Huen and Kingma[13], consisting of liquid flecainide and cisapride. Cisapride promotes gastric emptying, thereby facilitating resorption of flecainide. In a small in-hospital study, 4 out of 6 patients converted to sinus rhythm following liquid flecainide in combination with cisapride. Another interesting possibility is concomitant use of a beta blocker, when there is arousal of the sympathetic nervous system. In particular, sotalol which also shows rapid sublingual resorption[16], may be advantageous alone or in combination with Class I drugs.

A potential advantage of episodic therapy is the possibility of self medication. This will also imply that administration may take place very early after onset of the attack. As many reports indicate, efficacy very strongly depends on the time delay until institution of therapy. Although this approach seems promising, it is still in its early phase of development and not ready for widespread use until formal clinical trials have proven its feasibility and safety.

Maintenance of sinus rhythm. Maintenance therapy with antiarrhythmic drugs is applied in patients with frequent symptomatic attacks of paroxysmal atrial fibrillation. The approach to the patient strongly depends whether there is normal or abnormal left ventricular function. Patients with normal left ventricular function can be treated with all the usual anti arrhythmic drugs including Class Ia and Class Ic, sotalol and amiodarone. In patients with abnormal left ventricular function, one should stay away from Class I and in particular Class Ic drugs. Under these circumstances amiodarone may even be the drug of first choice. If drug therapy fails, patients with normal sinus node function may be eligible for surgical therapy, either the 'corridor'[17,18] or the 'maze' procedure[19], provided that there is no severe structural heart disease. A success rate of 80% may be anticipated from this form of therapy[17,18]. However, the surgical approach is in its early phase of development and needs longer follow-up to establish its clinical use[19].

Figure 1.   MANAGEMENT OF PAROXYSMAL

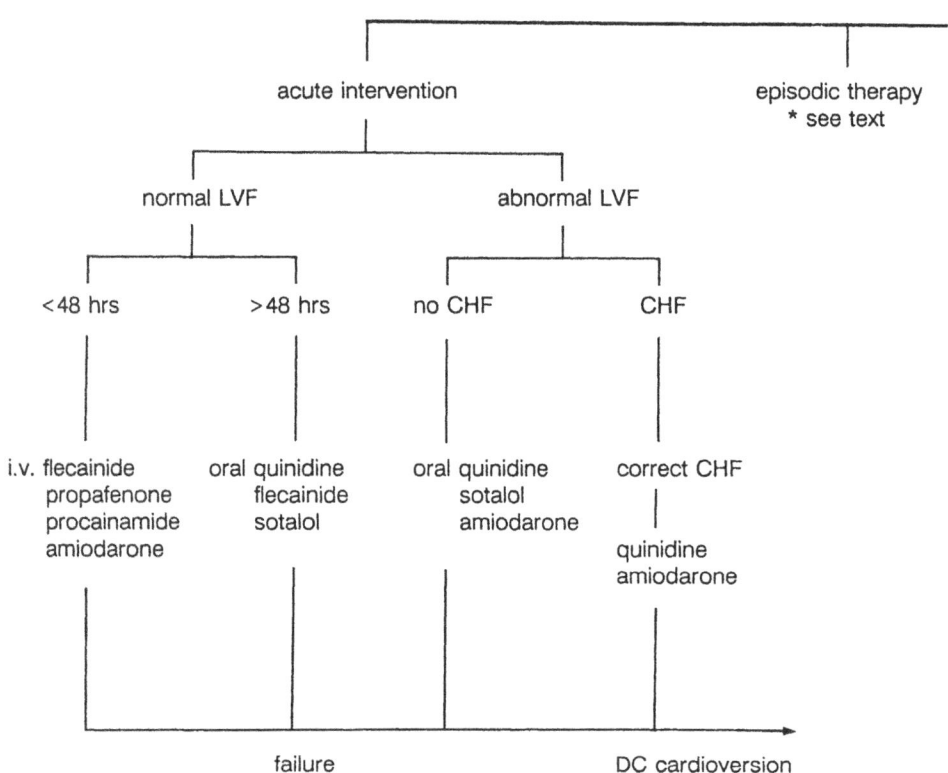

LVF = left ventricular function; SR = sinus rhythm; SN = sinus node; AF = atrial fibrillation;

Rate Control. When maintenance therapy fails to prevent relapses of atrial fibrillation and the patient is not eligible for surgical therapy, catheter ablation of the atrioventricular junction (AVJ ablation) followed by implant of a VVI rate responsive pacemaker, is applied to control heart rate. In particular patients with abnormal sinus node function and high ventricular rates during atrial fibrillation should be selected for this procedure. Patients with less frequent paroxysms of atrial fibrillation could even be treated with a DDI pacemaker, providing physiologic AV pacing during sinus rhythm which is inhibited on the atrial level during atrial fibrillation when VVI pacing is in operation.

ATRIAL FIBRILLATION

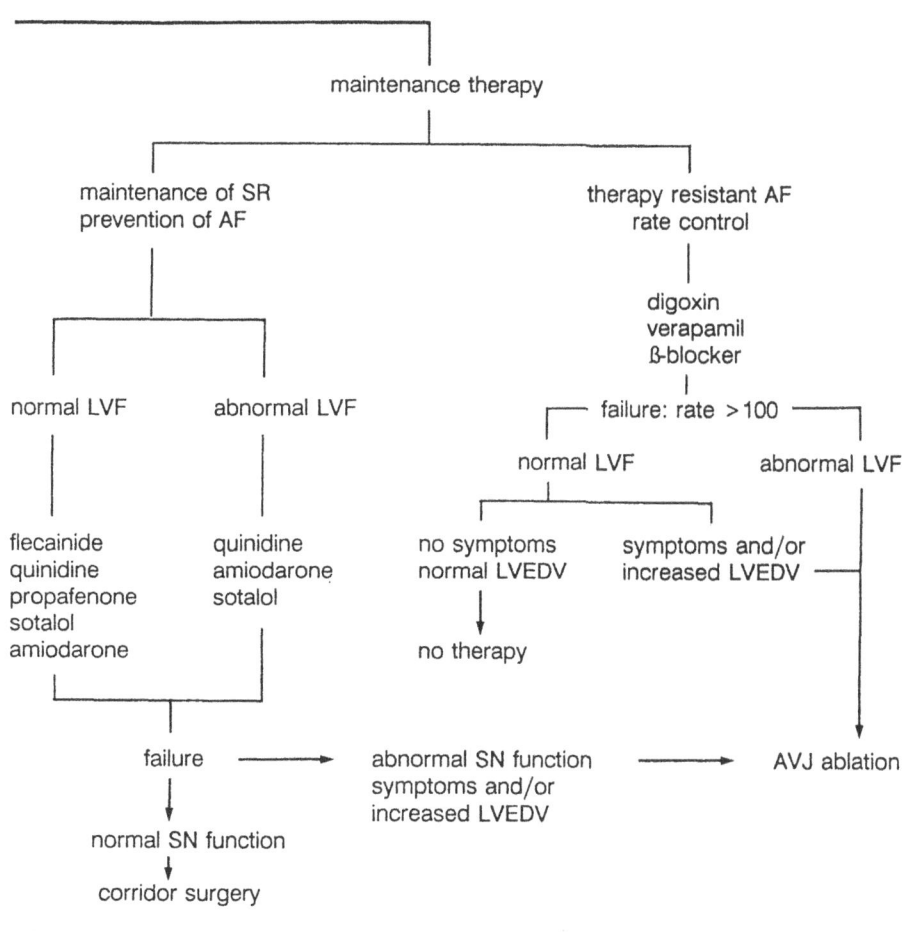

LVEDV = left ventricular enddiastolic volume; AVJ = atrioventricular junction.

In patients with drug resistant atrial fibrillation existing longer than 6 months, treatment will usually consist of control of heart rate. This is the only group of patients in which digitalis is still the therapy of choice. In all other previously discussed categories of patients the use of digitalis has declined. Patients with chronic atrial fibrillation and normal left ventricular function with a heart rate above

90 bpm should receive additional therapy, even when asymptomatic. If digitalis, verapamil or ß-blocker fail to reduce ventricular rate, symptomatic patients can be treated with AVJ ablation and subsequent pacemaker implant. Patients without symptoms and high ventricular rates should have regular echocardiographic follow-up for signs of left ventricular dysfunction. If left ventricular function worsens AVJ ablation is the therapy of choice, even if the left ventricular dysfunction is asymptomatic. Patients with left ventricular dysfunction and a heart rate above 90 bpm, should be treated with rate slowing drugs. If heart rate does not decrease below 90 bpm in these patients, AVJ ablation followed by VVI pacemaker implant should be strongly considered.

CONCLUSIONS

Therapy of atrial fibrillation is changing because of a better understanding of the pathophysiologic mechanisms and the availability of effective drug therapy, catheter and surgical interventions. Quinine, and later quinidine has dominated the therapy of atrial fibrillation for more than 200 years, frequently combined with digitalis glycosides. Digitalis has been used for more than a century both alone and as adjunctive therapy next to quinidine. Still many physicians believe that digitalis is capable of preventing atrial fibrillation, although findings from electrophysiologic studies point in another direction which is parallelled by lack of clinical efficacy. Digitalis may even increase the number and duration of attacks due to its electrophysiological properties[20].

The prescription of digitalis preparations in the European Community varies from 20% in France and Germany to even 83% in the United Kingdom (U.K.), with respect to the total number of prescriptions for supraventricular arrhythmias. Class I and III antiarrhythmic drug prescriptions vary from 2% to 31% in the U.K. and France, respectively[21]. Although digitalis is a potential and even dangerous drug if not used with great caution, the same caution applies to many of the old and newer antiarrhythmic drugs. There is a growing awareness of the potential pro-arrhythmic effects of these drugs, which was reinforced by the meta analysis from Coplen, indicating excess mortality in the quinidine treated patients who were in sinus rhythm[22]. The risk of pro-arrhythmia seems especially prominent in patients with structural heart disease like those with a history of previous infarction[11]. A considerable number of patients with atrial fibrillation is known with this kind of structural heart disease and will carry a risk for proarrhythmia when treated with these classes of drugs. The question to be answered is, should atrial fibrillation be prevented at all? In favour is certainly the improvement of hemodynamics, but also prevention of embolism and the quality of life associated with sinus rhythm. Negative aspects include the necessity for long-term use of antiarrhythmic drugs with not infrequently a sub-optimal therapeutic effect, and side effects, in particular proarrhythmia. Negative inotropic effects add to the detrimental condition of patients with congestive heart failure.

These factors detract from the improved quality of life associated with sustained sinus rhythm and may even outbalance the benefits of this approach. Therefore careful selection of therapy is mandatory. However, one should not easily resign to ordinary treatment with digitalis instead of the pursuit of optimal therapy using an innovative approach. Many different treatment modalities have been discussed: from treatment of the patient with a single attack of paroxysmal atrial fibrillation to the patient with very frequent recurrent attacks for whom AVJ ablation therapy is available and even surgical therapy can be considered in order to restore and maintain sinus rate and rhythm. The patient with atrial fibrillation should be offered therapy, commensurate with his needs and our new insights in the use of old and new antiarrhythmic drugs and alternative forms of treatment.

References

[1]   Selzer A. Atrial fibrillation revisited. N Engl J Med 1982;306:1044-1045.
[2]   Godtfredsen J. Atrial fibrillation. Etiology, course, and prognosis: a follow-up study of 1212 cases. Copenhagen, Munksgaard, 1975.
[3]   Petersen P, Godtfredsen J. Atrial fibrillation: A review of course and prognosis. Acta Med Scand 1984;216:5-9.
[4]   Kannel WB, Abbott RD, Savage DD, McNamara PM. Coronary heart disease and atrial fibrillation: the Framingham study. Am Heart J 1983;106:389-396.
[5]   Petersen P, Boysen G, Godfredsen J, Andersen ED, Andersen B. Placebo-controlled, randomized trial of warfarin and asperin for prevention of tromboembolic complications in chronic atrial fibrillation: The Copenhagen AFASAK study. Lancet 1989;i:175-179.
[6]   Stroke Prevention in Atrial Fibrillation (SPAF) Study Group Investigators. Preliminary report of the stroke prevention in atrial fibrillation study. N Engl J Med 1990;322:863-868.
[7]   Boston Area Anticoagulation Trial for Atrial Fibrillation (BATAAF) Investigators. The effect of low-dose warfarin on the risk of stroke in patients nonrheumatic atrial fibrllation. N Engl J Med 1990;323:1505-1511.
[8]   Suttorp MJ, Kingma JH, Lie-A-Huen L, Mast EG. Intravenous flecainide versus verapamil for acute conversion of paroxysmal atrial fibrillation or flutter to sinus rhythm. Am J Cardiol 1989;63:693-696.

[9]   Suttorp MJ, Kingma JH, Jessurun ER, Lie-A-Huen L, Hemel van NM, Lie KI. The value of Class Ic antiarrhythmic drugs for acute conversion of paroxysmal atrial fibrillation or flutter to sinus rhythm. J Am Coll Cardiol 1990;16:1722-1727.

[10] Allessie MA, Kirchhof C. Termination of atrial fibrillation by Class Ic antiarrhythmic drugs, a paradox? In: Kingma JH, van Hemel NM, Lie KI (eds), Atrial fibrillation, a treatable disease? Kluwer Academic Publishers, Dordrecht, The Netherlands, 1992, this issue.

[11] Cardiac Arrhythmia Suppression Trial (CAST) investigators: Preliminary report: Effect of encainide or flecainide on mortality in a randomized trial of arrhythmia suppression after myocardial infarction. N Engl J Med 1989;111:107-111.

[12] Suttorp MJ, Jessurun ER, Kingma JH. Pharmacological cardioversion of paroxysmal atrial fibrillation or atrial flutter to sinus rhythm. In: Kingma JH, van Hemel NM, Lie KI (eds), Atrial fibrillation, a treatable disease? Kluwer Academic Publishers, Dordrecht, The Netherlands, 1992, this issue.

[13] Lie-A-Huen L, Kingma JH. Episodic treatment of paroxysmal atrial fibrillation. In: Kingma JH, van Hemel NM, Lie KI (eds), Atrial fibrillation, a treatable disease? Kluwer Academic Publishers, Dordrecht, The Netherlands, 1992, this issue.

[14] Södermark T, Jonsson B, Olsson A, Orö L, Wallin H, Edhag O, Sjögren A, Danielsson M, Rosenhamer G. Effect of quinidine on maintaining sinus rhythm after conversion to atrial fibrillation or flutter. Br Heart J 1975;37:486-492.

[15] Borgeat A, Goy JJ, Meandly R, Kaufmann U, Grbic M, Sigwart U. Flecainide versus quinidine for cardioversion of atrial fibrillation to sinus rhythm. Am J Cardiol 1986;58:496-498.

[16] Edgar P. Personal communication. Internal report, Bristol Meyers Squibb, 1992.

[17] Defauw JJAM, van Hemel NM, Kingma JH, Jaarsma W, Vermeulen FEE, de Bakker JMT, Guiraudon GM. The 'corridor' operation as an alternative in the treatment of atrial fibrillation. In: Kingma JH, van Hemel NM, Lie KI (eds), Atrial fibrillation, a treatable disease? Kluwer Academic Publishers, Dordrecht, The Netherlands, 1992, this issue.

[18] Leitch JW, Klein GW, Yee R, Guiraudon GM. Sinus node atrioventricular node isolation. Long term results with the corridor operation for atrial fibrillation. J Am Coll Cardiol 1991;17:970-975.

[19] DiMarco JP. Surgical therapy for atrial fibrillation: a first step on what may be a long road. J Am Coll Cardiol 1991;17:976-977.

[20] Falk RH, Knowlton AA, Bernard SA, Gotlieb NE, Battinelli RN. Digoxin for converting recent onset atrial fibrillation to sinus rhythm. Am Int Med 1987;106:503-506.

[21] Anonymus. Personal communication marketing manager pharmaceutical industry on international prescription of antiarrhythmic medications, 1992.

[22] Coplen SE, Antman EM, Berlin JA, Hewitt P, Chalmers TC. Efficacy and safety of quinidine therapy for maintenance of sinus rhythm after cardioversion: a meta-analysis of randomized control trials. Circulation 1990;82:1106-1116.

[23] Suttorp MJ. Paroxysmal atrial fibrillation and atrial flutter: current concepts and new strategies. Thesis. University of Groningen, The Netherlands, 1992.

Developments in Cardiovascular Medicine

1. Ch.T. Lancée (ed.): *Echocardiology*. 1979   ISBN 90-247-2209-8
2. J. Baan, A.C. Arntzenius and E.L. Yellin (eds.): *Cardiac Dynamics*. 1980
     ISBN 90-247-2212-8
3. H.J.Th. Thalen and C.C. Meere (eds.): *Fundamentals of Cardiac Pacing*. 1979
     ISBN 90-247-2245-4
4. H.E. Kulbertus and H.J.J. Wellens (eds.): *Sudden Death*. 1980   ISBN 90-247-2290-X
5. L.S. Dreifus and A.N. Brest (eds.): *Clinical Applications of Cardiovascular Drugs*. 1980   ISBN 90-247-2295-0
6. M.P. Spencer and J.M. Reid: *Cerebrovascular Evaluation with Doppler Ultrasound*. With contributions by E.C. Brockenbrough, R.S. Reneman, G.I. Thomas and D.L. Davis. 1981   ISBN 90-247-2384-1
7. D.P. Zipes, J.C. Bailey and V. Elharrar (eds.): *The Slow Inward Current and Cardiac Arrhythmias*. 1980   ISBN 90-247-2380-9
8. H. Kesteloot and J.V. Joossens (eds.): *Epidemiology of Arterial Blood Pressure*. 1980
     ISBN 90-247-2386-8
9. F.J.Th. Wackers (ed.): *Thallium-201 and Technetium-99m-Pyrophosphate. Myocardial Imaging in the Coronary Care Unit*. 1980   ISBN 90-247-2396-5
10. A. Maseri, C. Marchesi, S. Chierchia and M.G. Trivella (eds.): *Coronary Care Units*. Proceedings of a European Seminar (1978). 1981   ISBN 90-247-2456-2
11. J. Morganroth, E.N. Moore, L.S. Dreifus and E.L. Michelson (eds.): *The Evaluation of New Antiarrhythmic Drugs*. Proceedings of the First Symposium on New Drugs and Devices, held in Philadelphia, Pa., U.S.A. (1980). 1981   ISBN 90-247-2474-0
12. P. Alboni: *Intraventricular Conduction Disturbances*. 1981   ISBN 90-247-2483-X
13. H. Rijsterborgh (ed.): *Echocardiology*. 1981   ISBN 90-247-2491-0
14. G.S. Wagner (ed.): *Myocardial Infarction*. Measurement and Intervention. 1982
     ISBN 90-247-2513-5
15. R.S. Meltzer and J. Roelandt (eds.): *Contrast Echocardiography*. 1982
     ISBN 90-247-2531-3
16. A. Amery, R. Fagard, P. Lijnen and J. Staessen (eds.): *Hypertensive Cardiovascular Disease*. Pathophysiology and Treatment. 1982   IBSN 90-247-2534-8
17. L.N. Bouman and H.J. Jongsma (eds.): *Cardiac Rate and Rhythm*. Physiological, Morphological and Developmental Aspects. 1982   ISBN 90-247-2626-3
18. J. Morganroth and E.N. Moore (eds.): *The Evaluation of Beta Blocker and Calcium Antagonist Drugs*. Proceedings of the 2nd Symposium on New Drugs and Devices, held in Philadelphia, Pa., U.S.A. (1981). 1982   ISBN 90-247-2642-5
19. M.B. Rosenbaum and M.V. Elizari (eds.): *Frontiers of Cardiac Electrophysiology*. 1983   ISBN 90-247-2663-8
20. J. Roelandt and P.G. Hugenholtz (eds.): *Long-term Ambulatory Electrocardiography*. 1982   ISBN 90-247-2664-6
21. A.A.J. Adgey (ed.): *Acute Phase of Ischemic Heart Disease and Myocardial Infarction*. 1982   ISBN 90-247-2675-1
22. P. Hanrath, W. Bleifeld and J. Souquet (eds.): *Cardiovascular Diagnosis by Ultrasound*. Transesophageal, Computerized, Contrast, Doppler Echocardiography. 1982
     ISBN 90-247-2692-1
23. J. Roelandt (ed.): *The Practice of M-Mode and Two-dimensional Echocardiography*. 1983   ISBN 90-247-2745-6
24. J. Meyer, P. Schweizer and R. Erbel (eds.): *Advances in Noninvasive Cardiology*. Ultrasound, Computed Tomography, Radioisotopes, Digital Angiography. 1983
     ISBN 0-89838-576-8
25. J. Morganroth and E.N. Moore (eds.): *Sudden Cardiac Death and Congestive Heart Failure*. Diagnosis and Treatment. Proceedings of the 3rd Symposium on New Drugs and Devices, held in Philadelphia, Pa., U.S.A. (1982). 1983   ISBN 0-89838-580-6
26. H.M. Perry Jr. (ed.): *Lifelong Management of Hypertension*. 1983
     ISBN 0-89838-582-2
27. E.A. Jaffe (ed.): *Biology of Endothelial Cells*. 1984   ISBN 0-89838-587-3

Developments in Cardiovascular Medicine

28. B. Surawicz, C.P. Reddy and E.N. Prystowsky (eds.): *Tachycardias*. 1984
    ISBN 0-89838-588-1
29. M.P. Spencer (ed.): *Cardiac Doppler Diagnosis*. Proceedings of a Symposium, held in Clearwater, Fla., U.S.A. (1983). 1983   ISBN 0-89838-591-1
30. H. Villarreal and M.P. Sambhi (eds.): *Topics in Pathophysiology of Hypertension*. 1984   ISBN 0-89838-595-4
31. F.H. Messerli (ed.): *Cardiovascular Disease in the Elderly*. 1984
    Revised edition, 1988: see below under Volume 76
32. M.L. Simoons and J.H.C. Reiber (eds.): *Nuclear Imaging in Clinical Cardiology*. 1984   ISBN 0-89838-599-7
33. H.E.D.J. ter Keurs and J.J. Schipperheyn (eds.): *Cardiac Left Ventricular Hypertrophy*. 1983   ISBN 0-89838-612-8
34. N. Sperelakis (ed.): *Physiology and Pathology of the Heart*. 1984
    Revised edition, 1988: see below under Volume 90
35. F.H. Messerli (ed.): *Kidney in Essential Hypertension*. Proceedings of a Course, held in New Orleans, La., U.S.A. (1983). 1984   ISBN 0-89838-616-0
36. M.P. Sambhi (ed.): *Fundamental Fault in Hypertension*. 1984   ISBN 0-89838-638-1
37. C. Marchesi (ed.): *Ambulatory Monitoring*. Cardiovascular System and Allied Applications. Proceedings of a Workshop, held in Pisa, Italy (1983). 1984
    ISBN 0-89838-642-X
38. W. Kupper, R.N. MacAlpin and W. Bleifeld (eds.): *Coronary Tone in Ischemic Heart Disease*. 1984   ISBN 0-89838-646-2
39. N. Sperelakis and J.B. Caulfield (eds.): *Calcium Antagonists*. Mechanism of Action on Cardiac Muscle and Vascular Smooth Muscle. Proceedings of the 5th Annual Meeting of the American Section of the I.S.H.R., held in Hilton Head, S.C., U.S.A. (1983). 1984   ISBN 0-89838-655-1
40. Th. Godfraind, A.G. Herman and D. Wellens (eds.): *Calcium Entry Blockers in Cardiovascular and Cerebral Dysfunctions*. 1984   ISBN 0-89838-658-6
41. J. Morganroth and E.N. Moore (eds.): *Interventions in the Acute Phase of Myocardial Infarction*. Proceedings of the 4th Symposium on New Drugs and Devices, held in Philadelphia, Pa., U.S.A. (1983). 1984   ISBN 0-89838-659-4
42. F.L. Abel and W.H. Newman (eds.): *Functional Aspects of the Normal, Hypertrophied and Failing Heart*. Proceedings of the 5th Annual Meeting of the American Section of the I.S.H.R., held in Hilton Head, S.C., U.S.A. (1983). 1984
    ISBN 0-89838-665-9
43. S. Sideman and R. Beyar (eds.): [3-D] *Simulation and Imaging of the Cardiac System*. State of the Heart. Proceedings of the International Henry Goldberg Workshop, held in Haifa, Israel (1984). 1985   ISBN 0-89838-687-X
44. E. van der Wall and K.I. Lie (eds.): *Recent Views on Hypertrophic Cardiomyopathy*. Proceedings of a Symposium, held in Groningen, The Netherlands (1984). 1985
    ISBN 0-89838-694-2
45. R.E. Beamish, P.K. Singal and N.S. Dhalla (eds.), *Stress and Heart Disease*. Proceedings of a International Symposium, held in Winnipeg, Canada, 1984 (Vol. 1). 1985   ISBN 0-89838-709-4
46. R.E. Beamish, V. Panagia and N.S. Dhalla (eds.): *Pathogenesis of Stress-induced Heart Disease*. Proceedings of a International Symposium, held in Winnipeg, Canada, 1984 (Vol. 2). 1985   ISBN 0-89838-710-8
47. J. Morganroth and E.N. Moore (eds.): *Cardiac Arrhythmias*. New Therapeutic Drugs and Devices. Proceedings of the 5th Symposium on New Drugs and Devices, held in Philadelphia, Pa., U.S.A. (1984). 1985   ISBN 0-89838-716-7
48. P. Mathes (ed.): *Secondary Prevention in Coronary Artery Disease and Myocardial Infarction*. 1985   ISBN 0-89838-736-1
49. H.L. Stone and W.B. Weglicki (eds.): *Pathobiology of Cardiovascular Injury*. Proceedings of the 6th Annual Meeting of the American Section of the I.S.H.R., held in Oklahoma City, Okla., U.S.A. (1984). 1985   ISBN 0-89838-743-4

Developments in Cardiovascular Medicine

50. J. Meyer, R. Erbel and H.J. Rupprecht (eds.): *Improvement of Myocardial Perfusion.* Thrombolysis, Angioplasty, Bypass Surgery. Proceedings of a Symposium, held in Mainz, F.R.G. (1984). 1985   ISBN 0-89838-748-5
51. J.H.C. Reiber, P.W. Serruys and C.J. Slager (eds.): *Quantitative Coronary and Left Ventricular Cineangiography.* Methodology and Clinical Applications. 1986
ISBN 0-89838-760-4
52. R.H. Fagard and I.E. Bekaert (eds.): *Sports Cardiology.* Exercise in Health and Cardiovascular Disease. Proceedings from an International Conference, held in Knokke, Belgium (1985). 1986   ISBN 0-89838-782-5
53. J.H.C. Reiber and P.W. Serruys (eds.): *State of the Art in Quantitative Cornary Arteriography.* 1986   ISBN 0-89838-804-X
54. J. Roelandt (ed.): *Color Doppler Flow Imaging and Other Advances in Doppler Echo-cardiography.* 1986   ISBN 0-89838-806-6
55. E.E. van der Wall (ed.): *Noninvasive Imaging of Cardiac Metabolism.* Single Photon Scintigraphy, Positron Emission Tomography and Nuclear Magnetic Resonance. 1987
ISBN 0-89838-812-0
56. J. Liebman, R. Plonsey and Y. Rudy (eds.): *Pediatric and Fundamental Electrocar-diography.* 1987   ISBN 0-89838-815-5
57. H.H. Hilger, V. Hombach and W.J. Rashkind (eds.), *Invasive Cardiovascular Therapy.* Proceedings of an International Symposium, held in Cologne, F.R.G. (1985). 1987   ISBN 0-89838-818-X
58. P.W. Serruys and G.T. Meester (eds.): *Coronary Angioplasty.* A Controlled Model for Ischemia. 1986   ISBN 0-89838-819-8
59. J.E. Tooke and L.H. Smaje (eds.): *Clinical Investigation of the Microcirculation.* Proceedings of an International Meeting, held in London, U.K. (1985). 1987
ISBN 0-89838-833-3
60. R.Th. van Dam and A. van Oosterom (eds.): *Electrocardiographic Body Surface Mapping.* Proceedings of the 3rd International Symposium on B.S.M., held in Nijmegen, The Netherlands (1985). 1986   ISBN 0-89838-834-1
61. M.P. Spencer (ed.): *Ultrasonic Diagnosis of Cerebrovascular Disease.* Doppler Techniques and Pulse Echo Imaging. 1987   ISBN 0-89838-836-8
62. M.J. Legato (ed.): *The Stressed Heart.* 1987   ISBN 0-89838-849-X
63. M.E. Safar (ed.): *Arterial and Venous Systems in Essential Hypertension.* With Assistance of G.M. London, A.Ch. Simon and Y.A. Weiss. 1987
ISBN 0-89838-857-0
64. J. Roelandt (ed.): *Digital Techniques in Echocardiography.* 1987
ISBN 0-89838-861-9
65. N.S. Dhalla, P.K. Singal and R.E. Beamish (eds.): *Pathology of Heart Disease.* Proceedings of the 8th Annual Meeting of the American Section of the I.S.H.R., held in Winnipeg, Canada, 1986 (Vol. 1). 1987   ISBN 0-89838-864-3
66. N.S. Dhalla, G.N. Pierce and R.E. Beamish (eds.): *Heart Function and Metabolism.* Proceedings of the 8th Annual Meeting of the American Section of the I.S.H.R., held in Winnipeg, Canada, 1986 (Vol. 2). 1987   ISBN 0-89838-865-1
67. N.S. Dhalla, I.R. Innes and R.E. Beamish (eds.): *Myocardial Ischemia.* Proceedings of a Satellite Symposium of the 30th International Physiological Congress, held in Winnipeg, Canada (1986). 1987   ISBN 0-89838-866-X
68. R.E. Beamish, V. Panagia and N.S. Dhalla (eds.): *Pharmacological Aspects of Heart Disease.* Proceedings of an International Symposium, held in Winnipeg, Canada (1986). 1987   ISBN 0-89838-867-8
69. H.E.D.J. ter Keurs and J.V. Tyberg (eds.): *Mechanics of the Circulation.* Proceedings of a Satellite Symposium of the 30th International Physiological Congress, held in Banff, Alberta, Canada (1986). 1987   ISBN 0-89838-870-8
70. S. Sideman and R. Beyar (eds.): *Activation, Metabolism and Perfusion of the Heart.* Simulation and Experimental Models. Proceedings of the 3rd Henry Goldberg Workshop, held in Piscataway, N.J., U.S.A. (1986). 1987   ISBN 0-89838-871-6

Developments in Cardiovascular Medicine

71. E. Aliot and R. Lazzara (eds.): *Ventricular Tachycardias*. From Mechanism to Therapy. 1987   ISBN 0-89838-881-3
72. A. Schneeweiss and G. Schettler: *Cardiovascular Drug Therapoy in the Elderly*. 1988   ISBN 0-89838-883-X
73. J.V. Chapman and A. Sgalambro (eds.): *Basic Concepts in Doppler Echocardiography*. Methods of Clinical Applications based on a Multi-modality Doppler Approach. 1987   ISBN 0-89838-888-0
74. S. Chien, J. Dormandy, E. Ernst and A. Matrai (eds.): *Clinical Hemorheology*. Applications in Cardiovascular and Hematological Disease, Diabetes, Surgery and Gynecology. 1987   ISBN 0-89838-807-4
75. J. Morganroth and E.N. Moore (eds.): *Congestive Heart Failure*. Proceedings of the 7th Annual Symposium on New Drugs and Devices, held in Philadelphia, Pa., U.S.A. (1986). 1987   ISBN 0-89838-955-0
76. F.H. Messerli (ed.): *Cardiovascular Disease in the Elderly*. 2nd ed. 1988   ISBN 0-89838-962-3
77. P.H. Heintzen and J.H. Bürsch (eds.): *Progress in Digital Angiocardiography*. 1988   ISBN 0-89838-965-8
78. M.M. Scheinman (ed.): *Catheter Ablation of Cardiac Arrhythmias*. Basic Bioelectrical Effects and Clinical Indications. 1988   ISBN 0-89838-967-4
79. J.A.E. Spaan, A.V.G. Bruschke and A.C. Gittenberger-De Groot (eds.): *Coronary Circulation*. From Basic Mechanisms to Clinical Implications. 1987   ISBN 0-89838-978-X
80. C. Visser, G. Kan and R.S. Meltzer (eds.): *Echocardiography in Coronary Artery Disease*. 1988   ISBN 0-89838-979-8
81. A. Bayés de Luna, A. Betriu and G. Permanyer (eds.): *Therapeutics in Cardiology*. 1988   ISBN 0-89838-981-X
82. D.M. Mirvis (ed.): *Body Surface Electrocardiographic Mapping*. 1988   ISBN 0-89838-983-6
83. M.A. Konstam and J.M. Isner (eds.): *The Right Ventricle*. 1988   ISBN 0-89838-987-9
84. C.T. Kappagoda and P.V. Greenwood (eds.): *Long-term Management of Patients after Myocardial Infarction*. 1988   ISBN 0-89838-352-8
85. W.H. Gaasch and H.J. Levine (eds.): *Chronic Aortic Regurgitation*. 1988   ISBN 0-89838-364-1
86. P.K. Singal (ed.): *Oxygen Radicals in the Pathophysiology of Heart Disease*. 1988   ISBN 0-89838-375-7
87. J.H.C. Reiber and P.W. Serruys (eds.): *New Developments in Quantitative Coronary Arteriography*. 1988   ISBN 0-89838-377-3
88. J. Morganroth and E.N. Moore (eds.): *Silent Myocardial Ischemia*. Proceedings of the 8th Annual Symposium on New Drugs and Devices (1987). 1988   ISBN 0-89838-380-3
89. H.E.D.J. ter Keurs and M.I.M. Noble (eds.): *Starling's Law of the Heart Revisted*. 1988   ISBN 0-89838-382-X
90. N. Sperelakis (ed.): *Physiology and Pathophysiology of the Heart*. (Rev. ed.) 1988   ISBN 0-89838-388-9
91. J.W. de Jong (ed.): *Myocardial Energy Metabolism*. 1988   ISBN 0-89838-394-3
92. V. Hombach, H.H. Hilger and H.L. Kennedy (eds.): *Electrocardiography and Cardiac Drug Therapy*. Proceedings of an International Symposium, held in Cologne, F.R.G. (1987). 1988   ISBN 0-89838-395-1
93. H. Iwata, J.B. Lombardini and T. Segawa (eds.): *Taurine and the Heart*. 1988   ISBN 0-89838-396-X
94. M.R. Rosen and Y. Palti (eds.): *Lethal Arrhythmias Resulting from Myocardial Ischemia and Infarction*. Proceedings of the 2nd Rappaport Symposium, held in Haifa, Israel (1988). 1988   ISBN 0-89838-401-X
95. M. Iwase and I. Sotobata: *Clinical Echocardiography*. With a Foreword by M.P. Spencer. 1989   ISBN 0-7923-0004-1

Developments in Cardiovascular Medicine

96. I. Cikes (ed.): *Echocardiography in Cardiac Interventions*. 1989
ISBN 0-7923-0088-2
97. E. Rapaport (ed.): *Early Interventions in Acute Myocardial Infarction*. 1989
ISBN 0-7923-0175-7
98. M.E. Safar and F. Fouad-Tarazi (eds.): *The Heart in Hypertension*. A Tribute to Robert C. Tarazi (1925-1986). 1989 ISBN 0-7923-0197-8
99. S. Meerbaum and R. Meltzer (eds.): *Myocardial Contrast Two-dimensional Echocardiography*. 1989 ISBN 0-7923-0205-2
100. J. Morganroth and E.N. Moore (eds.): *Risk/Benefit Analysis for the Use and Approval of Thrombolytic, Antiarrhythmic, and Hypolipidemic Agents*. Proceedings of the 9th Annual Symposium on New Drugs and Devices (1988). 1989 ISBN 0-7923-0294-X
101. P.W. Serruys, R. Simon and K.J. Beatt (eds.): *PTCA - An Investigational Tool and a Non-operative Treatment of Acute Ischemia*. 1990 ISBN 0-7923-0346-6
102. I.S. Anand, P.I. Wahi and N.S. Dhalla (eds.): *Pathophysiology and Pharmacology of Heart Disease*. 1989 ISBN 0-7923-0367-9
103. G.S. Abela (ed.): *Lasers in Cardiovascular Medicine and Surgery*. Fundamentals and Technique. 1990 ISBN 0-7923-0440-3
104. H.M. Piper (ed.): *Pathophysiology of Severe Ischemic Myocardial Injury*. 1990
ISBN 0-7923-0459-4
105. S.M. Teague (ed.): *Stress Doppler Echocardiography*. 1990 ISBN 0-7923-0499-3
106. P.R. Saxena, D.I. Wallis, W. Wouters and P. Bevan (eds.): *Cardiovascular Pharmacology of 5-Hydroxytryptamine*. Prospective Therapeutic Applications. 1990
ISBN 0-7923-0502-7
107. A.P. Shepherd and P.A. Öberg (eds.): *Laser-Doppler Blood Flowmetry*. 1990
ISBN 0-7923-0508-6
108. J. Soler-Soler, G. Permanyer-Miralda and J. Sagristà-Sauleda (eds.): *Pericardial Disease*. New Insights and Old Dilemmas. 1990 ISBN 0-7923-0510-8
109. J.P.M. Hamer: *Practical Echocardiography in the Adult*. With Doppler and Color-Doppler Flow Imaging. 1990 ISBN 0-7923-0670-8
110. A. Bayés de Luna, P. Brugada, J. Cosin Aguilar and F. Navarro Lopez (eds.): *Sudden Cardiac Death*. 1991 ISBN 0-7923-0716-X
111. E. Andries and R. Stroobandt (eds.): *Hemodynamics in Daily Practice*. 1991
ISBN 0-7923-0725-9
112. J. Morganroth and E.N. Moore (eds.): *Use and Approval of Antihypertensive Agents and Surrogate Endpoints for the Approval of Drugs affecting Antiarrhythmic Heart Failure and Hypolipidemia*. Proceedings of the 10th Annual Symposium on New Drugs and Devices (1989). 1990 ISBN 0-7923-0756-9
113. S. Iliceto, P. Rizzon and J.R.T.C. Roelandt (eds.): *Ultrasound in Coronary Artery Disease*. Present Role and Future Perspectives. 1990 ISBN 0-7923-0784-4
114. J.V. Chapman and G.R. Sutherland (eds.): *The Noninvasive Evaluation of Hemodynamics in Congenital Heart Disease*. Doppler Ultrasound Applications in the Adult and Pediatric Patient with Congenital Heart Disease. 1990
ISBN 0-7923-0836-0
115. G.T. Meester and F. Pinciroli (eds.): *Databases for Cardiology*. 1991
ISBN 0-7923-0886-7
116. B. Korecky and N.S. Dhalla (eds.): *Subcellular Basis of Contractile Failure*. 1990
ISBN 0-7923-0890-5
117. J.H.C. Reiber and P.W. Serruys (eds.): *Quantitative Coronary Arteriography*. 1991
ISBN 0-7923-0913-8
118. E. van der Wall and A. de Roos (eds.): *Magnetic Resonance Imaging in Coronary Artery Disease*. 1991 ISBN 0-7923-0940-5
119. V. Hombach, M. Kochs and A.J. Camm (eds.): *Interventional Techniques in Cardiovascular Medicine*. 1991 ISBN 0-7923-0956-1
120. R. Vos: *Drugs Looking for Diseases*. Innovative Drug Research and the Development of the Beta Blockers and the Calcium Antagonists. 1991 ISBN 0-7923-0968-5

Developments in Cardiovascular Medicine

The manufacturer's authorised representative in the EU is Springer
Nature Customer Service Centre GmbH, Europaplatz 3, 69115 Heidelberg,
Germany. If you have any concerns regarding our products, please
contact ProductSafety@springernature.com

Printed and bound by CPI Group (UK) Ltd, Croydon, CR0 4YY
24/04/2026
02096308-0007